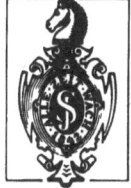

Raymond L. Hurt (Ed.)

# Management of Oesophageal Carcinoma

With 110 Figures

Springer-Verlag
London Berlin Heidelberg New York
Paris Tokyo Hong Kong

Raymond L. Hurt, MB, BS, FRCS
Consultant Thoracic Surgeon, North Middlesex Hospital, Edmonton,
London N18 1QX and St. Bartholomew's Hospital, London EC1A 7BE

ISBN-13: 978-1-4471-3155-7    e-ISBN-13: 978-1-4471-3153-3
DOI: 10.1007/978-1-4471-3153-3


British Library Cataloguing in Publication Data
Management of oesophageal cancer.
1. Man. Oesophagus. Cancer  I. Hurt, Raymond 616.99'432


Library of Congress Cataloging-in-Publication Data
Management of oesophageal carcinoma/Raymond Hurt (ed.).
p.  cm.    Includes bibliographies and index.

1. Esophagus—Cancer. 2. Esophagus—Surgery. I. Hurt, Raymond.
[DNLM: 1. Esophageal Neoplasms.   WI 250 M266]   RC280.E8M36   1989
616.99'432—dc19   DNLM/DLC                      for Library of Congress   89–6101
                                                                          CIP

Filmset by Wilmaset, Birkenhead, Wirral
Printed by Henry Ling Ltd, The Dorset Press, Dorchester
2128/3916-543210   Printed on acid-free paper

# Preface

> What you should put first in all the practice of our art is how to make the patient well; and if he can be made well in many ways, one should choose the least troublesome.
>
> *Hippocrates*

Cancer of the oesophagus was described in China over two thousand years ago as *Ye Ge*, which means dysphagia and belching. "Those discovered to suffer from oesophageal cancer in the autumn" it was said "will not live through the next summer". In the second century, Galen described "fleshy growths" as a cause of obstruction of the oesophagus which was associated with cachexia and a fatal outcome. Just over half a century ago the disease was thought to be beyond hope and help.

Cancer of the oesophagus has proved to be one of the most difficult types of malignant growth to treat successfully and even though dramatic developments in technique have occurred in the last 40 years there is still considerable controversy concerning the efficacy of treatment and the nature of that treatment, ranging from the pessimistic attitude that all therapy is merely palliative to the more radical approach of total oesophagectomy for selected cases in the hope of a permanent cure. No field of surgery has presented more dangers and difficulties and in none has the challenge been taken up with more persistent endeavour in the face of repeated failures. This endeavour was encouraged by pathological evidence that a large number of oesophageal carcinomas are technically resectable and that the likelihood of complete removal is greater than in carcinoma of the stomach. Furthermore, autopsy records showed that cancer of the oesophagus often remained a localised disease even in its terminal phase and that death occurred solely from cachexia or local complications. It was thought that cure might be possible once resection techniques had been perfected.

The oesophagus is without doubt an unforgiving organ – both to the patient with a carcinoma who will suffer from increasing dysphagia and ultimately an unpleasant death, and to the clinician who is called upon to attempt a cure or to alleviate symptoms. But the reward to the patient for the relief of those symptoms will be inestimable.

In many parts of the country the oesophagus is considered a no-man's-land – scorned by some surgeons as too difficult an area to enter, and entered into by other surgeons on an occasional basis, usually with disastrous results. There is continued controversy concerning the place of thoracic or general surgeons in the treatment of this disease – a subject which was extensively discussed by Allison and Temple in a lively debate held at the annual meeting of the Society of Thoracic Surgeons of Great Britain and Ireland in 1965 and published in *Thorax* the following year. Whatever views are held on this controversial subject, there can be no doubt that the infrequent operator on the oesophagus must be most actively discouraged. Oesophageal resection is an operation that is probably associated with the highest mortality rate of elective operations commonly performed in the United Kingdom and it has been shown recently that this mortality rate is directly related to the number of such operations carried out each year in a particular unit, and that the mortality rate of operation is unacceptably high in those surgical units in which only a few resections are performed and in which experience of postoperative thoracic care is minimal. This is not in the interests of the patient. Would it not, therefore, be wise for a strong plea to be made by the Surgical Royal Colleges, (or perhaps more than merely a plea – though it is recognised that this latter proposal is very controversial), that this type of operation be confined to a few well-publicised centres? Only by this means will an acceptable mortality rate for oesophageal resection be achieved throughout the country.

There is now *some* hope for *some* patients with oesophageal carcinoma and it is hoped that this book will show the scope of present-day methods of investigation and treatment of this dire disease and will play a small part in contributing to an improvement in its treatment – a malignant growth which accounts for almost four thousand deaths in the United Kingdom each year.

For those patients who are able to have a resection, a 5-year survival rate of 14%–18% should now be possible, with an operative mortality rate of 7%–18%. For the many remaining patients several palliative procedures for the relief of dysphagia are now available and this palliation must be provided if at all possible.

I am indebted to all the authors for the excellence of their contributions which have made the editorial work so much less arduous; to the early contributors for their patience in waiting for the publication of their material; to Fay Bendall for her compulsive attention to detail in her work as copy editor; to Mary Benstead for the line drawings which accompany Chapter 2; to Christine Murdock for her guidance through the intricacies of publication; and to Michael Jackson, Medical Editor, Springer for his unfailing courtesy and assistance at all times.

London                                                                 Raymond Hurt
1989

# Contents

# Contributors

S. J. Arnott, FRCS, FRCR
Consultant Radiotherapist, Radiotherapy Department, St. Bartholomew's Hospital, West Smithfield, London EC1A 7BE

R. S. Bonser, MB, FRCS
Senior Registrar in Cardiothoracic Surgery, Brompton Hospital,
Fulham Road, London SW3 6HP

Paula J. Cook-Mozaffari, MA, BLitt
Medical Research Council External Scientific Staff, ICRF, Cancer
Epidemiology Unit, Department of Community Medicine, Radcliffe
Infirmary, Woodstock Road, Oxford OX2 6HE

R. J. Donnelly, FRCS Ed
Consultant Thoracic Surgeon, Regional Adult Cardiothoracic Unit,
Broadgreen Hospital, Thomas Drive, Liverpool L14 3LB

P. Goldstraw, MB, FRCS, FRCSE
Consultant Thoracic Surgeon, Brompton Hospital, Fulham Road,
London SW3 6HP

D. F. N. Harrison, MD, MS, PhD, FRCS
Professor, The Institute of Laryngology and Otology, 330 Gray's Inn
Road, London WC1X 8EE

R. L. Hurt, MB, BS, FRCS
Consultant Thoracic Surgeon, North Middlesex Hospital, Edmonton,
London N18 1QX and St. Bartholomew's Hospital, London EC1A
7BE

R. M. Kirk, MS, FRCS
Consultant Surgeon, Royal Free Hospital, London, Pond Street,
London NW3 2QG

R. E. Lea, MBChB, FRCS Ed
Consultant Thoracic Surgeon, Wessex Cardiothoracic Unit, South-ampton General Hospital, Tremona Road, Southampton SO9 4XY

Alison M. McLean, MB, BChir, MRCP, FRCR
Consultant Radiologist, St. Bartholomew's Hospital, London EC1A 7BE

K. Matthewson, MB, BS, MRCP
Consultant Physician and Gastroenterologist, General Hospital, Hexham, Northumberland, NE46 1QJ

K. M. Pagliero, MB, BS, FRCS
Consultant Thoracic Surgeon, Royal Devon and Exeter Hospital (Wonford), Barrack Road, Exeter EX2 5DW

R. H. Reznek, MRCP, FRCR
Consultant Radiologist, St. Bartholomew's Hospital, West Smith-field, London EC1A 7BE

J. R. Salisbury, BSc, MB, BS, MRCPath
Senior Lecturer, Department of Morbid Anatomy, King's College School of Medicine and Dentistry, Denmark Hill, London SE5 8RX

A. Watson, MD, FRCS
Consultant Surgeon, Royal Lancaster Infirmary, Lancaster LA1 4RP

W. F. Whimster, MD, FRCP, FRCPath
Reader and Head of Department, Department of Morbid Anatomy, King's College School of Medicine and Dentistry, Denmark Hill, London SE5 8RX

# Chapter 1

# Historical Survey of Surgical Treatment

R. L. Hurt

That which is *New* at this time will one day be *Ancient*; as what
today is *Ancient* was once *New* . . . it is not *Length of Time* which
can give a value to *Things*; it is only their own *Excellency*.
(Belloste, The Hospital Surgeon, 1701)

Since the middle of the last century, surgeons have shown great courage and
enterprise in developing techniques for the resection of carcinoma of the
oesophagus – first for growths in the cervical oesophagus, then for growths at the
lower end of the oesophagus (by the abdominal route), and finally for growths in
the thoracic oesophagus. The history of the development of these techniques may
be divided, like Gaul, into three parts.

1. *1877–1912*: Early procedures in which no attempt had been made to restore
continuity between the pharynx and the stomach (except for carcinoma of the
cervical oesophagus).

2. *1913–1938*: Later procedures in which continuity had been restored, usually at
a subsequent operation, by a presternal tube of skin, stomach, jejunum or colon,
or an external rubber tube.

3. *1938 onwards*: The ideal procedure of excision and immediate restoration of
continuity within the chest or neck to allow normal swallowing.

The development of successful techniques was slow because of the inaccessibi-
lity of the oesophagus, both in the neck and in the thorax, the lack of a serous coat
to the oesophagus which made early anastomotic techniques hazardous, and the

situation of the oesophagus in an area where postoperative infection was especially dangerous and rapid in its spread.

# Nineteenth Century

"Surgeons have travelled a long rugged road to bring their craft to its present position. This road can be measured by milestones of triumph and progress; also by tombstones of tragedy and prejudice. The journey cannot be described as a particularly sentimental one, but rather as a struggle in which stern realism has usually obscured any elements of romance. Only the words of those who have lighted the way remain to show the romance of surgery. They are the words of earnest men, the strength of whose convictions exceeded the techniques available for its expression. These men stand poles apart from today's 'bright boys' who are so facile in wielding the techniques they have inherited." (E. D. Churchill, 1960)

Acknowledgement should also be made to the courage of those innumerable patients whose fortitude in the early days of thoracic surgery enabled progress to be maintained. This was in the face of much adversity which often lasted for several months during the complicated staged procedures necessary for the completion of the early operations.

The saga of the development of resection techniques began in Central Europe in the late nineteenth century, at a time when the Viennese School of Surgery was at its height. Theodor Billroth (Fig. 1.1), that giant among surgeons who was also a capable pianist, violinist, composer and music critic, as well as a personal friend of Brahms, began to investigate the possibility of the resection of the *cervical oesophagus* in dogs in Vienna in 1870. He was assisted by Czerny, who later, when Professor of Surgery in Heidelberg, achieved in 1877 the first successful resection of an oesophageal carcinoma. This carcinoma, an annular stricture a short distance below the pharynx in a 51-year-old woman, was excised by removing a segment of the cervical oesophagus containing the growth and bringing out the lower end onto the neck. Subsequent feeding was through a catheter inserted into this oesophagostomy and the patient was well and back at work five months later. She lived for a further seven months before dying from a recurrence of the tumour.

Two years later, in 1879, Billroth himself resected a more extensive carcinoma of the cervical oesophagus. After a preliminary tracheostomy, the carcinoma, together with the larynx and thyroid gland, were removed and a feeding oesophageal tube was left in place. Perhaps somewhat surprisingly there were no immediate complications and four weeks later the operation wound was "encouraged to close", with the hope that epithelialisation would produce a new oesophageal channel. Bougies were passed to maintain the lumen but alas two weeks later a bougie passed into the mediastinum and the patient died within three days from mediastinitis. Using this technique nine resections were reported up to 1885 by Bergmann (Berlin), Billroth, Czerny, Langenbeck (Berlin), Thiersch, Novarro, Israel and Iversen. There were five operative deaths and only

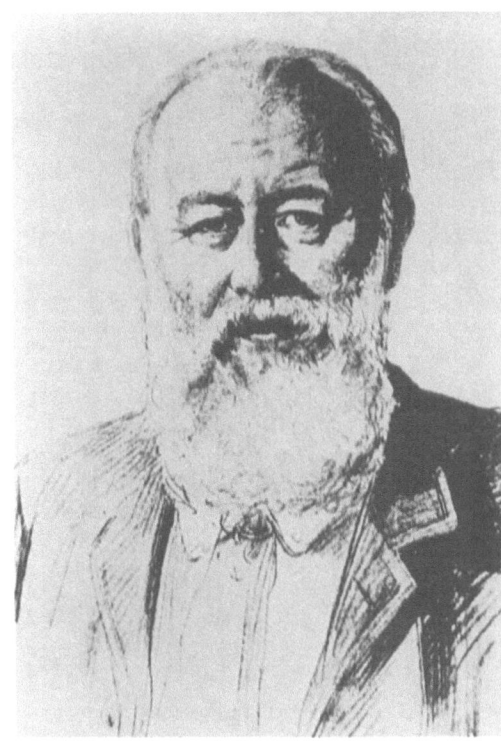

**Fig. 1.1.** Theodor Billroth 1829–1894. From Meade, History of Thoracic Surgery, 1961. Courtesy of Charles C Thomas, Publisher, Springfield, Illinois.

four patients survived operation for 3–12 months (von Mikulicz 1886). Doubtless many non-survivors were not reported.

A considerable advance was made in 1886 by von Mikulicz of Cracow University, Poland, who had also been a pupil of Billroth. He successfully reconstructed the cervical oesophagus by the use of skin flaps and his patient was able to swallow normally for about eleven months after operation before dying from a recurrence of the growth (von Mikulicz 1886). Karl Garré of Switzerland reported three successful resections in 1898, the first two by a Mikulicz-type of operation and the third by a new technique using healthy laryngeal mucous membrane as a pedicle graft to construct a new oesophagus. By the end of the nineteenth century Germany was clearly pre-eminent in the development of oesophageal resection and in the *Handbuch der Praktischen Chirurgia* edited by Bergmann, Bruns and Mikulicz (1899), the Viennese surgeon Lotheisen summarised the accepted views on the treatment of oesophageal carcinoma available at that time:

The treatment includes such operative procedures as oesophageal resection or oesophagotomy and gastrostomy. Non-operative methods are dilation with sounds or rubber catheters and the introduction of permanent intubation for feeding.

*Resection of the oesophagus*: Radical measures are rarely possible for the growth is not often so located as to be accessible for resection. Only in the cervical portion have any results – even transitory ones – been achieved by surgeons. Up to the present time only 15 cases of primary carcinoma of the

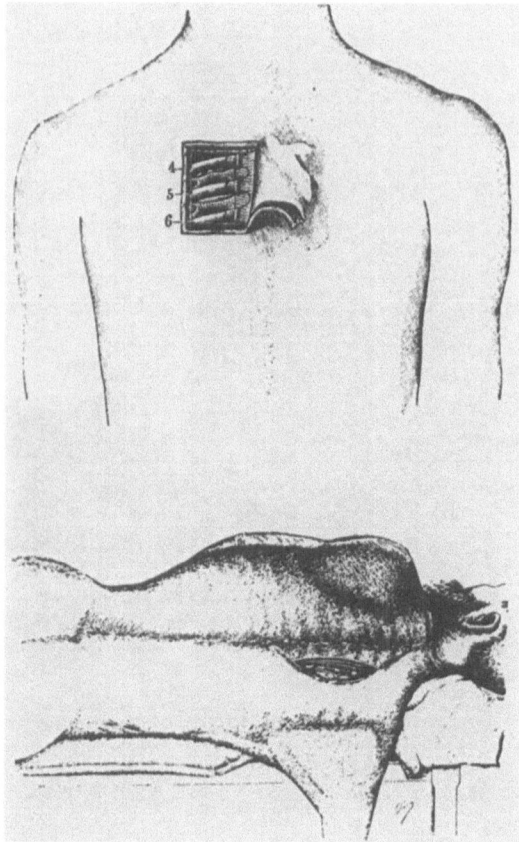

**Fig. 1.2.** Bryant's (1895) approach to the posterior mediastinum (above) and Potarca's (1898) approach to the intrathoracic oesophagus (below).

oesophagus have come to operation, of which numbers five terminated fatally. Resection is often followed by severe oesophageal stricture . . . This is particularly so if there is tension. (Quoted by L. A. Hochberg, 1960)

Resection of the *thoracic oesophagus* had been a very much more difficult problem for two reasons – firstly, the physiological and anaesthetic problems of operating inside the chest had not yet been solved and, secondly, the problem of mediastinal infection had not yet been overcome.

Nassiloff of St Petersburg must be given the credit for first suggesting in 1888 an extrapleural approach to the upper thoracic oesophagus "from the posterior part of the thorax outside the pleura by resecting four ribs". This study of dissections in cadavers, which was repeated by Bryant in 1895 in the USA and by Potarca in 1898 in Bucharest (Fig. 1.2), was originally proposed for the removal of foreign bodies and, indeed, in 1901 Enderlen of Heidelberg successfully removed a swallowed denture by this route. A logical extension of this work was for the resection of carcinoma. It had been thought that this extrapleural approach would reduce the hazard of mediastinal and pleural infection but in fact most subsequent operations were by the transpleural route.

# Early Twentieth Century

From 1900 onwards there were two approaches to the problem of resection of the thoracic oesophagus: (1) excision of the growth, together with a cervical oesophagostomy and a feeding gastrostomy, followed *later* by the use of an external rubber tube (Torek operation) or the construction of a presternal tube of skin, stomach, jejunum or colon; or (2) resection of the growth and an *immediate* anastomosis of the oesophagus to the mobilised stomach brought up into the chest.

1. *Torek operation.* A successful resection and the use of a cervical oesophagostomy was not accomplished till 1913 by Franz Torek (Fig. 1.3) in New York, who resected an oesophageal carcinoma situated at the level of the aortic arch in a 67-year-old woman by a left transpleural approach, a route which had first been attempted by both Mikulicz and Fauré 10 years earlier but without success. The aortic arch was retracted anteriorly after division of the upper intercostal arteries. The lower end of the oesophagus was invaginated like an appendix stump, the upper end, together with the carcinoma, brought out through a cervical incision, the carcinoma resected and the remainder of the oesophagus tunnelled under the skin to make an oesophagostomy on the anterior chest wall at the second interspace. During this operation there was considerable concern at the necessity for the division of the cardiac branches of the vagus nerve. During previous

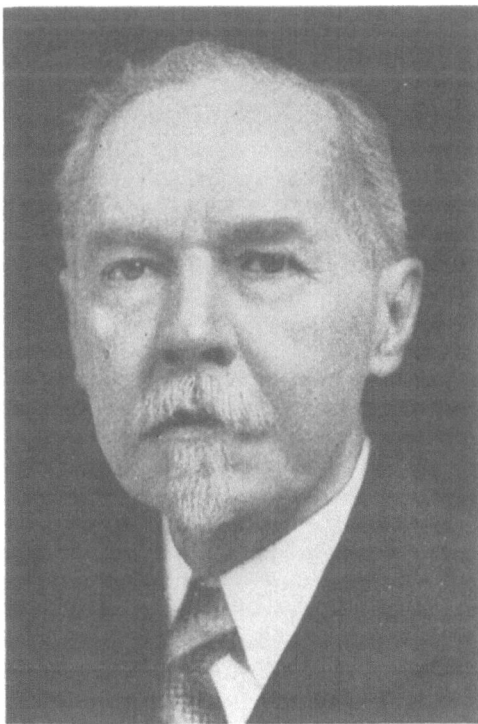

**Fig. 1.3.** Franz Torek 1861–1938. From Nissen, Pages in the History of Chest Surgery, 1960, Courtesy of Charles C Thomas, Publisher, Springfield, Illinois.

attempted operations these nerves had first been anaesthetised with the local application of cocaine "to prevent the dreaded vagal collapse". However, in Torek's operation no such problem occurred. At the end of the operation, which had lasted 2 hours 27 minutes, she was given a hot whisky and strychnine enema. Eight days later the cervical oesophagostomy and a gastrostomy which had been performed at a previous operation were joined by a rubber tube (Fig. 1.4). She refused to have any plastic reconstruction of an antethoracic oesophagus and remained well for 13 years, until she died from natural causes at the age of 80 years. The tumour was a squamous cell carcinoma. Torek was never able to repeat this successful operation although he was in the audience 25 years later when Garlock presented his report in 1938 of three consecutive successful resections using the Torek technique. Even so the operative mortality remained very high and in 1941 Oschner and DeBakey wrote that out of 58 reported cases only 17 had survived operation, an operative mortality of 70.6%. Most operations had been performed through the left chest though Wookey (1940), anticipating Lewis' later work, advocated a right sided approach, as also did Fauré in 1903, 10 years before Torek's first successful operation.

2. *Resection and immediate anastomosis.* The second approach to the resection of the thoracic oesophagus, resection and immediate anastomosis, proved to be an even greater problem and many years passed before a successful operation was performed. Contrary to what is usually stated in historical reviews on this subject, the first intrathoracic resection of a carcinoma of the oesophagus with immediate restoration of continuity was carried out in Moscow by Dobromysslov in 1901. The case was exceptional, however, in that the growth was a short one, a resection of only 3–4 cm of oesophagus was necessary and a direct end-to-end

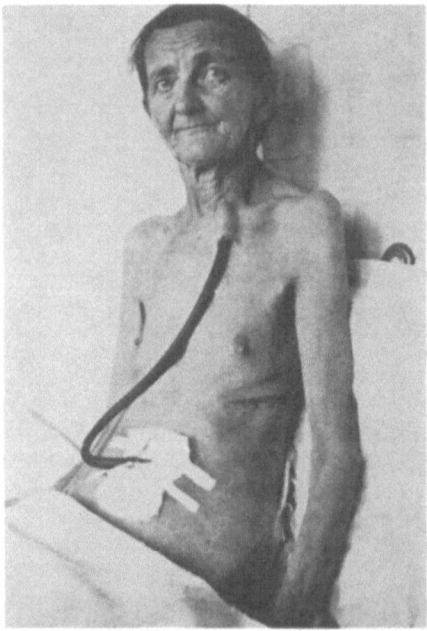

**Fig. 1.4.** Photograph of Franz Torek's patient who had the first resection of a carcinoma of the middle third of the oesophagus in 1913.

anastomosis was possible. The site of anastomosis was covered by a pedicled skin flap, hinged posteriorly.

## Early Attempts at Resection and Anastomosis

In 1881 Bloch carried out animal experiments and used the stomach to replace the thoracic oesophagus. Further animal studies were carried out by Biondi in 1895 at the University of Sienna and he successfully anastomosed the oesophagus directly to the stomach. This work, which involved extraction of the thoracic oesophagus through the neck, was repeated in 1898 by Levy, who nevertheless was of the opinion that such an operation was not applicable to man because of the inherent danger of opening the pleura "I must understandably refrain from suggesting that the deep seated cancer of the oesophagus in humans be removed in the same manner as I have torn out the oesophagus in dogs." He considered that the extrapleural approach described by Nassiloff, Bryant and Potarca in 1888–1898 was preferable.

In the same year, Ludwig Rehn reported from Germany two cases of stricture of the oesophagus (one a carcinoma) in which the stricture was opened, a tube passed through and the oesophagus sutured over the tube. Although both patients succumbed, he was the first surgeon to approach the oesophagus directly through the chest by an extrapleural route and he paved the way for future attempts. Until then the mere proximity of the heart had been considered a contraindication to operation on this part of the oesophagus.

In 1903 and 1905 Gossett in Paris and Sauerbruch in Germany carried out animal experiments and cadaver dissections ("recherches cadaverique" as Gossett described this latter work!) and anastomosed the oesophagus and stomach side-to-side and end-to-end respectively. Sauerbruch (a former assistant to Mikulicz) attempted this operation in three patients but the tumours were all found to be inoperable. Carl Beck, who emigrated from Germany and became Professor of Surgery in New York, must be given the credit for the first demonstration by animal experiments in 1905 that the greater curvature of the stomach could be made into a tube long enough to reach high in the chest. This was a very great advance in operative technique and its use as a human presternal conduit was reported in 1914 by Jianu in Hungary. In 1913 Willy Meyer, another German emigrant to New York, used this technique to bypass inoperable carcinoma and he suggested its use within the chest to replace the lower oesophagus after resection. He was so elated by this success that he wrote that "this appears to have advanced by another great step the surgery of the oesophagus, which is now making headway by leaps and bounds"(!). This technique has recently been re-introduced by Heimlich of New York as the "reversed gastric tube" operation in which the newly fashioned tube of stomach is brought up to the neck either in front of the sternum, within the chest immediately behind the sternum or through the posterior mediastinum.

The first successful resection of a carcinoma at the lower end of the oesophagus by the abdominal route was carried out by Voelcker of Heidelberg in 1908 through a left subcostal incision. The oesophagus was pulled down into the abdomen, the carcinoma resected and an oesophago-gastric anastomosis made. Of the three patients operated on, only one survived.

## Alternative Procedures

Despite these early successes, alternative procedures were proposed. In 1907 Roux of Lausanne used a loop of jejunum as the lower part of a presternal conduit, the upper part being made from a skin tube. This operation was originally devised for benign stricture but was subsequently used for carcinoma and in 1946 was reported by Rienhoff at Johns Hopkins Hospital, Baltimore as an intrathoracic procedure within the mediastinum. In 1949, Crafoord reported Yudin's (1944) experience in Russia of 200–300 cases of jejunal loop used as a presternal or retrosternal conduit to replace the oesophagus. In 1911 Kelling of Dresden used for the first time the transverse colon as the lower portion of an antethoracic oesophagus – a staged operation which was almost successful.

By 1910, only very few successful resections for carcinoma of the oesophagus had been carried out, progress had been very slow and most of the work had been carried out in Continental Europe. But the tide was beginning to turn. In 1913, Wolfgang Denk of Vienna described a "pull-through" operation performed in cadavers in which the oesophagus was removed without opening the chest. The cervical oesophagostomy and gastrostomy which were a consequence of this operation would later be joined by an antethoracic skin tube, but up to 1941 the procedure proved to be associated with a prohibitively high operative mortality and only three out of 32 reported cases had survived operation (Oschner and DeBakey 1941). Denk himself did not have a success, but the procedure, which avoided the considerable hazard at that time of opening the chest, was later developed and first performed successfully by Grey Turner in England. The direct approach of a thoraco-abdominal incision for oesophageal resection had been suggested by two New York surgeons, Janeway and Green, in 1910, and in 1913 (the same year as Denk's report) Zaaijer of Leiden performed two successful staged transpleural resections of carcinoma at the lower end of the oesophagus using the Sauerbruch negative pressure chamber as an aid to anaesthesia. He brought the upper end of the oesophagus onto the chest wall in the axilla, which had previously been mobilised by a 6th to 12th rib thoracoplasty to shorten the distance between the chest wall and the oesophageal bed.

### 1913 – An Eventful Year

The year 1913 was an eventful year and marked four major advances in the development of surgery for carcinoma of the oesophagus – Torek's momentous resection of a middle third carcinoma, Denk's description of his "pull-through" operation in cadavers, Zaaijer's two successful staged transpleural resections of lower third carcinoma and Meyer's use of a tube made from the greater curve of the stomach as a presternal conduit.

### Further Developments

In 1915 Meyer wrote that only 5 patients had so far had successful resections of a thoracic oesophageal carcinoma – by Ack (Munich), Kummell (Hamburg),

Sauerbruch (Berlin), Voelcker (Heidelberg) and Zaaijer (Leiden), "each one by a different plan". This was not strictly true, as Torek had already described his successful operation in 1913, but it did accurately describe the "state of the art" of oesophageal resection at that time and showed the lack of uniformity of technique. Ach's remarkable one-stage Torek type operation of a gastrostomy, transpleural resection of lower end of oesophagus and upper portion of stomach, mobilisation of upper oesophagus into the neck and production of an oesophagostomy in the third intercostal space, had been carried out in 1 hour 25 minutes!

In 1920 Kirschner, who had previously demonstrated by animal experiments that the blood vessels on the left side of the stomach could be safely divided without jeopardising its blood supply, described an operation for benign stricture of the oesophagus in which the mobilised stomach was brought up subcutaneously to the neck for anastomosis to the divided upper end of the cervical oesophagus. At the lower end of the divided oesophagus a Roux-en-Y jejunal anastomosis was made. His first patient survived but three subsequent patients succumbed and no further reports of this operation were made until the work of Ong (1973), who described successful operations in 14 patients. Yudin (1944) had considered the operation to be associated with too high a risk because of the necessity for an extra anastomosis to the jejunum. Nevertheless, Kirschner's original work undoubtedly led to the later development of mobilisation of the stomach and intrathoracic oesophago-gastric anastomosis.

Further reports of oesophageal resection appeared in the literature, some of which involved multiple staged operations. In 1921, for example, Lilienthal of New York described a staged extrapleural approach to a short carcinoma at the lower end of the oesophagus which was resected and continuity restored by the use of a pedicled skin flap. Hedblom of the Mayo Clinic resected a carcinoma of the lower end of the oesophagus in 1922 by a staged procedure involving a preliminary 7-rib thoracoplasty to facilitate an upper axillary thoracic oesophagostomy, which was later joined by a rubber tube to a gastrostomy made from a tube of the greater curve of the stomach. Both these patients survived these complicated procedures. In 1925, Rovsing described two cases in which he had successfully created an antethoracic oesophagus by the use of skin flaps.

By 1933 very little further progress had been made and most attempted operations had failed because of postoperative infection, either in the mediastinum or in the lungs. Eggers, for example, reported five resections in 1933 by the Torek technique, though only two patients survived operation.

## Successful Transpleural Resection

Continued attempts to improve and simplify the operative technique met with little success until the Japanese work of Oshawa at the Imperial University in Kyoto was reported, though it received little publicity in the Western world despite the large amount of research which had clearly been carried out. He performed the first successful transthoracic oesophagectomy and oesophago-gastric anastomosis for oesophageal carcinoma and had regularly used since 1925 "free thoracotomy" without the use of positive pressure respiration for anaesthesia, which in some cases was entirely by the use of procaine. In 1933 he reported nineteen patients whose lower third oesophageal carcinomas had been resected and a primary anastomosis carried out, though only eight patients survived operation.

Even at this time the importance of postoperative underwater seal drainage was not universally accepted. In Torek's first case, for example, no pleural drain was used nor was one used in any of Oshawa's cases. In 1939 there was also still considerable controversy concerning whether or not the diaphragm should be paralysed by phrenic crush at operation as "a quiet diaphragm is desirable during the time of healing of the anastomosis" (Bird 1939), and even in 1948 Garlock advised that the phrenic nerve should be crushed "to put the left leaf of the diaphragm at rest"! Naturally, as is now recognised, this encouraged postoperative lung complications, one of the major causes of postoperative mortality.

In 1937/38, however, dramatic developments occurred in the United States. Exteriorisation, skin flaps, the use of Green, Janeway or Murphy buttons for anastomosis, "pull-through" methods and staged procedures had all produced their own individual problems, but with the introduction of improved anaesthetic techniques and the use of sulphonamides to counter infection, a return to less complicated surgery became possible. Until this time operation had been restricted to removing the growth by the least hazardous method, and in the unlikely event of the patient recovering from the resection, to restoring continuity at a later date (Bird 1939). "Fear of the pleura will in a few years pass into the limbo of forgotten things, there to keep company with the fear of the peritoneum which for so long haunted the minds of surgeons". These words were written by Antonin Gosset in 1903 and although he must have been surprised how many years were to pass by, he lived to see his prophesy vindicated by the time he died in 1944. It was only shortly before this that it was appreciated that there was no necessity to induce an artificial pneumothorax one week before operation. "The bold early experiments in oesophageal surgery were followed by decades spent in trying to circumvent rather than face the dangers" (Lewis 1946). What was required was a return to straightforward resection with anastomosis and this now became a reality.

In 1938 Marshall of Boston and Adams and Phemister of Chicago separately reported successful transpleural resections for carcinoma of the lower oesophagus with a primary oesophago-gastric anastomosis. Adams and Phemister are generally credited with priority but in fact this honour should go to Marshall who carried out the resection in July 1937. Adams and Phemister's patient, whose operation for a squamous cell carcinoma was carried out 6 months later in January 1938, survived for 10 years, even though the coeliac glands were involved by growth. Until this time only 30 successful resections by 13 different surgeons had been reported in the USA, and only Torek's first case had survived for more than 5 years (Adams and Phemister 1938). Of these 30 operations 17 had been during the previous three years. Torek's later cases succumbed soon after operation from mediastinal or less commonly from pulmonary infection, as did those of most other surgeons using the same technique. Also in 1938 Garlock reported three consecutive successful resections of a carcinoma of the thoracic oesophagus, though by the Torek technique. Nissen, at the University of Basle, had reported in 1937 a successful oesophageal resection with immediate oesophago-gastric anastomosis, albeit for benign stricture.

During the next 10 years a dramatic fall in operative mortality occurred. Oschner and DeBakey, in a review of the literature up to 1940, collected 191 resections with an operative mortality of 59–91%, depending on the operative technique used (average 72%), but by 1948 Sweet was able to report the greatly reduced mortality of only 16.5% for 181 resections of middle and lower third oesophageal carcinoma by partial oesophago-gastrectomy.

## Two Milestones – 1913 and 1938

The years 1913 and 1938 stand out as two milestones in the history of the surgery for carcinoma of the oesophagus – 1913 the year of the pioneering operations of Denk, Meyer, Torek and Zaaijer, and 1938 the year of the successful achievement in the Western world of primary transpleural oesophageal resection, together with Garlock's three consecutive successful Torek operations. Indeed, in 1938 oesophageal surgery emerged from the wilderness and became an established and satisfactory procedure. This was after a period of 40 years of exploration and the development of elaborate and ingenious methods to overcome the problems of operation on a septic organ within the sterile environment of the mediastinum and pleural cavity.

# United Kingdom

Until World War II progress in the United Kingdom had been less dramatic. In 1909 Evans of the Westminster Hospital, London resected a carcinoma of the cervical oesophagus which had involved the larynx in a 63-year-old patient. The upper oesophagus was brought out as a cervical oesophagostomy and this was subsequently joined to a gastrostomy by a rubber tube which the patient herself inserted before each meal. She was still well 25 years later (Ogilvie 1960).

In 1911, Sir Arbuthnot Lane at Guys Hospital successfully resected a carcinoma which involved the upper oesophagus and back of the larynx. He restored continuity by the use of a skin flap. A similar type of operation was carried out on a 62-year-old man by Wilfred Trotter in two stages in 1925, with survival of the patient for 10 years (Pilcher 1937). In 1920 Logan Turner, of Edinburgh, resected a localised carcinoma from the back of the larynx and posterior pharyngeal wall, leaving the larynx itself intact. The patient was subsequently fed through a tube inserted into a cervical oesophagostomy.

*Professor Grey Turner.* The history of oesophageal surgery in the United Kingdom must always be associated with Professor Grey Turner (Fig. 1.5), firstly in Newcastle-upon-Tyne before his move south to London to the Postgraduate Medical School at Hammersmith. His comment in 1931 that "surgery for carcinoma of the oesophagus has usually been considered the most unsatisfactory subject in the whole realm of surgery" epitomised surgical opinion at that time. He had used Denk's technique of oesophageal resection without thoracotomy (the "pull-through" technique) and had three long-term successes out of the 25 cases which were reported by Ogilvie in his Grey Turner lecture in 1959. His

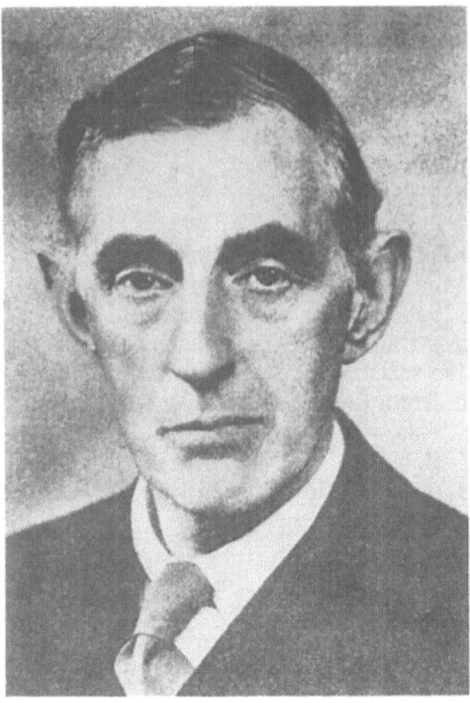

**Fig. 1.5.**   George Grey Turner 1877–
1951. From Meade, History of Thoracic
Surgery, 1961. Courtesy of Charles C
Thomas, Publisher, Springfield, Illinois.

operability rate was 44% and the operative mortality was 40%. His first successful
operation was in 1933 on a 58-year-old North Country miner who had a
carcinoma at the junction of the middle and lower third of the oesophagus. Two
months later oesophageal continuity was restored by a presternal channel formed
by a skin tube above and a jejunal loop below (Turner 1933). The patient lived for
19 months without obvious recurrence before dying from uraemia, though at post
mortem there was a small plaque of carcinoma in the stomach. The problems that
were encountered in those early days are well shown by his description of his first
operation in 1927. Whilst mobilising the oesophagus from below "it was
necessary to introduce the whole hand into the posterior mediastinum and to
practise the manoeuvres of the obstetrician separating a retained placenta". The
withdrawal of the oesophagus "was followed by a gush of blood but this soon
stopped. As a precaution a large pack of gauze was temporarily thrust into the
posterior mediastinum. The removal of the gauze pack disclosed an enormous
yawning cavern, in and out of which air rushed with a terrifying and disconcerting
noise. Fortunately all bleeding appeared to have ceased. It was not possible to
draw together what had been the oesophageal aperture but it was effectively
closed by applying the left lobe of the liver over it like the lid of a box, fixing it
there by a stout suture" (Turner 1931). This whole operation, which was
completed in two hours, was before the introduction of modern thoracic
anaesthesia, readily available blood transfusion or a proper understanding of the
use of underwater seal drainage tubes after thoracotomy, and the patient
unfortunately succumbed from infection one week later. His last successful case

was in 1945 and the patient was alive and without recurrence 14 years later (Ogilvie 1960). Grey Turner was, without any doubt, a great pioneer although, perhaps not surprisingly, his "pull-through" technique was not attempted by many other surgeons, either in the United Kingdom or the USA and a transpleural approach with the creation of a presternal oesophagus was the preferred technique (Allison 1943; Taylor 1945). H. A. Kidd of Kingston Hospital, London reported two successful operations by the "pull-through" procedure in 1943.

*Other Workers.* Abel, who gave a Hunterian lecture in 1926 on various proposed experimental approaches to oesophageal resection, mainly by a posterior mediastinal extrapleural approach, and Sir Heneage Ogilvie were other workers in this field. O'Shaughnessy (who died so tragically in 1940 during the British evacuation at Dunkirk) and Raven published in 1934 a masterly paper on techniques for the surgical exposure of the oesophagus. In 1935 Tudor Edwards removed the whole oesophagus from a woman 57 years of age for a lower third oesophageal carcinoma. An extended Torek type of operation was performed through a left thoracotomy in two hours, under a spinal anaesthetic supplemented by oxygen administered by a face mask. It had been intended to restore continuity between the cervical oesphagostomy and the gastrostomy by a presternal skin tube but unfortunately the patient died from metastases seven months later before this could be carried out. Other successful Torek operations were reported by Muir (1936), Allison (1943), Franklin (1942) and Brock (1943) in the United Kingdom and by King (1936) in Melbourne.

## Successful Intrapleural Resection and Primary Anastomosis

In 1941, Vernon Thompson at the London Hospital carried out the first successful intrapleural resection in the United Kingdom of a carcinoma of the lower third of the oesophagus with immediate restoration of oesophageal continuity. This great advance was repeated two years later by Oswald Tubbs at St Bartholomew's Hospital and by G. H. Steel at Guildford, by Ivor Lewis in 1944 and by Dickson Wright at St Mary's Hospital in 1945. The risk of anastomotic leak was still thought to be considerable, however, and because of this Hermon Taylor preferred a presternal anastomosis and reported three successful resections by this technique in 1945.

In 1946, Ivor Lewis (Fig. 1.6) of the North Middlesex Hospital, London presented his work on the right-sided approach for carcinoma of the middle third of the oesophagus, an operation which has now become a standard procedure (Franklin 1977). A preliminary laparotomy to mobilise the stomach was followed by a right thoracotomy. This allowed good access to the middle third of the oesophagus for resection of the carcinoma and an immediate oesophago-gastric anastomosis. He reported two successful operations carried out by this technique in 1944 and 1945. This procedure was a development of an unsuccessful operation reported by Ogilvie in 1938 at a time when the technical details of oesophago-gastric anastomosis had not been perfected and the oesophagus had merely been intussuscepted into a tunnel on the gastric wall over a rubber tube.

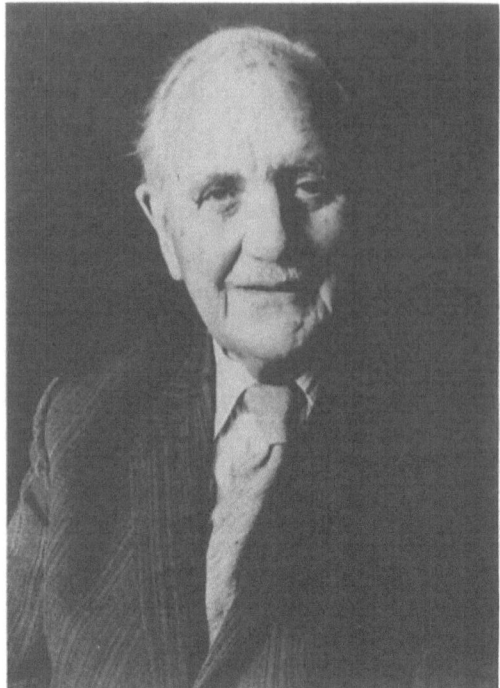

**Fig. 1.6.**   Ivor Lewis 1895–1982.

# The Modern Era

The modern era commenced immediately after World War II (1945), by which time anaesthetic and anastomotic techniques, control of infection and postoperative management had all improved to such an extent that primary resection and anastomosis became possible with an acceptable morbidity and mortality rate. The Torek type of operation, a major advance in its time, was no longer carried out. It had prolonged the patient's life in a few cases but it had also often prolonged his misery, even though some patients had been able to come to terms with its problems.

By 1954 Garlock of New York was able to report 75 resections of carcinoma of the thoracic oesophagus, using a thoraco-abdominal approach and a supra-aortic or infra-aortic anastomosis, with an operative mortality of 33%. Sweet at Harvard University had even better results – 120 resections of middle third growths and 167 resections of lower third growths, with operative mortality rates of 25% and 12% respectively.

In Japan, where the incidence of carcinoma of the oesophagus is very high, Nakayama (Oshawa's successor in the Chiba University Hospital) gained enormous experience and in 1954 reported 399 resections, by a left thoraco-abdominal approach for lower third growths and a right thoraco-abdominal approach for middle third growths. By 1959 he had carried out 953 resections, with an overall operative mortality rate of only 5.8%. The oesophago-gastric anastomosis had usually been carried out anterior to the sternum and this accounted for the very low mortality: in those cases in which an intrathoracic anastomosis had been carried out the mortality rate was 15%.

*At the present time* it is generally agreed that carcinoma at the lower end of the oesophagus should be resected through a left thoraco-abdominal approach. Growths in the middle third of the oesophagus are the subject of considerable controversy – the Lewis right-sided approach or a left-sided approach with an anastomosis above the aortic arch are the most favoured, though other techniques are possible (see Chap. 8). Carcinoma at the upper end of the oesophagus, together with postcricoid carcinoma, has always been a much more difficult surgical problem because of the proximity of the larynx, and growths at this level have usually been treated by radiotherapy. Recently, however, there has been a renewal of interest in surgical resection (see Chap. 7) following the work of Wookey (of Toronto) who reported in 1942 four patients successfully treated by pharyngo-laryngectomy with restoration of oesophageal continuity by skin flaps, and of Raven (of London) who in 1954 reported 23 consecutive successful operations using the same technique, eight of whom survived 9–51 months.

During recent years three major developments in the technique of oesophageal resection have occurred and three new procedures to restore continuity of the oesophagus have been introduced.

1. *Three-stage Oesophagectomy.* It had been shown by Garlock in 1944 that the fundus of the stomach could be brought up to the neck with preservation of its blood supply. This concept was developed by McKeown who extended the Lewis two-stage operation by bringing the stomach up to the neck as a third stage for anastomosis to the cervical oesophagus. This made any subsequent leak a much less serious complication, since contamination of the pleural cavity would be less likely to occur and any fistula would be likely to heal spontaneously without any further operation. An anastomosis in the neck may also be carried out after a left thoraco-abdominal resection (see Chap. 8).

2. *Mechanical Stapler.* The use of the mechanical stapler has dramatically reduced the time required both for mobilisation of the stomach and also for oesophago-gastric anastomosis. It may also have reduced the incidence of anastomotic leak (see Chap. 10).

3. *Transhiatal Oesophagectomy without Formal Thoracotomy.* It is somewhat surprising, and certainly associated with much controversy, that a development of the Denk/Grey Turner "pull-through" operation has recently been introduced in which the oesophagus is mobilised from above and below without opening the chest, so as to enable the stomach to be drawn up through the posterior mediastinum and anastomosed to the upper oesophagus in the neck. At present this operation is considered to be essentially a palliative procedure aimed at the relief of dysphagia. The possibility of cure remains to be seen (see Chap. 9).

4. *Colon Interposition.* Ascending, transverse and descending segments of colon, with preservation of their blood supply, have all been used for oesophageal replacement, and in the United Kingdom Allison from Oxford and Belsey from Bristol have been the foremost advocates of this technique. The present opinion is that an isoperistaltic transplant of the left colon and left half of the transverse colon, with preservation of the left colic artery, is the procedure of choice if the stomach cannot be used for reconstruction of the oesophagus (see Chap. 8).

5. *Jejunal Interposition.* The alternative technique of jejunal interposition has been increasingly used for oesophageal reconstruction if the stomach or colon cannot be used. The operation was originally described by Roux in 1907, was re-introduced by Rienhoff in 1946 but was associated with a prohibitively high postoperative morbidity and mortality rate until the technique was further developed by Allison (Allison and Da Silva 1953) (see Chap. 8).

6. *Free Graft of Jejunum.* It is now possible to use a free graft of jejunum to replace the cervical oesophagus, using a microvascular technique for anastomosis of the jejunal vessels to the superior thyroid artery and internal jugular vein.

## Present-day Surgical Statistics for Resection of Lower and Middle Third Oesophageal Carcinoma

The 5-year-survival rate after resection for oesophageal carcinoma is unfortunately poor and indeed it has been said by some authorities that all resections are only palliative. However, they are not as bad as those reported recently in the review of published series from the world literature by Earlam and Cunha-Melo (1980). In this review, a mean operative mortality of 29% and a mean 5-year-survival rate of 4% were quoted. These figures are grossly misleading, for they include series (15 out of 122) published *prior to 1961*, and many of the operations would therefore have been carried out up to 40 years ago, during which time there have been dramatic improvements in the control of postoperative infection! Furthermore, at least 21 authors reported an experience of fewer than 30 resections.

An operative mortality rate of 7%–18% and a 5-year-survival rate of 14%–18% is the standard to be expected in 1989 (Table 1.1).

**Table 1.1.** Surgical results of resection for oesophageal carcinoma

| Reference | No. cases | Mortality (%) | Two-year survival (%) | Five-year survival (%) |
|---|---|---|---|---|
| Dark *et al.* (1981) | 449 | 7.6 | – | 18 |
| Griffith and Davis (1980) | 211 | 11.4 | – | 15 |
| Jackson *et al.* (1979) | 216 | 18.0 | 25 | 14 |
| Lea (1987) | 205 | 10.0 | – | 15 |
| McKeown (1979) | 392 | 12.2 | – | – |

# References

Abel AL (1926) Treatment of carcinoma of the oesophagus. Br J Surg 14:131–159
Adams WE, Phemister DB (1938) Carcinoma of lower thoracic esophagus. J Thorac Surg 7:621–632
Allison PR (1943) Report of four cases of oesophageal carcinoma treated by excision. Br J Surg 30:132–141

Allison PR, Da Silva LT (1953) The Roux loop. Br J Surg 41:173–180
Beck C (1905) Demonstration of specimens illustrating a method of formation of a pre-thoracic oesophagus. IMJ 7:463
Belloste (1706) In: The hospital surgeon. S and F Sprint, London. Quoted by Hochberg (1960)
Belsey RHR (1965) Reconstruction of the oesophagus with left colon. J Thorac Cardiothorac Surg 49:33–55
Billroth CAT (1871) Uber die Resektion des Oesophagus. Arch Klin Chir 13:65–69
Billroth CAT (1879) Totalextirpation des Ganzenoesophagus vom pharynx bis zum Sternum; ein Totalextirpation des Ganzenlarynx mit des Ganzen Schilddruse. Verhandl Dtsch Ges Chir 8:7–9
Biondi D (1895) Experimental intrathoracic oesophago-gastrostomy. Policlinico [Suppl], p 964
Bird CE (1939) Recent advances in surgery of the esophagus. Surgery 6:772–801
Bloch (1881) Experimentelles zur Lungenresektion. Dtsch Med Wochenschr 7:634
Brock RC (1943) Report of clinical meeting. Proc R Soc Med 37:38
Bryant JD (1895) The surgical technique of entry to the posterior mediastinum. Trans Am Surg Assoc 13:443–459
Churchill ED (In: Foreword to Hochberg LA (1960)). Thoracic surgery before the 20th century. Vantage Press, New York
Churchill ED, Sweet RH (1942) Transthoracic resection of tumours of the stomach and esophagus. Ann Surg 115:897–917
Crafoord C (1949) Discussion of paper by Harrison. J Thorac Surg 18:325
Czerny V (1877) Neue Operationen; Resektion des Oesophagus. Zentralbl Chir 4:433–434
Dark JF, Mousalli H, Vaughan R (1981) Surgical treatment of carcinoma of the oesophagus. Thorax 36:891–895
Denk W (1913) Zur Radikaloperation des Oesophaguskarzinoms. Zentralbl Chir 40(2):1065–1068
Dobromysslov (1901) Ein Fall von Transpleuraler Oesophagectomie ein Brustabschnitte. Zentralbl Chir, p. 1 (quoted by Meade (1961))
Earlam R, Cunha-Melo JR (1980) Oesophageal squamous cell carcinoma. I. A critical review of surgery. Br J Surg 67:381–390
Edwards AT (1935) Transpleural removal of total oesophagus. Proc R Soc Med 29:188
Eggers C (1933) Experiences with carcinoma of the oesophagus. J Thorac Surg 2:229–246
Enderlen (1901) Ein Beitrag zur Chirurgie des Hinteren Mediastinum. Dtsch Zeitschr Chir 61: 441–495
Evans A (1932) A rubber oesophagus. Br J Surg 20:388–392
Fauré JL (1903) Cancer de la portion thoracique de l'oesophage. Extirpation du neoplasme par la voie mediastinin posterior droite. Combinée a une incision cervicale. Bull Mem Soc Chir 29:122–134
Franklin RH (1942) Two cases of successful removal of the thoracic oesophagus for carcinoma. Br J Surg 30:141–146
Franklin RH (1977) Advancing frontiers of oesophageal surgery. Ann R Coll Surg Engl 59:284–287
Garlock JH (1938) The surgical treatment of the thoracic esophagus. Surg Gynecol Obstet 66:534–548
Garlock JH (1944) Re-establishment of esophago-gastric continuity following resection of esophagus for carcinoma of middle third. Surg Gynecol Obstet 78:23–28
Garlock JH (1948) Progress in the surgical treatment of carcinoma of the esophagus and upper stomach. Surgery 23:906–911
Garlock JH, Klein S (1954) Surgical treatment of carcinoma of esophagus and cardia. Ann Surg 139:19–34
Garré K (1898) Uber oesophagusresektion und oesophagoplastik. Arch Klin Chir 57:719–722
Gossett A (1903) De l'oesophago-gastrostomie transdiaphragmatique. Rev Chir 28:694–707
Green N, Janeway HH (1910) Artificial respiration and intrathoracic oesophageal surgery. Ann Surg 52:58–66
Griffith JL, Davis JT (1980) A twenty year experience with the surgical management of carcinoma of the oesophagus and gastric cardia. J Thorac Cardiovasc Surg 79:447–452
Hedblom C (1922) Combined transpleural and transperitoneal resection of the thoracic oesophagus and cardia for carcinoma. Surg Gynecol Obstet 35:284–287
Heimlich HJ (1966) Elective replacement of the oesophagus. Br J Surg 53:913–916
Hochberg LA (1960) Thoracic surgery before the 20th century. Vantage Press, New York
Jackson JW, Cooper DKC, Guvendick L, Reece-Smith H (1979) Surgical management of malignant tumours of oesophagus and cardia. Br J Surg 66:98–104
Janeway HH, Green NW (1910) Cancer of esophagus and cardia. Ann Surg 52:67–82
Jianu A (1914) Uber Oesophagoplastik. Dtsch Chir 131:397–403
Kelling (1911) Oesophagoplastik mit Hilfe des Querkolon. Zentralbl Chir 38:1209–1212

Kidd HA (1943) Excision of the oesophagus for malignant growth by the abdominal cervical route. Br J Surg 30:340–344

King ESJ (1936) Oesophagectomy for carcinoma of the thoracic oesophagus. Br J Surg 23:521–529

Kirschner MB (1920) Eines Neues Verfahren der Oesophagoplastik. Arch. Klin Chir 114:606–626

Lane WA (1911) Excision of a cancerous segment of the oesophagus: restoration of the oesophagus by means of a skin flap. Br Med J i:16–17

Levy W (1898) Versuche uber die Resektion der Speiserohre. Arch Klin Chir 56:839–892

Lewis I (1946) Surgical treatment of carcinoma of the oesophagus. Br J Surg 34:18–31

Lilienthal H (1921) Carcinoma of thoracic oesophagus – extrapleural resection and plastic. Ann Surg 74:259–279

Lotheissen (1899) In: von Bergman E, von Bruns P, Mikulicz J (1899) Handbuch der praktischen Chirurgie. F Enke, Stuttgart

Marshall SF (1938) Carcinoma of the esophagus: successful resection of lower end of esophagus with re-establishment of esophageal gastric continuity. Surg Clin North Am 18:643–648

McKeown KC (1976) Total three-stage oesophagectomy for cancer of the oesophagus. Br J Surg 63:259–262

Meade RH (1961) A history of thoracic surgery. Charles C Thomas, Illinois

Meyer W (1913) Oesophagoplasty. Ann Surg 58:289–295

Meyer W (1915) Resection of cardia for carcinoma. Ann Surg 62:693–709

Muir EG (1936) Resection of the lower oesophagus and cardia. Lancet II:75

Nakayama K (1954) Approach to midthoracic esophageal carcinoma for its radical surgical treatment. Surgery 35:574–589

Nakayama K (1959) Statistical review of 5-year survivals after surgery for carcinoma of esophagus and cardiac portion of stomach. Surgery 45:883–889

Nassiloff II (1888) Oesophagotomia et resectio oesophagi endothoracica. Vrach St Petersburg 9:481–482

Nissen R (1937) Die transpleurale Resektion der Kardia. Dtsch Zeitschr Chir 249:311–316

Ogilvie WH (1938) Intrathoracic reconstruction of lower oesophagus. Br J Surg 26:10–22

Ogilvie WH (1960) The surgery of the oesophagus. Br J Surg 47:457–466

Ong GB (1973) The Kirschner operation – a forgotten procedure. Br J Surg 60:221–227

Oschner A, DeBakey M (1941) Surgical aspects of a carcinoma of the esophagus. J Thorac Surg 10:401–445

O'Shaughnessy L, Raven RW (1934) Surgical exposure of the oesophagus. Br J Surg 22:365–377

Oshawa T (1933) The surgery of the oesophagus. Arch Jap Chir 10:604–695 (quoted by Bird (1939))

Potarca J (1898) Du mediastinum posterieur et en particular trajat des plèvres mediastinales posterieures. Presse Méd 2:296–300

Raven RW (1954) Cancer of the oesophagus. Chir Thorac 7:3–23

Rehn L (1898) Operationen an dem Brustabschnitt der Speiserohre. Verh Dtsch Ges Chir 21:448–470

Rienhoff WF (1946) Intrathoracic oesophagojejunostomy for lesions of the upper third of the oesophagus. South Med J 39:928–940

Roux C (1907) L'oesophago-jejuno-gastrome, nouvelle operation pour retrecissement infrachisable de l'oesophage. Semaine Méd 27:37

Rovsing T (1925) Antethoracic oesophagoplasty. A new method. Ann Surg 81:52–58

Sauerbruch F (1905) Experimentelle Beitrage zur Oesophagus-chirurgie. Verh Dtsch Ges Chir 34:140–149

Steel GH (1943) Carcinoma of the oesophagus. Lancet II:797–798

Sweet RH (1944) Discussion of paper by Garlock. J Thorac Surg 13:423–424

Sweet RH (1948) Treatment of carcinoma of the esophagus and cardiac end of stomach by surgical extirpation. Surgery 23:952–975

Sweet RH (1950) Thoracic surgery. Mosby, St Louis

Sweet RH (1954) Late results of surgical treatment of carcinoma of the esophagus. JAMA 155:422–425

Taylor H (1945) An operation for removal of carcinoma of the oesophagus with pre-sternal oesophagogastrostomy. Br J Surg 32:394–399

Thompson VC (1945) Carcinoma of the oesophagus: resection and oesophago-gastrostomy, Br J Surg 32:377–380

Torek F (1913) The first successful case of resection of the thoracic portion of the esophagus for carcinoma. Surg Gynecol Obstet 16:614–617

Trotter W (1925) Reported by R. Pilcher (1937) In: Carcinoma of the cervical oesophagus. Lancet I:73–76

Tubbs OS (1943) Report in clinical section of the Royal Society of Medicine. Proc R Soc Med 37:39

Turner GG (1931) Some experiences in the surgery of the esophagus. N Engl J Med 205:657–674

Turner GG (1933) Excision of thoracic oesophagus for carcinoma. Lancet II:1315–1316

Turner L (1920) Carcinoma of the post-cricoid region of the upper end of the oesophagus. Proc R Soc Med (Section of Laryngology) 13:199–202

Voelcker (1908) Uber Extirpation der Cardia wegen Carcinoms. Verh Dtsch Ges Chir 37:126–129

von Mikulicz J (1886) Ein Fall von Resektion des Carcinomatosen Oesophagus mit Plastichen ersatz des Exeidirten Stuckes. Prag Med Wochenschr 11:93–94

Wookey H (1940) The surgical treatment of mid-oesophageal carcinoma. Br J Surg 27:696–705

Wookey H (1942) Surgical treatment of carcinoma of the pharynx and upper esophagus. Surg Gynecol Obstet 75:499–506

Wright D (1945) Report in Clinical Section of the Royal Society of Medicine. Proc R Soc Med 38:131

Yudin SS (1944) The surgical construction of 80 cases of artificial esophagus. Surg Gynecol Obstet 78:561–583

Zaaijer JH (1913) Erfolgreiche transpleurale Resektion eines Cardia-carcinoms. Beitr Klin Chir 83:419

*Chapter 2*

# Surgical Anatomy

R. L. Hurt

## Embryology

The oesophagus arises from the primitive foregut. It commences as a short tube which extends from the tracheal groove above to the fusiform dilatation of the foregut below, which 20 days after fertilisation will develop into the stomach. An external ridge develops on the 23rd day on its anterior wall and deep to this an internal groove, the laryngo-tracheal sulcus, forms which gradually extends caudally. This groove deepens and is pinched off by lateral ridges to form a tube situated ventral to the oesophagus. The tube later widens to form the bilobed lung bud. By the 36th day separation of the two tubes is complete. The primitive oesophagus lies on the posterior aspect of the septum transversum and is embedded in visceral mesoderm. The oesophagus rapidly lengthens during the sixth and seventh weeks as the larynx ascends and the heart and lung buds descend. During this time the oesophagus temporarily becomes obliterated due to its elongation and also because of a proliferation of the endodermal lining cells. Recanalisation of the oesophagus gradually occurs and the lining epithelium changes to a stratified squamous type, possibly as a result of metaplasia and possibly due to migration of cells from the oral cavity. Foci of columnar cells may persist, however, and this may explain the occasional development of an adenocarcinoma of the oesophagus. The visceral mesoderm differentiates into muscular and connective tissue layers between the 6th and 12th week. The left and right gastric nerves come to lie anterior and posterior to the oesophagus as the stomach rotates to the right.

# Adult Anatomy

The oesophagus is 20–25 cm in length, extending from the pharynx at the level of the lower border of the sixth cervical vertebra (or inferior margin of the cricoid cartilage) to the stomach opposite the eleventh thoracic vertebra.

Three constrictions are visible on radiological and endoscopic examination of the oesophagus: (1) a constriction at the upper end due to the cricopharyngeus muscle, (2) a left lateral indentation due to the aortic arch together with an anterior indentation due to the left main bronchus, and (3) a constriction at the lower end at its entrance into the stomach.

At the upper end of the oesophagus there is the upper oesophageal sphincter, composed mainly of the cricopharyngeus muscle, running transversely across the posterior wall of the oesophagus and connecting the two lateral borders of the cricoid cartilage. Inferiorly, this muscle blends with the circular and longitudinal muscle fibres of the upper oesophagus. At the lower end of the oesophagus, at its entrance into the stomach, there is a complex sphincter mechanism, composed partly of circular muscle fibres in the wall of the oesophagus itself, and also partly of fibres of the right crus of the diaphragm, the angle of insertion of the oesophagus into the stomach, and the presence of a short length of oesophagus below the diaphragm (and therefore within the abdomen) where the pressure is positive and approximates the walls of the oesophagus.

The oesophagus is essentially a midline structure, but in the neck it is slightly deviated to the left, in the upper and mid thorax slightly to the right and in the lower thorax again slightly to the left. These deviations are of surgical importance in that the cervical oesophagus is more easily approached from the left, the upper and middle oesophagus from the right and the lower oesophagus from the left.

At its upper end the longitudinal muscle of the oesophagus is attached to the cricoid cartilage. Thereafter the oesophagus is loosely attached by areolar tissue containing elastin fibres throughout its passage through the neck and mediastinum into the abdomen. There are accessory slips of smooth muscle fibres between the oesophagus and the trachea, left main bronchus, pericardium and aorta. This loose attachment permits vertical movement of the oesophagus during respiration and peristalsis.

At the lower end of the oesophagus there is said to be a phreno-oesophageal ligament fixing the lower oesophagus to the diaphragm – the importance, and indeed even existence, of this ligament is subject to considerable controversy! At operation, the author has never been able to convince himself of its presence.

## Anatomical Relationships

### Cervical Segment

The oesophagus is situated between the trachea anteriorly and the pre-vertebral layer of cervical fascia which covers the longus cervicis muscle posteriorly (Fig. 2.1). There is loose areolar tissue between the oesophagus and the membranous wall of the trachea. On each side, laterally, is the carotid sheath containing the carotid vessels and vagus nerve, with the inferior thyroid artery and lobes of the

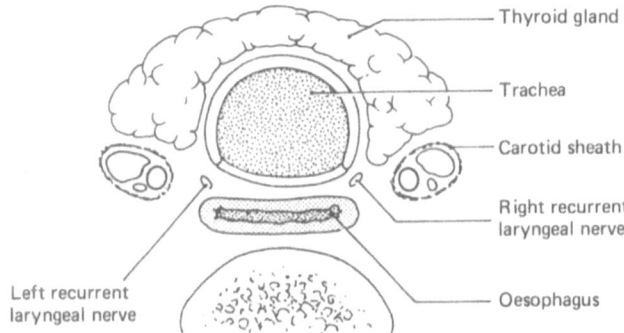

**Fig. 2.1.**  Transverse section in lower part of neck.

thyroid gland more anteriorly. The recurrent laryngeal nerve is situated on each side in the groove between the trachea and oesophagus. As the oesophagus descends it gradually passes slightly to the left.

## Thoracic Segment

Within the chest the trachea continues to be an immediate anterior relation until it bifurcates at the level of the fifth thoracic vertebra (Fig. 2.2). The left main bronchus then crosses in front of the oesophagus and this is the commonest site for a malignant oesophago-bronchial fistula. Thereafter, the oesophagus lies

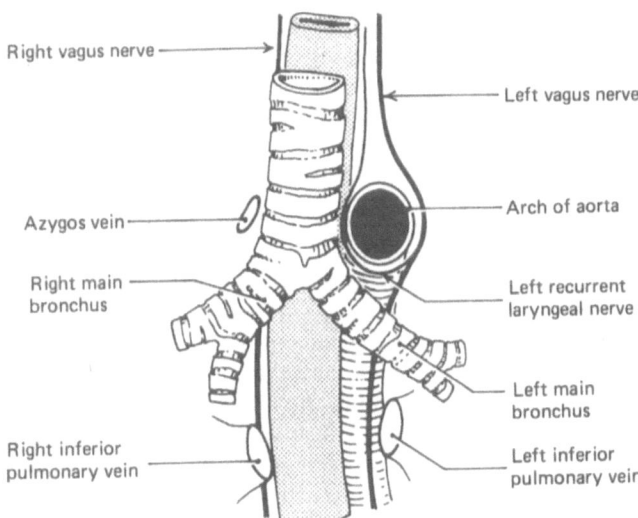

**Fig. 2.2.**  Relationships of thoracic oesophagus viewed from the front.

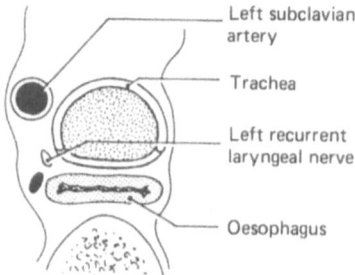

Left subclavian artery

Trachea

Left recurrent laryngeal nerve

Oesophagus

**Fig. 2.3.a** Transverse section above tracheal bifurcation. **b** Transverse section at level of tracheal bifurcation.

a

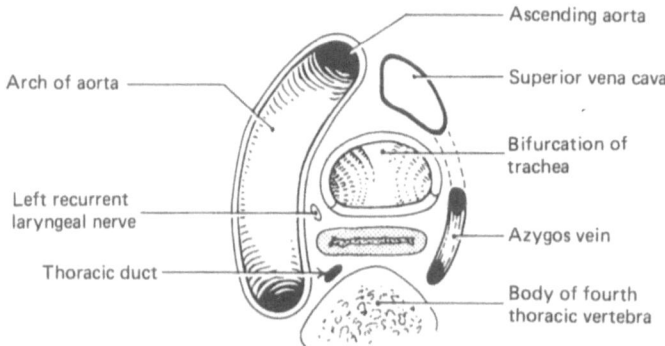

Arch of aorta

Left recurrent laryngeal nerve

Thoracic duct

Ascending aorta

Superior vena cava

Bifurcation of trachea

Azygos vein

Body of fourth thoracic vertebra

b

behind the pericardium and left atrium (Fig. 2.3). In the superior and posterior mediastinum the oesophagus lies on the prevertebral fascia covering the longus cervicis muscle.

At mid-oesophageal level on the right side the azygos vein arches forwards close to the oesophagus above the right hilum to enter the superior vena cava. On the left side at the same level is the aortic arch passing in front of the oesophagus and leading to the descending aorta, which initially is to the left and then subsequently behind the oesophagus, until at the level of the diaphragm it is behind and to the right.

As the oesophagus descends it passes to the right and is in close contact with the right mediastinal pleura.

The *thoracic duct* passes up from the cysterna chyli in front of the body of the second lumbar vertebra beneath the right crus. It enters the thorax on the right side of the aorta through the aortic opening in the diaphragm and proceeds upwards through the posterior mediastinum to the right of the midline between the azygos vein and the aorta. At the level of the seventh thoracic vertebra the duct passes obliquely upwards to reach the left side of the mediastinum at the level of the fifth thoracic vertebra. It passes behind the oesophagus at this level and then passes upwards in close proximity to the left subclavian artery and along the left border of the oesophagus to the neck, where it enters the junction of the internal jugular and subclavian veins. Occasionally, there is an extra terminal branch which enters the vein on the right side of the neck. In about 50% of individuals two or more ducts are present at some stage in its course through the mediastinum. Van Pernis (1949), in a study of 1081 cadavre dissections, found that there was always a single duct from the cisterna chyli to the level of the eighth thoracic vertebra, though this was disputed by Kausel et al. (1957). There are, in addition, numerous other connections between the main thoracic duct and the azygos, intercostal and lumbar veins.

The *vagus nerves* pass downwards through the chest on each side of the oesophagus until the lower end where the left vagus becomes anterior and the right posterior. The left recurrent laryngeal nerve arises from the vagus and hooks around the arch of the aorta close to the obliterated ductus arteriosus before passing up to the larynx in the groove between the oesophagus and trachea. The right recurrent laryngeal nerve arises from the vagus at a higher level in front of the first part of the subclavian artery. It hooks under it and then passes up to the larynx, as on the left side, in the groove between the oesophagus and the trachea.

## Abdominal Segment

The oesophagus passes through the diaphragm anterior and to the left of the aorta. Within the abdomen it is covered by peritoneum and lies behind the oesophageal groove in the left lobe of the liver. The anterior and posterior vagal nerve trunks are closely applied to the abdominal portion of the oesophagus.

## Structure of the Oesophagus

The oesophagus is composed of a loose external layer, a double layer of muscle, a submucous layer and a relatively tough mucous layer.

1. *External layer.* The external layer is a condensation of the mediastinal fascia and it contains elastin fibres, some of which penetrate the muscular wall to surround the muscle bundles. This loose external layer facilitates mobilisation of the oesophagus.

2. *Muscle layer.* The muscle is in two layers – an outer longitudinal layer and an inner circular layer. The *outer longitudinal muscle* is thicker than the inner layer and at the upper end is continuous with the cricoid cartilage, except for a small area posteriorly where it separates into two longitudinal bundles, causing a weak area at the back of the upper end of the oesophagus known as Killian's dehiscence, the site of origin of a pharyngeal pouch. At the lower end the longitudinal muscle is continuous with the longitudinal fibres of the stomach. The *inner circular muscle* is thicker at the lower end of the oesophagus. It is continuous above with the inferior constrictor muscle of the pharynx and below with the oblique muscle fibres of the stomach.

The upper one-third of the oesophagus contains striated muscle, the middle third striated and smooth muscle and the lower third smooth muscle fibres.

3. *Submucous layer.* The submucous layer comprises loose areolar tissue containing elastin fibres, within which are blood vessels.

4. *Mucosal layer.* The mucosal layer is a grey, tough layer composed of stratified squamous epithelium beneath which is the muscularis mucosa. It is loosely attached to the muscle layer and is arranged in longitudinal folds. It is of

considerable strength and because there is no peritoneal coat, *the integrity of any anastomosis lies in the mucosal layer*, not the muscle layer. At the lower end of the oesophagus the epithelium becomes columnar – the exact point of change may not correspond to the anatomical oesophago-gastric junction. Furthermore, columnar (gastric) epithelium may be present in the lower oesophagus – due to "ectopic" gastric epithelium of developmental origin or the effects of reflux oesophagitis.

## Blood Supply

### Arterial Supply

The arterial supply (Fig. 2.4) of the *cervical oesophagus* is mainly by branches from the inferior thyroid arteries, though there are additional arterial twigs from

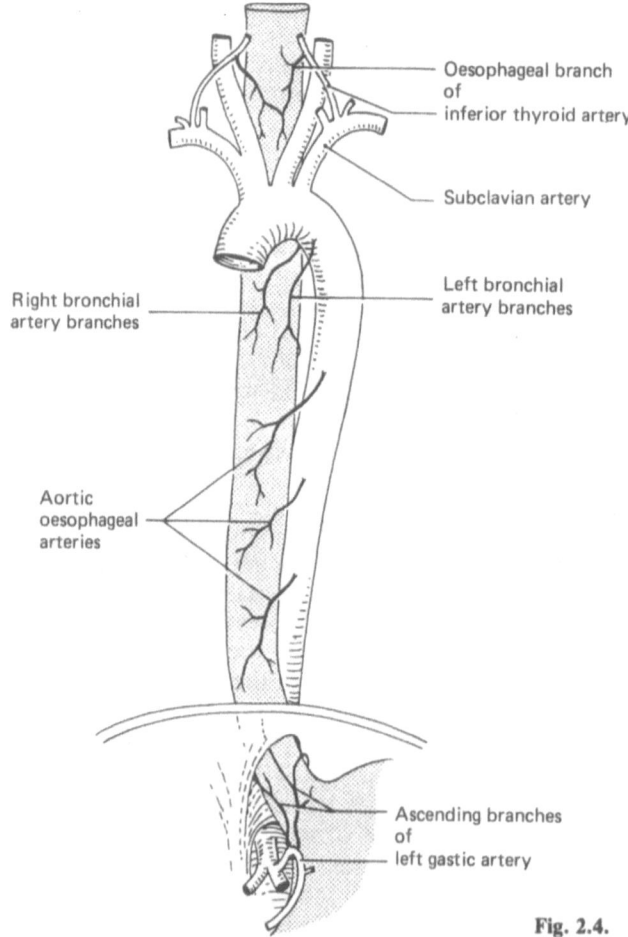

**Fig. 2.4.**   Arterial supply of oesophagus.

the common carotid, superior thyroid, costo-cervical trunk and vertebral arteries. The *thoracic oesophagus* is supplied by branches from the bronchial arteries and directly from the aorta. The *abdominal oesophagus* is supplied by branches from the left and right gastric and phrenic arteries (Shapiro et al. 1950; Swigart et al. 1950; Williams and Payne 1982).

## Venous Drainage

The venous drainage (Fig. 2.5) is more complex (Butler 1951). Subepithelial channels run longitudinally to drain into the inferior thyroid and vertebral veins above, the azygos and hemiazygos veins in mid thorax, and the left gastric veins below the diaphragm. These channels also pass through the muscle layers and form a peri-oesophageal plexus, the longest trunks of which accompany the vagus nerves.

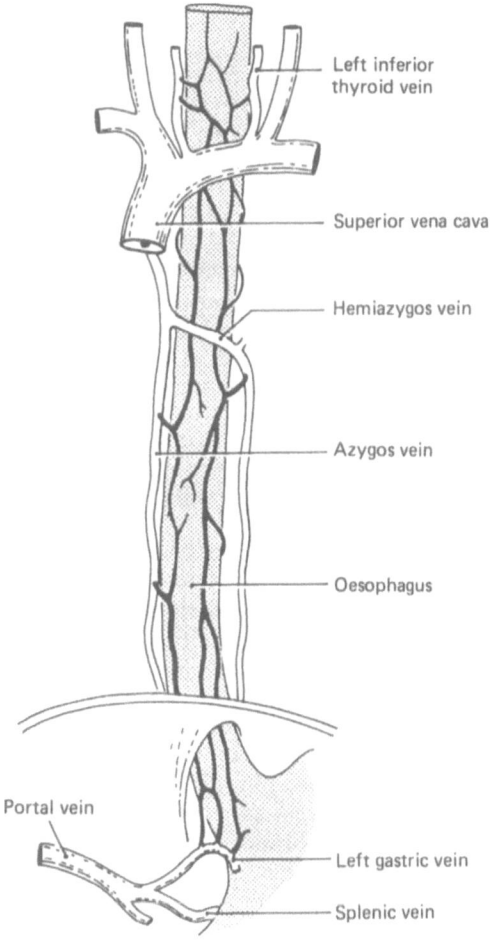

Left inferior thyroid vein

Superior vena cava

Hemiazygos vein

Azygos vein

Oesophagus

Portal vein

Left gastric vein

Splenic vein

**Fig. 2.5.**   Venous drainage of oesophagus.

## Lymphatic Drainage

The oesophagus contains numerous lymphatic channels which run independently of its blood supply. These channels form mucosal and submucosal networks which freely communicate with each other, and at the lower end of the oesophagus directly join those of the stomach. The submucosal network is especially prominent and the lymph travels considerable distances along this plane in a vertical direction before passing through the muscle layers to reach the draining lymph nodes.

The lymph nodes draining the oesophagus (Fig 2.6) are divided into three groups:

1. Those in close proximity to the oesophagus – from above downwards, the internal jugular nodes, posterior tracheal and para-oesophageal (superior mediastinal) nodes, inferior pulmonary ligament nodes, hiatal and cardiac lymph nodes

2. Lymph nodes in the mediastinum a short distance from the actual growth

3. More distant lymph nodes – the deep cervical, supraclavicular, tracheobronchial and coeliac nodes

The lymph drainage from the upper two-thirds of the oesophagus is essentially upwards to the neck, whereas from the lower one-third it is downwards towards the stomach.

*In considering the extent and feasibility of resection* it is important to remember two points.

1. The submucous spread of the carcinoma is always *much* greater than would be expected from the external appearance of the growth

2. Carcinoma of the oesophagus at *all* levels may spread relatively early to the supraclavicular lymph nodes, which may then be palpable. Furthermore, 30% of middle third growths and 50% of lower third growths spread directly and in their early stages to glands *below* the diaphragm.

## Nerve Supply

The oesophagus is innervated by the sympathetic and parasympathetic systems through two plexuses containing groups of ganglion cells, one situated between the two muscle layers (Auerbach's plexus) and the other in the submucous layer (Meissner's plexus).

The *sympathetic supply* in the neck is from the pharyngeal plexus, in the thorax from the superior and inferior cervical ganglia, and at the lower end from the left greater splanchnic nerve, the coeliac plexus and from plexuses around the left gastric and inferior phrenic arteries.

The *parasympathetic supply* in the neck is from branches of the recurrent laryngeal nerve, branches of the ninth and tenth cranial nerves and the cranial root of the eleventh nerve; in the thorax from the vagus nerves which lie on either side of the oesophagus and form a plexus around it; and at the lower end again from the vagi, which are joined by branches of the splanchnic nerves.

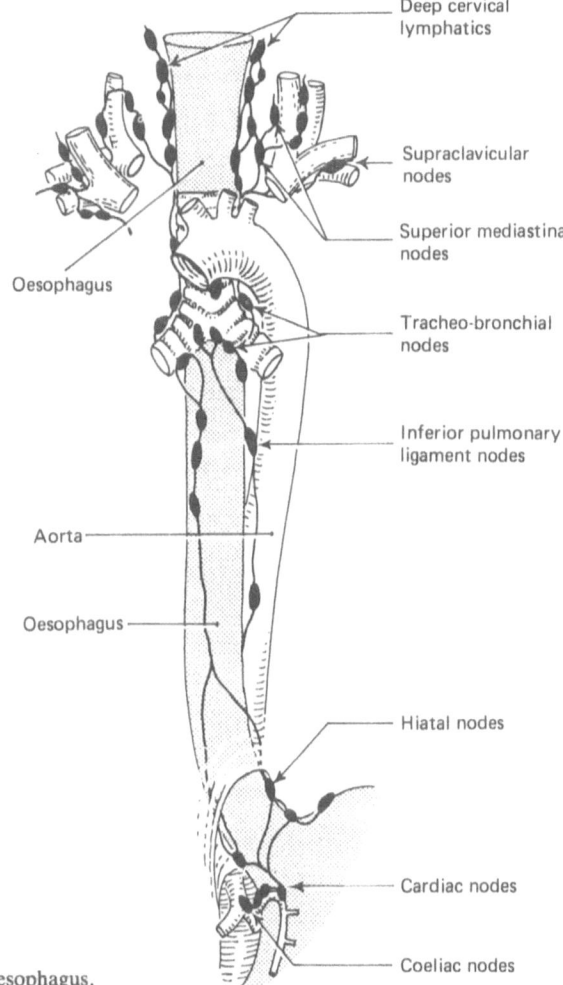

Deep cervical
lymphatics

Supraclavicular
nodes

Superior mediastinal
nodes

Oesophagus

Tracheo-bronchial
nodes

Inferior pulmonary
ligament nodes

Aorta

Oesophagus

Hiatal nodes

Cardiac nodes

Coeliac nodes

**Fig. 2.6.**   Lymphatic drainage of oesophagus.

Stimulation of the sympathetic nerves reduces peristalsis and increases contraction of the sphincter, whereas stimulation of the parasympathetic nerves has the opposite effect.

# References

Butler H (1951) The veins of the oesophagus. Thorax 6:276–296
Kausel HW, Reeve TS, Stein AA, Allen RD, Stranahan A (1957) Anatomic and pathological studies of the thoracic duct. J Thorac Surg 34:631–642
Shapiro AL, Robillard GL (1950) The esophageal arteries: their configurational anatomy and variations in relation to surgery. Ann Surg 131:171–185

Swigart LL, Siekert RG, Hambley WC, Anson BJ (1950) The oesophageal arteries: anatomic study of 150 specimens. Surg Gynecol Obstet 90:234–243
Van Pernis PA (1949) Variations of the thoracic duct. Surgery 26:806–809
Williams OB, Payne WS (1982) Observations on esophageal blood supply. Mayo Clin Proc 57:448–453

*Chapter 3*

# Epidemiology and Predisposing Factors

P. Cook-Mozaffari

## Worldwide Occurrence

### Incidence in Men

Cancer of the oesophagus has a pattern of incidence that is remarkable in many respects. It is rare in most western populations but occurs frequently in parts of Asia and Africa (Table 3.1, Figs 3.1, 3.2). In certain restricted localities it has an exceptionally high incidence; in Kazakhstan and northern Iran, for example, the incidence rates are the highest observed in general populations for any type of cancer anywhere in the world. They are comparable with the incidence rates that have been observed in known high-risk groups – with the lung cancer rate, for example, among life-long heavy smokers in London.

Sharp gradients of frequency occur between regions only a few hundred miles apart. Between Gurjev town at the head of the Caspian Sea in Kazakhstan and the towns in Georgia, 500 miles away, the incidence of cancer of the oesophagus drops 70-fold for men and 230-fold for women (Doll 1969). In China, there is a 60-fold decrease for men and a 90-fold decrease for women between the northeast of Henan Province and parts of Shanxhi Province 300 miles to the north (Coordinating Group 1974). Similar, but slightly less extreme, gradients have been reported from northern Iran (Mahboubi et al. 1973); from southern and East Africa (within the Transkei, between Natal and southern Mozambique, and between western Kenya and Uganda) (Prates and Torres 1965; Schonland and Bradshaw 1968; Ahmed and Cook 1969; Rose 1973; Rose and McGlashan 1975). Worldwide, the range of incidence between different regions of the world, at around

**Table 3.1.**  Annual truncated incidence rates and estimated incidence rates (for the age group 35–64 years) for cancer of the oesophagus (age standardised using the World Standard Population)

| Area | References | Incidence per 100 000 men aged 35–64 years | Male/female incidence |
|---|---|---|---|
| Western Europe | | | |
| West Germany (Hamburg) | 3 | 3.7 | 3.4 |
| Austria | 4 | 4.9[a] | 6.5 |
| Belgium | 4 | 6.2[a] | 4.9 |
| Netherlands (3 provinces) | 1 | 2.5 | 3.2 |
| UK (average of 6 registries) | 3 | 5.6 | 1.4 |
| Ireland | 4 | 8.0[a] | 1.4 |
| Switzerland (average of 3 registries) | 14 | 11.6 | 1.9 |
| France | 4 | 25.5[a] | 18.2 |
| France | | | |
|    Normandy and Brittany | 5 | 40.8[a,b] | 25.0 |
|    Doubs | 14 | 20.3 | (14.5) |
| Northern Europe | | | |
| Iceland | 3 | 3.4 | 1.8 |
| Sweden | 3 | 3.5 | 3.2 |
| Norway | | | |
|    Urban | 3 | 4.6 | 7.7 |
|    Rural | 3 | 1.9 | 3.8 |
| Denmark | 3 | 3.7 | 4.1 |
| Finland | 3 | 8.1 | 1.8 |
| Eastern Europe | | | |
| East Germany | 3 | 3.8 | 5.4 |
| Poland | | | |
|    Warsaw City | 3 | 9.7 | 4.0 |
|    4 rural areas | 3 | 4.9 | 8.2 |
| Hungary (Vas) | 3 | 2.7 | (9.0) |
| Czechoslovakia (Slovakia) | 14 | 4.3 | 7.2 |
| Bulgaria | 4 | 2.5[a,b] | 2.0 |
| Rumania (Banat Region) | 3 | 2.3 | 7.7 |
| Western Soviet Union (towns) | | | |
| Belorussia | 4 | 9.3[a,b] | 3.6 |
| Estonia | 4 | 15.0[a,b] | 7.2 |
| Latvia | 4 | 11.6[a,b] | 9.9 |
| Lithuania | 4 | 5.2[a,b] | 2.4 |
| Moldavia | 4 | 9.1[a,b] | 5.7 |
| Ukraine | 4 | 10.7[a,b] | 3.5 |
| RSFSR | 4 | 24.1[a,b] | 9.8 |
| Georgia | 4 | 7.9[a,b] | 5.1 |
| Armenia | 4 | 9.1[a,b] | 6.3 |
| Azerbaidjan | 4 | 28.6[a,b] | 1.7 |
| Southern Europe | | | |
| Portugal | 4 | 11.5[a] | 3.7 |
| Spain (average of 2 registries) | 14 | 7.8 | (8.2) |
| Italy | 4 | 6.5[a] | 5.7 |
| Italy (Varese) | 14 | 11.2 | 11.2 |
| Malta | 3 | 3.4 | (8.5) |
| Yugoslavia (Slovenia) | 3 | 9.6 | 16.0 |
| Middle East | | | |
| Israel | | | |
|    Jews born in Israel | 14 | 2.2 | (1.7) |
|    Jews born in Africa/Asia | 14 | 2.7 | 1.4 |

**Table 3.1.** *(continued)*

| Area | References | Incidence per 100 000 men aged 35–64 years | Male/female incidence |
|---|---|---|---|
| Jews born in Europe/America | 14 | 1.6 | 1.5 |
| non-Jews | 3 | (2.7) | (4.5) |
| Kuwait (Kuwaitis) | 15 | 4.8[b] | 1.2 |
| Bahrain (Bahrainis) | 16 | 10.9 | 1.4 |
| Iran | | | |
| Gonbad | 8 | 206.4 | 0.8 |
| NE Gonbad | 8 | 515.6 | 1.1 |
| Central Gonbad | 8 | 217.7 | 0.7 |
| Sn Gonbad | 8 | 151.6 | 1.2 |
| Gorgan | 8 | 123.9 | 1.1 |
| Northern Gorgan | 8 | 173.7 | 0.9 |
| Southern Gorgan | 8 | 104.1 | 0.9 |
| Central Mazandaran | 8 | 62.8 | 1.4 |
| Western Mazandaran | 8 | 44.5 | 2.0 |
| Gilan | 8 | 48.7 | 3.4 |
| Azerbaidjan (Ardebil) | 8 | 109.8 | 2.1 |
| Central Soviet Asia (towns) | | | |
| Kazakhstan | 4 | 64.9[a,b] | 1.3 |
| Gurjev | 4 | 547.2[b] | 1.6 |
| Uzbekistan | 4 | 48.6[a,b] | 2.3 |
| Turkmenistan | 4 | 110.5[a,b] | 1.1 |
| Kirighizia | 4 | 23.6[a,b] | 2.4 |
| Tajikstan | 4 | 32.5[a,b] | 10.5 |
| Far East | | | |
| Pakistan | | | |
| Karachi | 15 | 8.0 | (1.0) |
| Hyderabad | 15 | 3.0 | (0.7) |
| India | | | |
| Bombay | 3 | 21.0 | 1.0 |
| Ahmedabad | 15 | 18.9 | 1.6 |
| Bangalore | 15 | 14.7 | 1.1 |
| Madras | 15 | 11.2 | 1.9 |
| Burma (Rangoon) | 15 | 22.3 | 2.1 |
| Singapore | | | |
| Chinese | 3 | 30.0 | 3.3 |
| Malay | 3 | (4.4) | (0.5) |
| Indians | 3 | 7.9 | (0.8) |
| Japan | | | |
| Miyagi | 3 | 20.1 | 5.0 |
| Okayama | 3 | 4.9 | (1.8) |
| Osaka | 3 | 11.2 | (3.6) |
| Korea | 15 | 4.7 | 10.0 |
| Hong Kong | 14 | 33.8 | 3.8 |
| China | | | |
| Beijing | 17 | 33.9[a] | 2.3 |
| Shanghai | 17 | 42.1[a] | 3.0 |
| Tainjin | 17 | 30.9[a] | 1.8 |
| Hebei | 17 | 86.1[a] | 2.3 |
| Shanxi | 17 | 104.3[a] | 1.7 |
| Hunyuan and Tatung | 6 | 3.9[b] | 2.3 |
| Nei Mongol | 17 | 39.5[a] | 2.2 |
| Liaoning | 17 | 18.8[a] | 2.5 |

*(Table 3.1 continued on next page)*

**Table 3.1.**  *(continued)*

| Area | References | Incidence per 100 000 men aged 35–64 years | Male/female incidence |
|---|---|---|---|
| Jilin | 17 | 17.1[a] | 2.7 |
| Heilongjiang | 17 | 13.8[a] | 2.2 |
| Shaanxi | 17 | 89.2[a] | 2.9 |
| Gansu | 17 | 40.7[a] | 2.6 |
| Ningxia | 17 | 57.3[a] | 3.0 |
| Qinghai | 17 | 42.3[a] | 2.4 |
| Xingjiang | 17 | 50.8[a] | 1.6 |
| Shandong | 17 | 51.9[a] | 2.5 |
| Jiangsu | 17 | 111.0[a] | 1.7 |
| Zhejiang | 17 | 42.3[a] | 2.4 |
| Anhui | 17 | 79.6[a] | 2.1 |
| Jiangxi | 17 | 24.6[a] | 2.0 |
| Fujian | 17 | 93.7[a] | 1.9 |
| Henan | 17 | 126.8[a] | 1.9 |
| Yangcheng and Hehpih | 6 | 236.6[a,b] | 1.6 |
| Hubei | 17 | 64.9[a] | 2.5 |
| Hunan | 17 | 12.8[a] | 2.2 |
| Guangdong | 17 | 40.8[a] | 1.8 |
| Guangxi | 17 | 14.4[a] | 2.0 |
| Sichuan | 17 | 61.1[a] | 1.8 |
| Guizhou | 17 | 8.0[a] | 2.3 |
| Yunnan | 17 | 4.7[a] | 2.0 |
| Xizang | 17 | 23.6[a] | 1.7 |
| Canada | | | |
|   Average of 7 registries | 3 | 4.8 | 4.0 |
|   Eskimos | 15 | 29.5 | (1.7) |
| Eastern and Central USA | | | |
|   Connecticut | 3 | 9.4 | 3.8 |
|   New York State | 3 | 6.6 | 3.0 |
|   Michigan | | | |
|     Detroit, white | 14 | 6.6 | 2.8 |
|     Detroit, black | 14 | 29.3 | 2.7 |
| Western USA | | | |
|   Utah | 3 | 4.1 | 5.9 |
|   Nevada | 3 | 5.0 | 2.3 |
|   California | | | |
|     Alameda, white | 3 | 7.2 | 2.3 |
|     Alameda, black | 3 | 19.8 | (4.0) |
|     San Francisco Bay, white | 3 | 6.4 | 1.8 |
|     San Francisco Bay, black | 3 | 27.9 | 2.8 |
|     San Francisco Bay, Chinese | 3 | 12.5 | (7.8) |
| Southern USA | | | |
|   Texas | | | |
|     El Paso, Spanish | 3 | (3.1) | 3.1/0.0 |
|     El Paso, other white | 3 | 2.7 | (2.1) |
|   New Mexico | | | |
|     Spanish | 3 | 2.4 | (4.8) |
|     Other white | 3 | 4.0 | 3.1 |
|     American Indian | 3 | (4.6) | 4.6/0.0 |
|   Georgia | | | |
|     Atlanta, white | 14 | 4.7 | 2.8 |
|     Atlanta, black | 14 | 45.8 | 5.9 |

**Table 3.1.** *(continued)*

| Area | References | Incidence per 100 000 men aged 35–64 years | Male/female incidence |
|---|---|---|---|
| Louisiana | | | |
| New Orleans, white | 14 | 6.5 | 5.4 |
| New Orleans, black | 14 | 31.2 | 4.3 |
| Caribbean | | | |
| Puerto Rico | 3 | 29.6 | 2.7 |
| Cuba | 3 | 7.4 | 2.6 |
| Jamaica | 3 | 13.0 | 2.3 |
| Costa Rica | 15 | 6.1 | 2.4 |
| Martinique | 15 | 22.5 | 4.0 |
| Curacao | 9 | 44.4[b] | 18.7 |
| Netherlands Antilles | 14 | 14.5 | 2.3 |
| South America | | | |
| Colombia (Cali) | 3 | 7.3 | 4.1 |
| Bolivia (La Paz) | 15 | 2.3 | (5.0) |
| Venezuela | 4 | 4.8[a] | 1.0 |
| Brazil | | | |
| Recife | 3 | 10.5 | 5.5 |
| São Paulo | 3 | 22.0 | 7.3 |
| Uruguay | 4 | 23.6[a] | 2.8 |
| Africa (blacks) | | | |
| Senegal (Dakar) | 14 | (0.5) | (0.7) |
| Nigeria (Ibadan) | 2 | (2.5) | (8.3) |
| Uganda (Kyadondo) | 1 | 5.5 | 1.6 |
| Kenya (C. Nyanza) | 10 | 106.0[c] | 11.8 |
| S. Africa | | | |
| Cape Province | 2 | 77.0 | 2.2 |
| Transkei South (Butterworth) | 11 | 180.7[b] | 2.3 |
| Transkei North (Bizania) | 11 | 26.2[b] | 2.3 |
| Natal | 2 | 93.1 | 3.5 |
| Johannesburg | 12 | 54.5[c] | 4.2 |
| Mozambique (Lourenço Marques) | 1 | 11.8 | 11.8/0.0 |
| Zimbabwe (Bulawayo) | 2 | 94.9 | 3.3 |
| Africa (other) | | | |
| S. Africa | | | |
| Cape Province (white) | 2 | 9.0 | 6.4 |
| Cape Province (coloured) | 2 | 21.3 | 21.3/0.0 |
| Natal (Indian) | 2 | (14.7) | 0.6 |
| Oceania | | | |
| Australia | 4 | 5.0[a] | 2.9 |
| New Zealand | | | |
| Maori | 14 | 12.1 | (6.1) |
| Non-Maori | 14 | 7.3 | 2.7 |
| Hawaii | | | |
| Hawaiian | 14 | 22.7 | (4.6) |
| Caucasian | 14 | 4.4 | 1.2 |
| Chinese | 14 | 11.0 | (5.2) |
| Japanese | 14 | 4.7 | (15.6) |
| Filipino | 14 | 6.4 | (4.6) |
| Fiji | | | |
| Fijians | 13 | 4.2 | 4.2/0.0 |
| Indians | 13 | 4.5 | 3.5 |
| New Caledonia (Melanesians) | 15 | 22.0 | 22.0/0.0 |

*(Table 3.1 continued on next page)*

**Table 3.1.** *(continued)*

| Area | References | Incidence per 100 000 men aged 35–64 years | Male/female incidence |
| --- | --- | --- | --- |

[a]Estimate from mortality data (Doll 1969).
[b]Estimate from a different age group.
[c]Adjusted for under-reporting.
  (Incidence based on fewer than 10 cases.)

**References**
 1 Doll et al. (1966)
 2 Doll et al. (1970)
 3 Waterhouse et al. (1976)
 4 Doll (1969)
 5 Estimate from Tuyna (1969, personal communication)
 6 Estimate from Coordinating Group, Chinese (1974)
 7 Estimate from Miller (1978)
 8 Mahboubi et al. (1973)
 9 Estimate from IARC Annual Report (1970)
10 Ahmed and Cook (1969)
11 Estimate from Rose and McGlashan (1975)
12 Estimate from Robertson et al. (1971)
13 Estimate from Boyd et al. (1973)
14 Waterhouse et al (1982)
15 Parkin (1986)
16 Hamadeh (1988)
17 Chinese Atlas of Cancer Mortality (1979)

500-fold, is greater than the range for almost any other commonly occurring type of cancer. Cancer of the lung, for example, shows only a 40-fold variation between the highest and lowest recorded incidence levels; cancer of the stomach, 20-fold; cancer of the colon, 10-fold variation (Doll 1967). Comparisons are for the age group 35–64 years for which the figures are most reliable (Doll and Cook 1967).

The highest rates in Asia occur in peoples of Turko-Mongolian origin (Kazakhs, Turkomans, Karakalpaks, Uzbeks and Yakuts) (Kolycheva 1980) and not in peoples of Indo-European origin (Persians, Tadjiks, Pathans and Slavs) (Nugmanov and Kolycheva 1970; Sobin 1969; Mahboubi et al. 1973). However, there is considerable variation in incidence within these groups and there are Turko-Mongolian peoples that have rates lower than the highest rates for Indo-Europeans in Central Asia. Similarly, within populations of purely Chinese origin (eastern and southern Provinces of China (Fig. 3.1)) there is a wide variation in risk.

Over most of Europe incidence is low, but moderately high rates have been reported from Normandy and Brittany in northern France (Tuyns and Massé 1973) and from northern Italy (Cislaghi et al. 1978). Data by canton within Normandy and Brittany show a concentration of highest rates within certain small areas (Tuyns and Vernhes 1981) giving sharp gradients similar to those that have been recorded in Asia and Africa.

Incidence is low in the white populations of the USA, Canada, Africa, Australia and New Zealand. American blacks, however, have a risk of the disease that is between two and ten times higher than that in whites who live in the same areas. In the Caribbean and South America both black and white populations have moderate levels of incidence. In Asia there are reports of moderate incidence from India, Burma, Singapore and Japan.

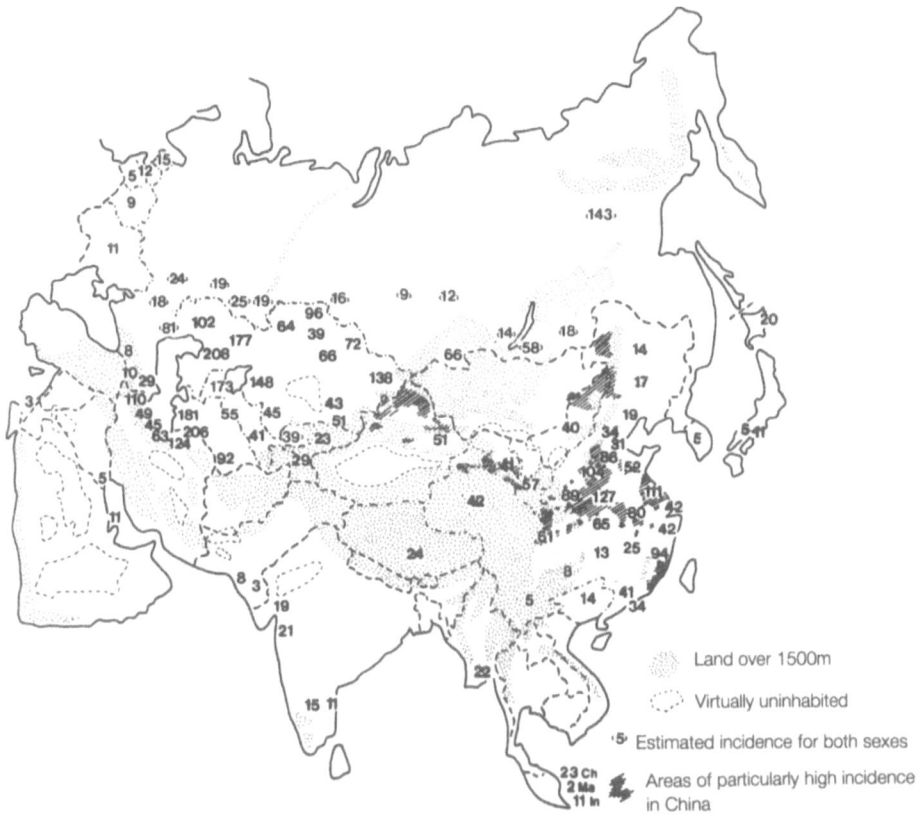

**Fig. 3.1.** Estimated incidence of cancer of the oesophagus in Asia for men at ages 35–64 years (per 100 000) at periods between 1960 and 1980. (Data for areas of particularly high incidence in China are taken from the Chinese Atlas of Cancer Mortality 1979.)

A problem in epidemiological investigations of cancer of the oesophagus has been that the highest reported incidence levels occur in economically less advanced countries, where routinely collected incidence or mortality data are not available. Histology records often give an inaccurately low impression of frequency because over much of rural Africa and Asia doctors rarely attempt to take a biopsy from inaccessible tumours (Burkitt et al. 1968; Mahboubi et al. 1973). In view of this, special surveys have been mounted in areas where an exceptional incidence has been suspected, and tumours diagnosed on radiological or even on clinical grounds alone have been included. In the Transkei region of South Africa, a village-to-village search was mounted over a period of years to identify all cases of cancer of the oesophagus (Burrell 1962, 1969; Rose 1973). In northern Iran, technicians were sent each month, again over a period of years, to several hundred doctors to collect information about newly diagnosed cases (Mahboubi et al. 1973). In the latter survey, a check was made on completeness of reporting by collecting information not just about cancer of the oesophagus but about all malignant tumours. The incidence of cancer at other sites showed a very

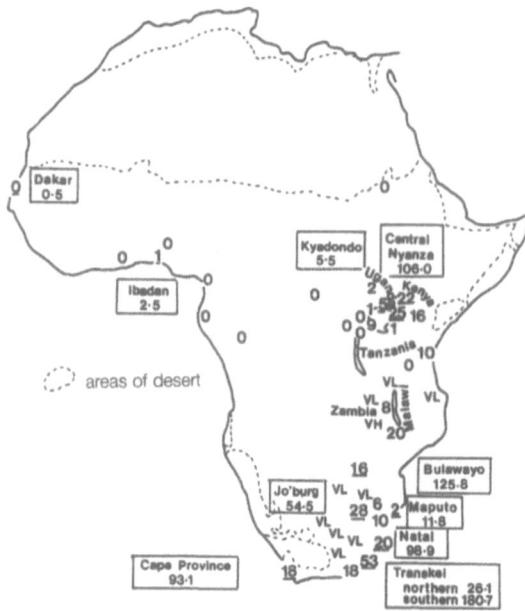

**Fig. 3.2.**   Estimated incidence of cancer of the oesophagus in Africa for men at ages 35–64 years (per 100 000) (figures in boxes) and proportional frequency of cancer of the oesophagus in men expressed as a proportion of all male cancer (figures on the map). The letters VH and VL stand for a frequency that was "very high" or "very low", using information from centres where insufficient data were available for the calculation of percentages. Data are for periods between 1960 and 1980.

similar level across all regions in contrast to the gradients observed for cancer of the oesophagus.

Expense limits the area that can be covered by such intensive incidence investigations and the pattern of cancer occurrence in wide tracts of rural Africa has been outlined using less rigorous survey methods. In the absence of population data, the frequency of one type of cancer has been expressed as a proportion of the number of tumours at other sites (Cook and Burkitt 1971) or relative to the number of hospital beds or admissions (Oettlé 1963). In both surveys, data were collected by postal questionnaire; in East Africa the forms were sent out monthly over a period of years. The information of this type for cancer of the oesophagus is summarised in Fig. 3.2. Two features are of particular interest. In the first place, there are clearly several other gradients of frequency in addition to those that have been defined in the incidence surveys described above; between Johannesburg and rural areas of the northern Transvaal; between southern Malawi and southern Tanzania and the adjacent areas of eastern Zambia; and between Central Nyanza in Kenya and northern Tanzania. It is of interest that, as in Asia, sharp gradients of frequency are found within a single ethnic group, as occurs, for example, between the Luo of Central Nyanza and the Luo of North Mara in Tanzania.

The second striking feature of the occurrence of cancer of the oesophagus in Africa is the very low incidence of the disease in all areas of West Africa for which data are available.

## Incidence in Women

Most of the descriptions of patterns of frequency so far have been for men. The ratio of male to female incidence is given in the right-hand column of Table 3.1 and it can be seen that, whereas the rates for women sometimes show the same high frequency, they often occur at a much lower level. Furthermore, although in one or two areas of very high incidence the female risk is marginally higher than that for men, there is no example of a high incidence in women unaccompanied by a high incidence in men.

In the exceptionally high incidence areas of Central Soviet Asia, Iran and China, where the incidence in men and women is nearly equal, there is a steeper decline of risk for women than for men as one passes into the adjacent areas of lower incidence. In Africa, the same differential decline occurs between the south and the north of Transkei, but in southern Malawi, Bulawayo and Kenya a high incidence in men is accompanied by rates in women that are ten to twelve times lower. In Normandy and Brittany, cancer of the oesophagus is outstandingly a disease of men, with a sex ratio of over 25:1.

## Changing Frequency with Time

Well-documented increases in incidence have been recorded for both sexes among blacks in the USA, in the population of England and Wales and for men in Normandy and Brittany (Cutler and Devesa 1973; Audigier et al. 1975; Chilvers et al. 1979). In England and France the increases have been modest, but amongst black men of working age in the USA a sharp increase over time has given rates that are now second only to those for lung cancer in several urban centres (Waterhouse et al. 1982). Similarly, in South Africa there are indications that the disease has come up like an epidemic from being very rare in the 1930s to being one of the commonest types of cancer diagnosed at some centres by the 1960s and 1970s. The most reliable reports are from Johannesburg where, at the principal African hospital, cancer of the oesophagus represented 2% of all tumours diagnosed in men in the 1930s (Berman 1935), 10% in the early 1950s, and 20% in the early 1960s (Robertson et al. 1971; Cook-Mozaffari 1980), by which time the oesophagus had become the most common individual site for cancer development in men. The earlier figure for Johannesburg (Berman 1935) seems to represent a genuinely low incidence in that it was based on all cases diagnosed, not only on histology records, and tumours at other internal sites were well represented in the series. Similar reports of a dramatic rise in frequency come from Durban and from the Transkei (Schonland and Bradshaw 1969; Burrell 1962; Rose 1973).

The increases in southern Africa appear to be affecting also areas where until the early 1960s (Oettlé 1963) the disease was little known. By the mid-seventies moderate frequencies had been reported from Swaziland, the Transvaal and Botswana (Keen 1971; Sutherland 1968; Macrae and Cook 1975). Recent data from Swaziland indicate a further increase over time to the point where cancer of the oesophagus amongst men is now second in frequency (at 17.5% of all malignancies) only to cancer of the liver (20.8%) (Peers and Keen 1986).

In East Africa there is also some indication of increases over time. The pathology records at the large central hospital in Nairobi, Kenya, showed cancer of the oesophagus representing fewer than 0.1% of all tumours diagnosed in the mid 1930s (Vint 1935) compared with around 16% in the late 1960s (Cook and Burkitt 1971) and, whereas doctors at small mission hospitals may never take an oesophageal biopsy, it seems less likely that this would be the practice at a central government hospital. In Uganda, as in the lower-frequency areas of southern Africa, cancer of the oesophagus is beginning to be seen more commonly (Templeton 1973).

There is no evidence concerning recent change in the exceptionally high incidence areas of Iran and Soviet Central Asia. In northern China in the 1920s and 1930s several missionary doctors reported cancer of the oesophagus as one of the types of cancer most commonly diagnosed (Davies 1924; Gear 1935) while the Chinese epidemiologists who have more recently been investigating the disease say that it has been known in the high-incidence areas for over 2000 years (Kaplan and Tsuchitani 1978). In Iran a medical text from the twelfth century describes and illustrates cancer of the oesophagus, which indicates that there, too, it may be of long-standing origin (Elgood 1951).

## Frequency amongst Migrants

Data from the Singapore Cancer Registry give information on whether patients were born in China or in Singapore and on the regional origin of patients from within China (Shanmugaratnam et al. 1983). Incidence is highest in the Teochew and Hokkien groups who come from high incidence areas within Guangdong and Fujian Provinces and lowest in the Cantonese who come from the low-incidence area south of Guangdong. Comparison with rates shown in the Chinese Atlas of Cancer Mortality (1979), however, suggests that the rates for Singapore are lower than those in the home regions of China and this is consonant with the fact that, in Singapore, amongst Chinese born in Singapore the rates are around three times lower than the rates among those born in China. It would be of interest to know whether rates amongst Singapore Chinese who were born in China are lower than those for Chinese who remained in China but the data are not presented in sufficient detail to permit such comparison.

Studies from the USA show rates among people of Chinese and Japanese origin who were born in China or Japan that are two to three times higher than rates among white Americans, and rates among those who were born in the USA that are similar to those for white Americans (King and Locke 1980; Locke and King 1980). Again, however, it is not possible to compare rates among first generation immigrants to the USA with rates in the home territories because the precise regional origin of patients is not known.

## Frequency in Specific Population Groups

Studies from the USA have shown a low risk for cancer of the oesophagus among Seventh Day Adventists and Mormons (Wynder et al. 1959; Enstrom 1980; Lyon et al. 1980) and a higher risk amongst Catholics than amongst Jews (Wynder and Bross 1961). The latter finding was repeated in a recent study from Los Angeles (Mack et al. 1985).

Routinely published data from England and Wales show a gradient of increasing risk with decreasing socio-economic status, with the lowest rates in professional workers and the highest rates in unskilled labourers (Registrar General, 1971; Office of Population Censuses and Surveys, 1978). A similar gradient has been demonstrated in the USA from a study of median rental values (Graham et al. 1960).

# Aetiology

## Genetic Factors

The only clearly defined genetic association for cancer of the oesophagus is with tylosis – originally described in Liverpool when 18 cases occurred in several generations of two families (Howel-Evans et al. 1958). A possible association exists with coeliac disease where an increased incidence has been observed both in patients (Harris et al. 1967: Holmes et al. 1976) and among male relatives of patients (Stokes et al. 1976). However, neither association can account for more than a few of the cases that occur throughout the world.

Various case-control studies from China and Central Asia in earlier years suggested a greater risk of oesophageal cancer among family members of patients than among controls, and these studies might indicate a genetic effect. However, such studies are notoriously difficult to interpret in view of the problems of recall bias. For example, a recent study from Iran reported more cases among the blood relatives of Turkoman patients than among non-blood relatives (Ghadirian 1985) but no controls were included that would have permitted a check on the extent to which the concerns of blood relatives were remembered better than those of non-blood relatives.

## Environmental Factors

The wide range of incidence for cancer of the oesophagus between different parts of the world and within groups of common ethnic origin together with the changes of incidence that have been observed following migration strongly indicate that environmental factors are responsible for the majority of cases that occur. It has been suggested that the sharp gradients of incidence that have been observed reflect the multiplicative effect of several factors acting together rather than the dominant effect of a single risk factor as occurs with cigarette smoking in the aetiology of cancer of the lung (Day et al. 1982). A number of environmental factors have been identified as playing a role in the development of cancer of the oesophagus.

### Alcohol, Tobacco and Other Substances Smoked or Chewed

*Europe and America.* Detailed questioning of patients (Craver 1932; Mosebech and Videback 1955) and analysis of cancer rates associated with different occupations (Young and Russell 1926; Versluys 1949) have long indicated a role for alcohol and sometimes for tobacco in the development of cancer of the oesophagus. Formal case-control and cohort studies have subsequently confirmed an effect for both factors (Steiner 1956; Schwartz et al. 1962; Martinez 1969; Hakulinen et al. 1974) and have elucidated the way in which the two act together to increase risk. A study in the USA showed a clear dose-response for both factors independently and a substantial increase in risk for heavy consumers of both alcohol and tobacco (Wynder and Bross 1961). Seventy per cent of male oesophageal cancer patients had taken more than '3 units' of alcohol daily while only 26% of controls had imbibed at this level. There was a five-fold increase in risk compared with non-smokers and non-drinkers for those who, in addition to taking 3 or more units of alcohol, had also smoked more than 20 cigarettes a day, and a six-fold increase in risk for those who had consumed alcohol and smoked cigars or a pipe.

A more recent study from Brittany in France has shown a clearly multiplicative effect of the two factors (Tuyns et al. 1977) with a relative risk of over 130 for those who smoked more than 20 g of tobacco and drank more than 120 g of ethanol a day compared with those who smoked less than 10 g of tobacco and drank less than 40 g of ethanol. As in several previous studies it appears that the effect of alcohol with little tobacco smoking is greater than the effect of smoking accompanied by little alcohol intake, with a dose response that is exponential for alcohol and less than linear for tobacco (Day and Muñoz 1982). However, data from the USA are thought to indicate that heavy alcohol intake without smoking has little effect (Wynder et al. 1975).

Studies from various parts of the world suggest that different alcoholic drinks have differing effects, with spirits carrying a greater risk than wine or beer (Wynder and Bross 1961; Martinez 1969; Tuyns 1970; Pequignot and Tuyns 1975; Hirayama 1979). In Brittany and Normandy there is an indication of a geographical association with the frequency of home distillation (Barrelier 1974).

It has been estimated that, in Europe, North America and the Caribbean, alcohol and tobacco together probably account for around 90% of cases of oesophageal cancer and that these two factors can explain most of the increases that have occurred over time, most of the regional variation and most of the variation between different cultural, socio-economic and occupation groups (Day and Muñoz 1982). This is almost certainly true for men but it is not clear that the attributable risk is as high for women. In the American study by Wynder and Bross (1961), for example, 41% of the female patients were non-smokers and 43% rarely or never drank.

*Africa.* Studies from southern Africa also suggest that alcohol and tobacco are risk factors in the development of oesophageal cancer, at least among urban residents in that area. In Durban and Johannesburg it has been shown that the greatest elevation of risk occurred for those who consumed both spirits and beer and who smoked pipe tobacco either in pipes or in hand-rolled cigarettes (Bradshaw and Schonland 1969, 1974). In neither study did there appear to be any risk associated with the smoking of commercial cigarettes alone at any level of alcohol consumption. In a more recent study from Natal, both commercial cigarettes and pipe-smoking emerged as major risk factors (van Rensburg et al. 1985). The role of alcohol is not clear in the latter study as figures are not given for the consumption of beer or of commercial spirits but only for home-made spirits.

In a population study from the Transkei, one of the areas where there was a long tradition of pipe-smoking, it was found that 78% of men and 7% of women smoked and drank in the high-incidence southern areas compared with only 25% and 1% in the low-incidence northern areas (Bradshaw et al. 1983). Also, a higher proportion of the population drank spirits in the high-incidence than in the low-incidence areas. A previous study had noted the swallowing of dottle (intshonga) from the pipe stem and the chewing of residue (isixaxa) from the bowl of the pipe (Rose 1978), substances which were found to be mutagenic (Hewer et al. 1978), but the population survey showed that only 2–3% of the population consumed intshonga or isixaxa (Bradshaw et al. 1983). It is not clear, however, how long the current levels of chewing, smoking or drinking have been extant in the Transkei and how relevant they are, therefore, to the pattern of oesophageal cancer observed in the 1960s and 1970s.

Information from East Africa suggested that there was no simple association in Africa with the quantity of alcohol consumed. A Liquor Commission in low-incidence Uganda established that illicit distilling was the third industry of the country after cotton and coffee (Uganda Government 1963) and legislation was passed to permit production of spirits by local distillers. Similarly, in West Africa, where the disease is rare, the drinking of palm wine is common. A study of the ingredients that were used to make the traditional beers and wines consumed in different parts of Africa pointed to a geographical and temporal association between the occurrence of cancer of the oesophagus and the use of maize as a major ingredient of beer (Cook 1971). During the previous 50 years in much of East and southern Africa maize had replaced the traditional millet and sorghum for beer-making. In Uganda, however, maize beer had only recently begun to usurp the traditional banana or millet brews.

Little information was available on smoking habits except that outside the areas of South Africa discussed above the smoking of cigarettes had been rare almost everywhere (Cook and Burkitt 1971). Both men and women in Central Nyanza in Kenya were said to have smoked pipes (as in the Transkei) but whereas the disease was common in both men and women in the Transkei it was some twelve times more common in men than in women in Central Nyanza (Cook 1971) and the role of pipe-smoking there is not clear. More information is needed on the frequency of smoking by men and women in different parts of Africa. It could be that areas of high alcohol intake but low oesophageal cancer incidence, such as Uganda, are areas where tobacco smoking had not been traditionally practised. In support of this hypothesis, it is known that in the mid 1960s most tobacco grown on large estates in low-incidence Uganda and Tanzania was consumed in high-incidence Kenya (O'Connor 1966).

*Middle East.* By the end of the 1960s, information was beginning to come from Iran that there were rural areas of very high incidence for both men and women in which the proscriptions of the Moslem religion concerning alcohol were still widely observed – especially by women (Kmet and Mahboubi 1972). The low intake of alcohol was confirmed in a subsequent case-control study (Mahboubi et al. 1978) and a series of epidemiological investigations was launched to investigate the role of other factors. Analysis of morphine metabolites from a small number of urine specimens collected during the population-study phase suggested a geographical association in northern Iran between opium intake and the occurrence of cancer of the oesophagus (Iran-IARC Joint Study Group 1977).

Fifty percent of the sample of men and women from the areas of highest incidence had consumed opium in the previous day or two. Subsequent enquiry in these regions indicated a high consumption of dross scraped from the inside of opium pipes and dross was found to be mutagenic whereas raw opium was not (Hewer et al. 1978; Malaveille et al. 1982). Preliminary results of a case-household/control-household study set up to measure morphine metabolites showed an elevated proportion of subjects from the high-incidence areas (in both case families and control families) having a high intake of opium compared with the subjects from the low-incidence areas. There was also a higher intake, of marginal statistical significance, among the family members of cases than among the family members of controls (Ghadirian et al. 1985). The oesophageal cancer patients themselves could provide no useful information on the use of opium since many will have been taking it to alleviate their symptoms. A higher intake among case-household members could indicate a long-term habituation by these households which had involved also the individuals who had subsequently developed cancer of the oesophagus. Unfortunately, this study was cut short by political events in Iran in 1979.

*Asia.* Early reports from China are conflicting about the role of alcohol (Kwan 1937; Cheng 1949; Wu et al. 1951; Li et al. 1962). The preliminary results of a case-control study currently underway show that only 24% of either patients or controls have ever drunk alcoholic beverages (Li et al. 1985). No mention is made in any studies of a possible role for opium products and its use is likely to have been severely restricted since the end of the Second World War.

Results from a case-control study in Singapore (de Jong et al. 1974) have shown moderate increases in risk associated with Chinese wine (Samsu) and with cigarette smoking. A prospective study from Japan (Hirayama 1971) showed an age-standardised (all-age) rate of 8.4 per 100 000 for non-smokers and non-drinkers compared with 10.8 and 9.2 for smokers of <20 and >20 cigarettes a day who did not drink alcohol daily and 26.2 and 27.1 for smokers at the two levels who took alcohol daily. Risk was highest for those who drank whisky and shochu (a local liqueur) and lowest for beer (Hirayama 1979). The 8.4 per 100 000 for non-smokers and non-drinkers in Japan is several times higher than the average figure of 2.8 per 100 000 for men in the general population of the UK, during a similar period (Doll et al. 1970), a figure which will largely be derived from cases among smokers and drinkers.

A study of over 600 patients and controls from the moderate-incidence city of Bombay in India showed that only 28.8% of male patients and none of the female patients were habitual drinkers (Jussawalla 1971). It was not thought that prohibition, which was currently in force in Bombay, led to serious underestimation of alcohol intake. Raised risks amongst men were observed for the following combined habits: smoking with alcohol use; the chewing of "pan" (betel quid with or without tobacco) with alcohol use; and especially for smoking with chewing (relative risk (RR) 36.2). Risks were highest for those who smoked the local "bidi" cigarettes, who drank the local, home-made brew that had a high content of raw spirits and, surprisingly, for those who chewed "pan" without tobacco (RR in combination with smoking 94.2). This was thought to occur because chewers who did not include tobacco in their quid habitually swallowed most of the juice produced from chewing whereas those who included tobacco would spit out the juice.

For women in Bombay the highest risks were associated with the individual habits of smoking "bidi" cigarettes and of chewing "pan" without tobacco (RRs 17.8 and 7.0). Thus, although oesophageal cancer is as common amongst women in Bombay as amongst men, a far lower proportion of cases can be explained by the consumption of alcohol, tobacco or betel quid.

## Dietary Deficiencies

As it became clear during the 1960s that the worldwide variation in the range of incidence for cancer of the oesophagus was too great to be explained simply in terms of alcohol and tobacco consumption and, indeed, that there were populations of exceptionally high incidence, such as the women of northeastern Iran, amongst whom the consumption of alcohol and tobacco was negligible, it seemed that the best way to generate new ideas would be to investigate the geographical clues and to examine in detail the environment and way of life of regions where sharp gradients of incidence had been observed (IARC Internal Report 1968). An international programme of research was entered upon in Iran to carry out work along these lines. Initial perusal of available environmental information showed a strong negative association with rainfall and partial correlations with the many variables dependent on rainfall, such as vegetation, soil types and crop patterns (Kmet and Mahboubi 1972).

The limits of what could be learned from published sources were quickly reached and a population survey was mounted to collect additional information. Field teams lived during the course of a year in some 40 villages around the south of the Caspian Sea and carried out detailed dietary, sociological and physiological surveys on the general population of the area (Iran-IARC Joint Study Group 1977). This work focused attention on the very restricted diet of the highest incidence areas. For most of the year little besides home-baked bread, tea and sugar is consumed. The flocks of sheep and goats give milk for yoghurt in the spring before the pastures are scorched dry with the approach of summer. The bare steppe grasslands provide virtually no vegetables or fruit and the traditional diet of the Turkomans is almost completely lacking in either. Such a diet has very low levels of animal protein, vitamin A, riboflavin and vitamin C (Hormozdiari et al. 1975). Overt clinical signs of riboflavin deficiency are widespread (Kmet, McLaren and Siassi 1980).

A subsequent case-control study confirmed the risk attributable to a low intake of fruit and vegetables and demonstrated that within the generally poor rural communities of northern Iran it is those of the lowest economic status who are most at risk for cancer of the oesophagus (Cook-Mozaffari et al. 1979).

Case-control studies conducted in the USA and Puerto Rico had also shown an increased risk associated with low socio-economic status (Wynder and Bross 1961; Martinez 1969). However, the importance of the investigation in Iran, and of a subsequent study in Singapore (de Jong et al. 1974), both of which found an association with duration of schooling (shorter duration giving higher risk), was that they suggested a long-standing association with poverty. Poverty may thus itself be implicated in the development of the disease rather than occurring as the result of a debilitating addiction to, say, alcohol or opium (Day and Muñoz 1982).

Early reports from China had also indicated that oesophageal cancer patients were mostly from the "hard-working class" (farmers, peddlers or labourers (Lang 1938)) or from the "lower socio-economic level" (Wu et al. 1951). Subsequent dietary work in Linxian Country in the high-incidence Henan Province indicated a low intake of riboflavin (96% of subjects) and of retinol (43%) from the measurement of serum vitamin levels (IARC Annual Report 1982). Comparison with a low-incidence county in Shandong Province showed that only riboflavin status was significantly different in the two areas (Thurnham et al. 1987).

Widespread oesophagitis was demonstrated in high-incidence areas of China (Muñoz et al. 1982) as had previously been found in Iran (Crespi et al. 1979) and an intervention trial was carried out in Huixian Province of China to determine whether combined treatment with retinol, riboflavin and zinc would result after one year in a lower prevalence of precancerous lesions (Muñoz et al. 1985). The preliminary results showed no difference between the treated and the placebo populations in the frequency of histologically diagnosed precancerous lesions. Subsequent analysis showed that increases in blood retinol and serum riboflavin levels (the latter not reaching statistical significance) were associated with a reduced prevalence of precancerous lesions but that the changes had occurred independently of treatment (Wahrendorf et al. 1987). It was also found that the prevalence of micronucleated cells in the oesophagus as an indicator of chromosomal aberrations was reduced in the treatment group as compared to the placebo group (Muñoz et al. 1987a) and that vitamin treatment reduced the abnormal cell proliferation in the upper layers of the epithelium (IARC Biennial Report 1986/ 1987). A second intervention trial is underway in Linxian County in China to investigate further the role of vitamin deficiency in the development of cancer of the oesophagus (Yang et al. 1985; Blot and Li 1985).

With the poor economic situation in most African countries, a restricted diet could clearly be a major background factor there in the development of cancer of the oesophagus. Low intakes of vitamin A and riboflavin, for example, are characteristic of the diet in the high-incidence areas of central and western Kenya (Cook-Mozaffari 1979). Van Rensburg (1981) has reemphasised the geographical association throughout Africa with the consumption of corn (maize) that was noted above (Cook 1971) and has suggested that the relevant factors are the dietary deficiencies engendered.

Studies from the USA suggest that, even in western populations where alcohol and tobacco are the dominant risk factors, dietary deficiency may play a part in the development of cancer of the oesophagus. Wynder and Bross (1961) found that patients consumed less butter, milk, eggs and green and yellow vegetables than controls. A case-control study conducted among black males in a part of Washington where excessive smoking and drinking were widespread also found that the patients were accustomed to eating more processed foods, more starchy foods and less red meat, chicken, eggs, fruit and vegetables (Pottern et al. 1985). Mettlin et al. (1980) found a decreased risk in New York associated with the consumption of fruit and vegetables. Furthermore, an excessive alcohol intake can result in nutritional deficiencies not only because of poor and irregular eating habits that accompany addiction but also because alcohol itself interferes with the absorption of other nutrients (Vitale and Coffey 1971; Theurer and Vitale 1976).

A precedent for a role of dietary deficiency in the development of cancer of the oesophagus had been established much earlier by studies which showed a high frequency of cancer of the upper oesophagus and hypopharynx in patients, particularly women, who had suffered from sideropenic dysphagia (the Plummer–Vinson syndrome) which was formerly common in much of northern Europe (Ahlbom 1936; Simpson 1939; Jacobsson 1948; Beveridge et al. 1965; Wynder 1971). It has been suggested that the relatively high rates for oesophageal cancer among women in northern areas of Norway and rural Wales might be remnants of a high prevalence of the Plummer–Vinson syndrome 40–50 years ago (Day and Muñoz 1982). Comparison of the site distribution of tumours in women from north Wales and from other regions covered by the Liverpool Cancer Registry did not suggest a preponderance in the upper third of the oesophagus but the proportion for whom site was unspecified was too high for conclusive results to emerge (Cook-Mozaffari, unpublished calculations).

Animal experiments have shown both that vitamin A and riboflavin can inhibit tumour development and that riboflavin deficiency can produce squamous metaplasia in the epithelium of the oesophagus in mice (Wynder and Klein 1965; Wynder and Chan 1970; overviews, Berg 1975; Day and Muñoz 1982).

An association that it was anticipated might be found in Iran was a link between oesophageal cancer and zinc deficiency as the symptoms of the latter had been reported from dry areas elsewhere in the country (Prasad et al. 1963). Zinc has an important role in maintaining the integrity of epithelial tissue and animal experiments have shown that zinc deficiency can promote the induction of oesophageal tumours (Fong and Newberne 1978). It is known that a high intake of bread rich in fibre, such as is eaten in the high-incidence areas of northern Iran, causes increased faecal excretion of zinc and other minerals (Reinbold et al. 1976) and this could exacerbate loss from sweating and from blood-loss through parasites so as to cause deficiency. However, the population study in northern Iran showed no difference in the zinc content of hair and nail samples between areas of high and low incidence (Iran-IARC Study Group 1977). Various studies have shown a lower concentration of zinc in tissues from patients than in those from controls, the latest being from China (Lin et al. 1977). However, it is not possible to tell whether the differences observed have preceded or followed the development of the malignant tumours. Day and Muñoz (1982) have noted that severe zinc deficiency has been observed in patients with coeliac disease who do not respond to gluten-free diets (Love et al. 1978) and have suggested that there may be an association between this and the increased incidence of oesophageal cancer that has been found in coeliac patients (Harris et al. 1967; Holmes et al. 1976).

## Carcinogenic Items of Diet

During the early years of research into cancer of the oesophagus in Africa interest centred on the possibly harmful contamination of home-made spirits distilled through old exhaust pipes and laced with metal polish (Burrell 1957; McGlashan 1969). However, these were features of distilling in urban areas and could not explain the high rural frequencies of cancer of the oesophagus. A more promising lead was the report that nitrosamines had been found in maize spirit from a high-incidence region of Zambia (McGlashan et al. 1968). This seemed to be a finding

of considerable importance because, not only were nitrosamines strongly carcinogenic, they were also the only group of chemicals known to cause oesophageal
tumours in experimental animals (Magee and Barnes 1967). However, at this
stage, the chemists were continually revising their techniques for measuring
nitrosamines and when spirit samples from high- and low-incidence areas in East
Africa were measured using more rigorous methods they showed no trace of
nitrosamine contamination (Collis et al. 1971). Re-analysis of the Zambia
samples led to the same conclusion (McGlashan et al. 1970). Subsequently, low
levels of nitrosamines were detected in home-made ciders and apple brandies
from Normandy and Brittany in France (IARC Annual Report 1975) and in a
variety of food samples from both the high- and low-incidence areas in Iran
(IARC Annual Report 1976). It was concluded that these probably represented a
general background level of contamination of little significance for cancer of the
oesophagus. Nonetheless, in view of the potent and specific activity of nitrosamines in experimental animals, research into their possible role and particularly
into their formation *in vivo* from ingested precursors has continued. Both tea,
which is widely consumed in northern Iran and vitamin C, which is lacking in
areas of high incidence, have been shown to inhibit the development of
nitrosamines in the stomach (Bogovski et al. 1972; Mirvish et al. 1972). Recent
work in China has suggested that inhabitants of a high-risk area were exposed to
more nitrates and N-nitrosamines than those living in a low-incidence area (Lu et
al. 1986) and subsequent investigation has shown an association between
mortality from cancer of the oesophagus and nitrosation potential of plasma
samples (IARC Biennial Report 1986/87). A negative association was apparent
with background ascorbate levels in plasma.

   From the Transkei there was a suggestion some years previously that
molybdenum deficiencies in the soil cause a build-up of nitrates in plants which
could be converted to nitrosamines in the stomach (Burrell et al. 1966). The soils
of high-incidence Linxian County in China are also low in molybdenum and its
addition to seeds before planting is said to have reduced considerably the nitrate
content of grains and increased the vitamin C content of vegetables (Kaplan and
Tsuchitani 1978).

   Intensive analysis of constituents of the diet in northern Iran for other known
carcinogens such as aflatoxins and polycyclic hydrocarbons showed very low
levels throughout the different incidence zones and no significant correlations
with incidence (IARC Annual Report 1975; Iran-IARC Joint Study Group
1977).

   Interest centred for some time on the possible fungal contamination of wheat
from storage in the underground pits that are characteristic of the high-incidence
areas of Iran and on the adulteration of bread with seeds from other plants.
Analysis of bread and wheat samples have demonstrated no carcinogenic
mycotoxins (Lacey and Booth 1980) but have shown a widespread admixture with
seeds other than wheat, some of which contained shikimic acid that has been
associated with tumour development in cattle from the eating of bracken fern
(Jarrett et al. 1978; Pamukbu and Price 1969). In Japan, where bracken fern is
commonly eaten as part of human diets, a case-control study showed a two-fold or
greater risk associated with its consumption (Hirayama 1979). However, shikimic
acid, which is widespread in plants, may not be the sole carcinogenic agent in
bracken fern (Berg 1975). It is thought that a more potent component needs to be
identified (Evans and Osman 1974). Subsequent testing showed no appreciable

mutagenic activity in bread and wheat samples from northern Iran (Bartsch et al. 1980).

In Linxian County in China, a maize bread cooked by steaming is the staple diet and on this a fungal mould is apparently widespread – grown during weeks of storage and relished as the preferred taste of bread (Coordinating Group 1974, 1975; Kaplan and Tsuchitani 1978; Yang 1980; Li 1982). Another commonly consumed dietary item is "pickled" (i.e. rotted in salt water) vegetables. Samples of pickled vegetables have been found to be mutagenic (Li 1981; Lu et al. 1981). A case-control study is underway to ascertain the risk associated with these dietary items as well as with numerous other factors (Li et al. 1985).

## Physical Trauma of Oesophageal Tissue

Cicatricial strictures of the oesophagus left after corrosive damage due to the swallowing of lye sometimes gives rise to malignant tumours (Vinson 1940). It is possible that other less dramatic damage can also increase the frequency of tumour development. It has repeatedly been suggested that the ingestion of hot food and drink increases risk (Watson 1933; Kwan 1937; Cheng 1949; Burrell 1957; Sato 1963). Segi (1975) found a geographical association in Japan between the consumption of a burning hot rice-tea gruel (chagayu) and the incidence of cancer of the oesophagus. At an individual level a case-control study showed a two-fold increase in risk for patients who had been frequent consumers of chagayu (Hirayama 1971). In Singapore, a three to fifteen-fold increase in risk was observed for patients who had preferred to take beverages burning hot (de Jong et al. 1974). Measurement of tea temperatures carried out in the late 1960s in Iran (Ghadirian 1987) suggested that tea was consumed at a higher temperature in high-incidence regions; while the nutrition survey found that a higher quantity of tea was taken there (Iran-IARC Joint Study Group 1977). However, in the case-control study both oesophageal and stomach cancer patients claimed to have drunk their tea hotter and it seemed that the developing gastrointestinal conditions may themselves have made patients more aware of the heat of foodstuffs (Cook-Mozaffari et al. 1977). Actual measurement of the rise in temperature at the lower end of the oesophagus, after swallowing measured quantities of coffee kept at a controlled temperature, showed that sip size rather than temperature was the controlling factor (de Jong et al. 1972) and this threw further doubt on the significance of temperatures assessed just before drinking. More recent support for the hypothesis that the consumption of excessively hot foodstuffs can increase risk has come from work in Brazil where daily intake of the plant infusion "maté", over a period of 40–50 plus years is associated with a two-fold increase in risk (Victoria et al. 1987) and where maté drinkers were twice as likely to develop oesophagitis as non-maté drinkers (Muñoz et al. 1987b). Evidence is discussed that suggests that maté does not have a carcinogenic effect per se but that it causes oesophagitis through thermal injury.

Another possible source of physical trauma to the oesophagus is the consumption of abrasive foodstuffs or contaminants of foodstuffs. Analysis of bread and wheat samples from high-incidence areas in Iran showed the frequent presence of abrasive seeds (Jarrett et al. 1978) that are known to cause gastric disturbances when they are included in cattle feed (Day 1980). Also, there were seeds with finely pointed silica fibres that could act as a stimulant to cell growth if lodged in the oesophagus (O'Neill et al. 1980). Silica fragments from millet bran were subsequently found in mucosa surrounding oesophageal tumours from patients in northern China (O'Neill et al. 1982). An earlier report from the Transkei in South Africa had also suggested that silica particles derived from the grinding stones used to prepare maize-flour might have an irritant effect on the oesophagus (Rose 1969).

# Conclusions

Several broad conclusions emerge from the wealth of epidemiological studies that have been conducted into the aetiology of cancer of the oesophagus. In the first place, relatively few cases seem to occur due to the action of a single, isolated carcinogenic agent. Rather, it appears that there is a complex of factors that may be present at different levels or substituted by equivalent factors in different parts of the world.

A necessary underlying factor may prove to be a heightening of susceptibility by dietary deficiency that is induced by the widespread intake of a poor diet from infancy in areas of high-incidence or, for certain individuals, by the harmful effects of alcohol on nutritional status in areas where alcohol is an important risk factor. A further heightening of susceptibility seems to occur in some areas from repeated small-scale irritation of the oesophageal mucosa by the ingestion of excessively hot food and drinks and of dry scratchy bread and cornmeal.

It can also be assumed that some specific carcinogenic agent or agents are involved in the development of cancer of the oesophagus. The failure to find any potent carcinogens at high levels in the highest-incidence areas suggests that perhaps a variety of weak carcinogenic agents may be acting on susceptible oesophageal tissue. These could occur, for example, in mouldy corn bread, opium residues, betel quid, maize beer, apple brandy or in a wealth of other substances as well as in tobacco. It is clear that tobacco smoke, which is mostly inhaled rather than swallowed, can offer only a weakly carcinogenic stimulus to the oesophagus and this is reflected in the low rates of oesophageal cancer that are found in western populations where smoking and lung cancer are both common. The same must be true in Iran for grains of opium dross as these are swallowed swiftly with tea so as to avoid the bitter taste.

The possibility has also been suggested that alcohol (Doll 1971) or hot tea (Day and Muñoz 1982) might act as solvents facilitating the passage of carcinogens to the basal layers of the oesophagus.

It would seem that where several of these factors are widespread in a region, they act multiplicatively to produce a very high incidence of cancer of the oesophagus and that the disappearance of any one element of the complex, as one moves to a neighbouring region, has a far more dramatic effect on lowering incidence than would occur in situations where that factor was acting alone.

# References

Ahmed N, Cook P (1969) The incidence of cancer of the oesophagus in West Kenya. Br J Cancer 23:302–312

Ahlbom HG (1936) Simple achlorhydric anaemia, Plummer–Vinson syndrome and carcinoma of the mouth, pharynx and oesophagus in women. Br Med J ii:331

Audigier JC, Tuyns AJ, Lambert R (1975) Epidemiology of oesophageal cancer in France. Digestion 13:209–213

Bartsch H, Malaveille C, Camus A et al. (1980) Validation and comparative studies on 180 chemicals with *S. typhimurium* strains and V79 Chinese hamster cells in the presence of various metabolizing systems. Mutation Res 76:1–50

Barrelier MT (1974) Le cancer de l'oesophage en Basse-Normandie. Thèse: Caen

Berg JW (1975) Diet. In: Fraumeni JF (ed) Persons at high risk for cancer. Academic Press, New York, pp 201–204

Berman C (1935) Malignant disease in the Bantu. S Afr J Med Sci 1:12–30

Beveridge BR, Bannerman RM, Evanson JM et al. (1965) Hypochromic anaemia. A retrospective study and follow-up of 378 in-patients. Q J Med 4:145–161

Blot WJ, Li J-Y (1985) Some considerations in the design of a nutrition intervention trial in Linxian, People's Republic of China. Natl Cancer Inst Monograph 69:29–34

Bogovski P, Castegnaro M, Pignatelli B, Walker EA (1972). The inhibiting effect of tannins on the formation of nitrosamines. In: Bogovski P, Preussmann R, Walker EA (eds) N-nitroso compounds. Analysis and formation. IARC Scientific Publications No 3, Lyon, pp 127–129

Boyd JT, Doll R, Gurd CH (1973) Cancer incidence in Fiji. Int J Epidemiol 2:177–187

Bradshaw E, Schonland M (1969) Oesophageal and lung cancer in Natal African males in relation to certain socio-economic factors. Br J Cancer 23:275–284

Bradshaw E, Schonland M (1974) Smoking, drinking and oesophageal cancer in African males of Johannesburg, South Africa. Br J Cancer 30:157–163

Bradshaw E, McGlashan ND, Harington JS (1983) Oesophageal cancer: smoking and drinking in Transkei. Institute of Social and Economic Research, Rhodes University, Grahamstown, South Africa (Occasional Paper No 27)

Burkitt DP, Hutt MSR, Slavin G (1968) Clinico-pathological studies of cancer distribution in Africa. Br J Cancer 22:1–6

Burrell RJW (1957) Oesophageal cancer in the Bantu. S Afr Med J 31:401–409

Burrell RJW (1962) Oesophageal cancer among the Bantu in the Transkei. J Natl Cancer Inst 28:495–514

Burrell RJW (1969) Distribution maps of oesophageal cancer among the Bantu in the Transkei. J Natl Cancer Inst 43:877–888

Burrell RJW, Roach WA, Shadwell A (1966) Oesophageal cancer in the Bantu of the Transkei associated with mineral deficiency in garden plants. J Natl Cancer Inst 36:201–209

Cheng PCL (1949) Carcinoma of the oesophagus. A statistical study of forty-three cases. Chin Med J 67:662–667

Chilvers C, Fraser P, Beral V (1979) Alcohol and oesophageal cancer: an assessment of the evidence from routinely collected data. J Epidemiol Commun Health 33:127–133

Chinese Atlas of Cancer Mortality (1979) Atlas of cancer mortality in the People's Republic of China. China Map Press, Peking

Cislaghi C, De Carli A, Morosini P, Puntoni R (1978) Atlante della mortalità per tumori in Italia 1970–72. Lega Italiana per la Lotta Contro i Tumori, Rome

Collis CH, Cook PJ, Foreman JK, Palframan JF (1971) A search for nitrosamines in East African spirit samples from areas of varying oesophageal cancer frequency. Gut 12:1015–1018

Cook P (1971) Cancer of the oesophagus in Africa. Br J Cancer 25:853–880

Cook PJ, Burkitt DP (1971) Cancer in Africa. Br Med Bull 27:14–20

Cook-Mozaffari P (1979) The epidemiology of cancer of the oesophagus. Nutr Cancer 1:51–61

Cook-Mozaffari PJ, Azordegan F, Day NE, Ressicaud A, Sabai C, Aramesh B (1979) Oesophageal cancer studies in the Caspian littoral of Iran: results of a case-control study. Br J Cancer 39:293–309

Cook-Mozaffari PJ (1980) The epidemiology and pathology of cancer of the oesophagus. In: Wright R (ed) Recent advances in gastrointestinal pathology. Saunders, Eastbourne, pp 267–284

Coordinating Group for Research on the Aetiology of Oesophageal Cancer of North China (1974) The epidemiology of oesophageal cancer in North China and preliminary results in the investigation of its aetiological factors. Peking

Coordinating Group for Research on the Aetiology of Oesophageal Cancer of North China (1975) The epidemiology and etiology of oesophageal cancer in North China. Chin Med J 1:167–183

Craver LF (1932) A clinical study of aetiology of gastric and oesophageal carcinoma. Am J Cancer 16:68–102

Crespi M, Muñoz N, Grassi A et al. (1979) Oesophageal lesions in northern Iran: a premalignant condition? Lancet II: 217–221

Cutler SJ, Devesa SS (1973) Trends in cancer incidence and mortality in the USA. In: Doll R, Vodopija I (eds) Host environment interactions in the etiology of cancer in man. IARC, Lyon, pp 15–34 (Scientific publications, no. 7)

Davies S (1924) Cancer in China. Br Med J i:131

Day NE (1980) Final Report for the contract NCI-CP-71048 between the NIH/NCI and IARC. IARC, Lyon

Day NE, Muñoz N (1982) Cancer of the oesophagus. In: Schottenfeld D, Fraumeni JF (eds) Cancer epidemiology and prevention. Saunders, New York

Day NE, Muñoz N, Ghadirian P (1982) Epidemiology of oesophageal cancer. A review. In: Correa P, Haenszel W (eds) Epidemiology of cancer of the digestive tract. Martinus Nijhoff, Netherlands

de Jong UW, Breslow N, Goh Ewe Hong J, Sridharan M, Shanmugaratnam K (1974) Aetiological factors in oesophageal cancer in Singapore Chinese. Int J Cancer 13:291–303

de Jong UW, Day NE, Mounier-Kuhn PL et al. (1972) The relationship between the ingestion of hot coffee and intra-oesophageal temperature. Gut 13:24–30

Doll R (1967) Prevention of cancer: pointers from epidemiology. Nuffield Provincial Hospitals Trust, London

Doll R (1969) The geographical distribution of cancer. Br J Cancer 23:1–8

Doll R (1971) Oesophageal cancer: a preventable disease? In: International seminar on the epidemiology of oesophageal cancer. Indian Cancer Society and UICC, Bangalore

Doll R, Cook P (1967) Summarizing indices for comparison of cancer incidence data. Int J Cancer 2:269–279

Doll R, Payne P, Waterhouse J (eds) (1966) Cancer incidence in five continents, vol I Springer-Verlag, Berlin Heidelberg New York

Doll R, Muir C, Waterhouse J (eds) (1970) Cancer incidence in five continents, vol II Springer-Verlag, Berlin Heidelberg New York

Elgood CA (1951) A medical history of Persia. Cambridge University Press, London

Enstrom JE (1980) Cancer mortality among Mormons in California during 1965–75. J Natl Cancer Inst 65:1073–1082

Evans IA, Osman MA (1974) Carcinogenicity of bracken and shikimic acid. Nature 250:435–466

Fernandez NA (1975) Nutrition in Puerto Rico. Cancer Res 35:3272–3291

Fong LYY, Newberne PM (1978) Nitrosobenzylmethylamine zinc deficiency and oesophageal cancer. In Griciute L, Lyle R (eds) Environmental aspects of N-nitroso compounds. IARC, Lyon, pp 503–516 (Scientific publications, no. 19)

Gear HS (1935) The incidence of tumours, benign and malignant, in hospital patients in China. Chin Med J 49:261–272

Ghadirian P (1985) Familial history of esophageal cancer. Cancer 56:2112–2116

Ghadirian P (1987) Thermal irritation and esophageal cancer in Northern Iran. Cancer 60:1909–1914

Ghadirian P, Stein GF, Gorodetzky C, Roberfroid MB, Mahon GAT, Bartsch H, Day NE (1985) Oesophageal cancer studies in the Caspian littoral of Iran: some residual results including opium use as a risk factor. Int J Cancer 35:593–597

Graham S, Levin M, Lilienfeld M (1960) The socio-economic distribution of various sites in Buffalo, NY, 1948–52. Cancer, 13:180–191

Hakulinen JS, Lehtimaki L, Lehtonen M, Tappo L (1974) Cancer morbidity among two male cohorts with increased alcohol consumption in Finland. J Natl Cancer Inst 52:1711–1714

Hamadeh R (1988) The impact of smoking in Bahrain. Doctoral thesis, University of Oxford

Harris OD, Cook WT, Thomson H et al. (1967) Malignancy in adult coeliac disease and idiopathic steatorrhoea. Am J Med 42:899–912

Hewer T, Rose E, Ghadirian P et al. (1978) Ingested mutagens from opium and tobacco pyrolysis products and cancer of the oesophagus. Lancet II:494–496

Higginson J, Oettlé (1960) Cancer incidence in the Bantu and Cape Coloured races of South Africa: a report of a cancer survey in the Transvaal (1953–1955). J Natl Cancer Inst 24:589–671

Hirayama T (1971) An epidemiological study of cancer of the oesophagus in Japan, with special reference to the combined effect of selected environmental factors. In: International seminar on the epidemiology of oesophageal cancer. Indian Cancer Society and UICC, Bangalore

Hirayama T (1979) Diet and cancer. Nutr Cancer 1:67–81

Holmes GKT, Stokes PL, Sorahan TM et al. (1976) Coeliac disease, gluten-free diet and malignancy. Gut 17:612–619

Hormozdiari H, Day NE, Aramesh R, Mahboubi E (1975) Dietary factors and oesophageal cancer in the Caspian littoral of Iran. Cancer Res 35:3493–3498

Howel-Evans W, McConnell RB, Clarke CA, Shepherd PM (1958) Carcinoma of the oesophagus with keratosis palmaris et plantaris (tylosis). Q J Med 27:413–431

IARC (1970) Annual Report. World Health Organisation, Lyon, France

IARC (1975) Annual Report. World Health Organisation, Lyon, France

IARC (1976) Annual Report. World Health Organisation, Lyon, France

IARC (1978) Annual Report. World Health Organisation, Lyon, France

IARC (1982) Annual Report. World Health Organisation, Lyon, France

IARC (1986/87) Biennial Report, World Health Organisation, Lyon, France

IARC (1968) Internal Report. Conference held to discuss future plans for research into the aetiology of cancer of the oesophagus. IARC, Lyon

Iran–IARC Joint Study Group (1977) Oesophageal cancer studies in the Caspian littoral of Iran: results of population studies – a prodrome. J Natl Cancer Inst 59:1127–1138

Jacobsson F (1948) Carcinoma of the tongue. A clinical study of 227 cases treated at Radiumhemmet 1931–1942. Acta Radiol 68:1–184

Jarrett WFH, McNeil PE, Grimshaw TR, Selman IE, McIntyre WIM (1978) High incidence of cattle cancer with a possible interaction between an environmental carcinogen and a papilloma virus. Nature 274:215–217

Jussawalla DJ (1971) Epidemiological assessment of aetiology of oesophageal cancer in greater Bombay. International seminar on epidemiology of oesophageal cancer, Bangalore, 4 Nov 1971 pp 2–30 (Monograph no. 1)

Kaplan HS, Tsuchitani PJ (eds) (1978) Cancer in China. Alan R Liss, New York

Keen P (1971) An apparent epidemic of oesophageal cancer in southern Africa. In: International seminar on the epidemiology of oesophageal cancer. Indian Cancer Society and UICC, Bangalore

King H, Locke FB (1980) Mortality among Chinese in the United States. J Natl Cancer Inst, 65:1141–1148

Kmet J, Mahboubi E (1972) Oesophageal cancer in the Caspian littoral of Iran: initial studies. Science 175:846–853

Kmet J, McLaren DS, Siassi F (1980) Epidemiology of oesophageal cancer with special reference to nutritional studies among the Turkoman of Iran. In: Tobin RB, Mehlman MA (eds) Advances in modern human nutrition. Pathotox, Illinois, pp 343–365

Kolycheva NI (1980) Epidemiology of cancer of the oesophagus in the USSR In: Levin D (ed) Joint USA/USSR monograph on cancer epidemiology in the USA and the USSR. pp 191–197. Department of Health and Human Services, Washington. NIH publication No. 80–2044

Kwan KW (1937) Carcinoma of the oesophagus: a statistical study. Chin Med J 52:237–254

Lacey J, Booth C (1980) Microbiological studies of cereal grains and other foodstuffs. In: Day NE (ed) Final report for the contract NCI-CP-71048 for studies on the aetiology of oesophageal cancer in the Caspian littoral of Iran. IARC, Lyon (internal report)

Lang KC (1938) Carcinoma of the oesophagus: Report of 59 cases. Chin Med J 53:57–63

Li J–Y (1982) Epidemiology of esophageal cancer in China. Natl Cancer Inst Monogr 62:113–120

Li J–Y, Chen Z–J, Ershow AG, Blot WJ (1985) A case-control study of esophageal cancer in Linxian, People's Republic of China. Natl Cancer Inst Monogr 69:5–7

Li KH, Kao JC, Qu YK (1962) A survey of prevalence of carcinoma of the oesophagus in North China. Chin Med J 81 (8):489–494

Li MH (1981) Studies of potential carcinogens in the diet of individuals of high risk for esophageal cancer. In: Marks PA (ed) Cancer research in the PRC and USA. Grune and Stratton, New York, pp 131–136

Lin HJ, Chan WC, Fong JJ et al. (1977) Zinc levels in serum, hair and tumours from patients with esophageal cancer. Nutr Report Int 15:6

Locke FB, King H (1980) Cancer mortality risk among Japanese in the United States. J Natl Cancer Inst 65:1149–1156

Love AHG, Elmes M, Golden NK et al. (1977) Zinc deficiency and coeliac disease. In: McNicholl B, McCarthy CF, Fottrell PF (eds) Perspectives in coeliac disease. MTP Press Lancaster, pp 335–342

Lu SH, Camus AM, Tomatis L et al. (1981) Mutagenicity of extracts of pickled vegetables collected in Linxian county, a high-incidence area for esophageal cancer in northern China. J Natl Cancer Inst 66:33–36

Lu SH, Ohshima H, Fu H et al. (1986) Urinary excretion of N-nitrosamino acids and nitrate by inhabitants of high and low risk areas for oesophageal cancer in northern China: endogenous formation of nitrosoproline and its inhibition by vitamin C. Cancer Res 46:1485–1491

Lyon JL, Gardner JW, West DW (1980) Cancer incidence in Mormons and non-Mormons in Utah during 1967–75. J Natl Cancer Inst 65:1055–1061

Mack TM, Berkel J, Bernstein L, Mack W (1985) Religion and cancer in Los Angeles County. Natl Cancer Inst Monogr No 69:235–245

Macrae SM, Cook BV (1975) A retrospective study of the cancer patterns among hospital in-patients in Botswana 1960–72. Br J Cancer 32:121–133

Magee PN, Barnes JM (1976) Carcinogenic nitroso compounds. Adv Cancer Res 10:168–193

Mahboubi E, Kmet J, Cook P, Day NE, Ghadirian P, Salmasizadeh S (1973) Oesophageal cancer studies in the Caspian littoral of Iran: the Caspian Cancer Registry. Br J Cancer 28:197–214

Mahboubi E, Day NE, Ghadirian P et al. (1978) The negligible role of alcohol and tobacco in the etiology of esophageal cancer in Iran – a case-control study. In: Nieburgs H (ed): Prevention and detection of cancer, part II. Detection. Marcel Dekker, New York, pp 1149–1159

Malaveille C, Friesen M, Camus AM et al. (1982) Mutagens produced by the pyrolysis of opium and its alkaloids as possible risk factors in cancer of the bladder and oesophagus. Carcinogenesis 3 (5):577–585

Martinez I (1969) Factors associated with cancer of the oesophagus, mouth and pharynx in Puerto Rico. J Natl Cancer Inst 42:1069–1094

McGlashan ND (1969) Oesophageal cancer and alcoholic spirits in central Africa. Gut 10:643–650

McGlashan ND, Walters CL, McLean AEM (1968) Nitrosamines in Africa: alcoholic spirits and oesophageal cancer. Lancet II:1017

McGlashan ND, Patterson RLS, Williams AA (1970) N-nitrosamines and grain-based spirits. Lancet II:1138

Mettlin C, Graham S, Priore R, Swanson M (1980) Diet and cancer of the oesophagus. Society for Epidemiologic Research, 13th annual general meeting, University of Minnesota, 18–20 June 1980

Miller RW (1978) Epidemiology. In: Kaplan HS, Tsuchitani PJ (eds) Cancer in China. Alan R Liss, New York

Mirvish SS, Wallcave L, Eagen M, Shubik P (1972) Ascorbate–nitrate reaction: possible means of blocking the formation of carcinogenic N-nitroso compounds. Science 177:65–68

Mosebech J, Videback A (1955) On the aetiology of oesophageal carcinoma. J Natl Cancer Inst 15:6

Muñoz N, Crespi M, Grassi A et al. (1982) Precursor lesions of oesophageal cancer in high-risk populations in Iran and China. Lancet I:876–879

Muñoz N, Wahrendorf J, Lu BJ, Crespi M et al. (1985) No effect of riboflavin, retinol and zinc on prevalence of precancerous lesions of oesophagus. Lancet III:111–114

Muñoz N, Hayashi M, Lu JB, Thurnham DI, Crespi M, Bosch FX (1987a) Effect of riboflavin, retinol and zinc on micronuclei of buccal mucosa and of oesophagus. J Natl Cancer Inst 79:687–691

Muñoz N, Victoria CG, Crespi M, Saul C et al. (1987b) Hot maté drinking and precancerous lesions of the oesophagus: an endoscopic survey in southern Brazil. Int J Cancer 39:708–709

Nugmanov SN, Kolycheva NI (1970) Age, sex and ethnic characteristics of patients with esophageal carcinoma in Kazakhstan. In: Epidemiology of malignant tumours. Alma Ata, pp 308–310

O'Connor AM (1966) An economic geography of East Africa. G Bell, London

Oettlé AG (1963) Regional variations in the frequency of Bantu oesophageal cancer cases admitted to hospitals in South Africa. S Afr Med J 37:434–439

Office of Population Censuses and Surveys (OPCS) (1978) Occupational mortality. The Registrar General's decennial supplement for England and Wales 1970–72. Her Majesty's Stationery Office, London (series DS No 1)

O'Neill CH, Hodges CM, Riddle PN et al. (1980) A fine silica contaminant of flour in the high oesophageal cancer area of Iran. Int J Cancer 26:617–628

O'Neill CH, Pan QQ, Clarke G et al. (1982) Silica fragments from millet bran in mucosa surrounding oesophageal tumours in patients in northern China. Lancet I:1202–1206

Pamukbu AM, Price JM (1969) Induction of intestinal and urinary bladder cancer in rats by feeding bracken fern (Pteris acquilina) J Natl Cancer Inst 43:275–281

Parkin DM (ed) (1986) Cancer occurrence in developing countries. IARC Scientific Publications No. 75, Lyon

Peers F, Keen P (1986) Swaziland Cancer Registry. In Parkin DM (ed) Cancer occurrence in developing countries. IARC Scientific Publication No. 75. IARC, Lyon

Pequignot G, Tuyns AJ (1975) Rations d'alcool consommées "declarées" et risques pathologiques. In: Symposium Franco-Britannique sur l'alcoolisme. INSERM Vol 54:23–40

Pottern LM, Morris LE, Blot WJ, Ziegler RG, Fraumeni JF (1985) Esophageal cancer among black men in Washington DC: alcohol, tobacco and other risk factors. J Natl Cancer Inst 67:777–783

Prasad AS, Sandstead HH, Schulert AR, el Rooby AS (1963) Urinary excretion of zinc in patients with the syndrome of anaemia, hepatosplenomegaly, dwarfism and hypogonadism. J Lab Clin Med 62:591–599

Prates MD, Torres FO (1965) A cancer survey in Lourenço Marques. J Natl Cancer Inst 35:729–757

Reinbold JG, Faradje B, Abadi P et al. (1976) Decreased absorption of calcium, magnesium, zinc and phosphorus by humans due to increased fibre and phosphorus consumption as wheat bread. J Nutr 106:493–504

Robertson MA, Harington JS, Bradshaw E (1971) The cancer pattern in Africans at Baragwanath Hospital, Johannesburg. Br J Cancer 25:377–384

Rose EF (1968) Carcinogenesis and oesophageal insults. S Afr Med J 42:334–336

Rose EF (1969) The interplay of factors determining a cancer pattern. Progr Exp Tumour Res Vol 12:95–101

Rose EF (1973) Oesophageal cancer in the Transkei: 1959–69. J Natl Cancer Inst 51:7–16

Rose EF (1978) Environmental risk factors associated with cancer of the oesophagus in Transkei. In: Silber W (ed): Carcinoma of the oesophagus, Balkema, Rotterdam, pp 91–98

Rose EF, McGlashan ND (1975) The spatial distribution of oesophageal carcinoma in the Transkei, South Africa. Br J Cancer 31:197–206

Sato T (1963) An approach method for finding causative agents of human cancer of environmental origin through the analyses of the relation between the distribution of the agents and the incidence rates of the cancer. Bull Inst Public Health, Tokyo 12:160–165

Schoenberg BS, Bailar JC, Fraumeni JF (1971) Certain mortality patterns of oesophageal cancer in the United States, 1930–1967. J Natl Cancer Inst 46:63–73

Schonland M, Bradshaw E (1968) Cancer in the Natal African and Indian 1964–66. Int J Cancer 3:304–316

Schonland M, Bradshaw E (1969) Oesophageal cancer in Natal Bantu: review of 516 cases. S Afr Med J 43:1029–1031

Schuyler A (1876) Turkistan. Rivington, London

Schwartz D, Flament R, Lellouch J et al. (1962) Resultats d'une étude retrospective. Rev Fr Études Cain Biol 7:590–604

Segi M (1975) Tea gruel as a possible factor for cancer of the oesophagus. Gan No Rinsho 66:199–202

Shanmugaratnam K, Lee HP, Day NE (1983) Cancer incidence in Singapore 1968–77. IARC, Lyon IARC scientific publications No. 47

Simpson RR (1939) Anaemia with dysphagia: a precancerous condition? Proc R Soc Med 32:1447–1474

Sobin LH (1969) Cancer in Afghanistan. Cancer 23:678–688

Steiner P (1956) Aetiology and histogenesis of carcinoma of oesophagus. Cancer 9:436–452

Stokes PL, Prior P, Sorahan TM et al. (1976) Malignancy in relatives of patients with coeliac disease. Br J Prev Social Med 30:17–21

Sutherland JC (1968) Cancer in a mission hospital in South Africa. Cancer 22:471–481

Templeton AC (ed) (1973) Tumours in a tropical country. Springer-Verlag, Berlin Heidelberg New York

Theurer RC, Vitale JJ (1976) Drug and nutrient interactions. In: Anderson CE, Coursin DB, Schneider HA (eds) Nutritional support for medical practice, Harper and Row, New York

Thurnham DI, Muñoz N, Wahrendorf J, Crespi M (1987) Aetiology of oesophageal cancer. Lancet I:1500

Tuyns A (1970) Cancer of the oesophagus: further evidence of the relation to drinking habits in France. Int J Cancer 5:152–156

Tuyns A, Jensen OM (1976) Aetiological factors in oesophageal cancer in France. In: IARC Annual Report 1976. IARC, Lyon, pp 35–40

Tuyns A, Massé LMF (1973) Mortality from cancer of the oesophagus in Brittany. Int J Epidemiol 2:242–245

Tuyns AJ, Pequignot G, Jensen OM (1977) Le cancer de l'oesophage en Ille-et-Villaine en fonctions de niveaux de consumption d'l'alcool et de tabac. Des risques qui se multiplient. Bull Cancer 64:45–60

Tuyns A, Vernhes JC (1981) La mortalitié par cancer de l'oesophage dans les départements du Calvados et de l'Orne. Gastroenterol Clin Biol 5:257–265

Uganda Government (1963) Report of the Spiritous Liquor Commission. Government Printer, Uganda

Vambery A (1869) Travels in Central Asia. John Murray, London

van Rensburg SJ, Bradshaw ES, Bradshaw D, Rose EF (1985) Oesophageal cancer in Zulu men, South Africa: a case-control study. Br J Cancer 51:399–405

Versluys JJ (1949) Cancer and occupation in the Netherlands. Br J Cancer 3:161–185

Victoria CG, Muñoz N, Day NE, Barcelos LB, Peccin DA, Braga NM (1987) Hot beverages and oesophageal cancer in southern Brazil: a case-control study. Int J Cancer 39:710–716

Vinson PP (1940) Diagnosis and treatment of diseases of the oesophagus. Baillière, Tindall and Cox, London

Vint FW (1935) Malignant disease in the natives of Kenya. Lancet II:628–630

Vitale JJ, Coffey J (1971) Alcohol and vitamin metabolism. In: Kissin B, Begleiter H (eds) Biology of alcoholism, vol 1. Biochemistry. Plenum Press, New York, pp 327–352

Wahrendorf J, Muñoz N, Lu JB et al. (1988) Blood retinol and zinc riboflavin status in relation to precancerous lesions of the oesophagus; findings from a vitamin intervention trial in the People's Republic of China. Cancer Res 48:2280–2283.

Waterhouse JAH (1974) Cancer handbook of epidemiology and prognosis. Churchill Livingstone, Edinburgh

Waterhouse J, Muir C, Correa P, Powell J (eds) (1976) Cancer incidence in five continents, vol III. IARC, Lyon (IARC scientific publication no. 15)

Waterhouse J, Muir C, Shanmugaratnam K, Powell J (1982) Cancer incidence in five continents, vol IV. IARC, Lyon (IARC scientific publication no. 42)

Watson WL (1933) Carcinoma of the oesophagus. Surg Gynecol Obstet 56:884–887

Wu YK, Luacks HH (1951) Carcinoma of the oesophagus or cardia of the stomach. Ann Surg 134:946–956

Wynder EL (1971) Etiological aspects of squamous cancers of the head and neck. JAMA 215:452–453

Wynder EL, Bross IJ (1961) A study of etiological factors in cancer of the esophagus. Cancer 14:389

Wynder EL, Chan PC (1970) The possible role of riboflavin deficiency in epithelial neoplasia. II. Effect on skin tumour development. Cancer 26:1221–1224

Wynder EL, Klein UE (1965) The possible role of riboflavin deficiency in epithelial neoplasia. I. Epithelial changes in mice in simple deficiency. Cancer 18:167–180

Wynder EL, Lemon FR, Bross IJ (1959) Cancer and coronary artery disease among Seventh Day Adventists. Cancer 5 (12):1016–1028

Wynder EL, Hoffmann D, Chan P et al. (1975) Interdisciplinary and experimental approaches: metabolic epidemiology. In: Fraumeni JR (ed) Persons at high risk of cancer: an approach to etiology and control. Academic Press, New York, pp 485–501

Yang C-S (1980) Research on esophageal cancer in China: a review. Cancer Res 40:2633–2644

Yang C-S, Sun Y, Yang Q, Miller KW et al. (1985) Nutritional status of the high esophageal cancer risk population in Linxian, People's Republic of China: effects of vitamin supplementation. Natl Cancer Inst Monogr 69:23–27

Young M, Russell WT (1926) An investigation into the statistics of cancer in different trades and professions. Her Majesty's Stationery Office, London

# Chapter 4

# Endoscopic Diagnosis and Intubation

K. M. Pagliero

Oesophagoscopy is an essential part of the investigation of carcinoma of the oesophagus, both for confirmation of diagnosis and also for assessment of the extent of the tumour. It may also be required for the relief of obstruction.

Rigid oesophagoscopy has a time-honoured place which has been much eroded in the last 15 years by the advent of the fibreoptic instrument. The choice must belong to the operator and many who have grown up with the rigid instrument feel comfortable with it and stick with it. For those taking up the procedure for the first time, the fibreoptic endoscope is recommended. Its flexibility makes it less likely to traumatise the oesophagus at vulnerable points, such as cervical osteophytes (Fig. 4.1) or diverticula. For the same reason, it is better tolerated under local anaesthesia whereas full general anaesthesia is usually advised for rigid instrumentation. The rigid oesophagoscope allows a larger biopsy to be obtained.

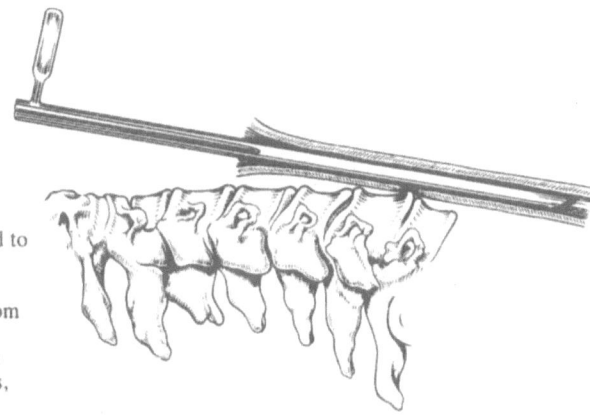

**Fig. 4.1.** Care must be exercised to prevent oesophageal damage on prominent cervical osteophytes. Reproduced, with permission, from Jackson JW, Cooper DKC (eds) (1986) Operative Surgery by Rob and Smith, 4th edn. Butterworths, London.

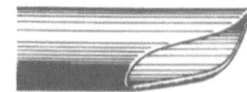

**Fig. 4.2.** The rigid oesophagoscope. Reproduced, with permission, from Jackson JW, Cooper DKC (eds) (1986) Operative Surgery by Rob and Smith, 4th edn. Butterworths, London.

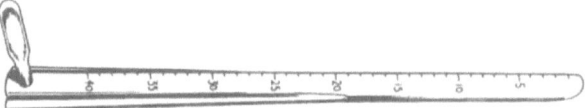

In practice, the two methods are complementary and ideally any endoscopic service should be equipped with both instruments and the expertise to use them.


# Technique


### Rigid Oesophagoscope

Some surgeons pass the rigid oesophagoscope (Fig. 4.2) under local anaesthesia and sedation; however, full general anaesthesia is generally advised. The upper head is towelled to prevent spilled oesophageal or gastric fluids from getting into the eyes. The endoscopist should wear gloves to guard against possible contamination. One hand is introduced into the mouth in such a way as to form a shield to the upper incisor teeth (Fig. 4.3). The endoscope is then passed into the mouth and any manipulation is performed using the thumb as a fulcrum rather than the teeth. Under direct vision the endoscope is advanced to the cricopharyngeal sphincter and this may be more easily achieved with the head horizontal or even slightly flexed. As the beak of the endoscope is passed gently through the cricopharyngeal sphincter it should be slightly elevated to lift the larynx forward and direct the instrument away from the cervical spine. Having negotiated the sphincter in this way further advancement is relatively easy but should be accompanied by increasing neck extension to keep the instrument in the line of the oesophagus.


### Fibreoptic Oesophagoscope

The flexible instrument (Fig. 4.4) is well tolerated with local anaesthesia (gargled Xylocaine gel) and intravenous sedation (e.g., Diazepam). Where therapeutic manoeuvres such as bougienage or intubation are also to be performed, general anaesthesia may be preferred.

Under sedation the patient is best positioned lying on his side. A mouth guard is inserted to protect the endoscope from being bitten as it is advanced towards the cricopharyngeal sphincter. At this point the patient is asked to swallow to relax the sphincter. As he does so the instrument is advanced into the upper oesophagus. Its continued passage is under direct vision aided by gentle insufflation with air and manipulation of the flexion controls of the instrument.

**Fig. 4.3.** Passage of the rigid oesophagoscope should use the operator's thumb as a fulcrum and not the patient's incisor teeth. Reproduced, with permission, from Jackson JW, Cooper DKC (eds) (1986) Operative Surgery by Rob and Smith, 4th edn. Butterworths, London.

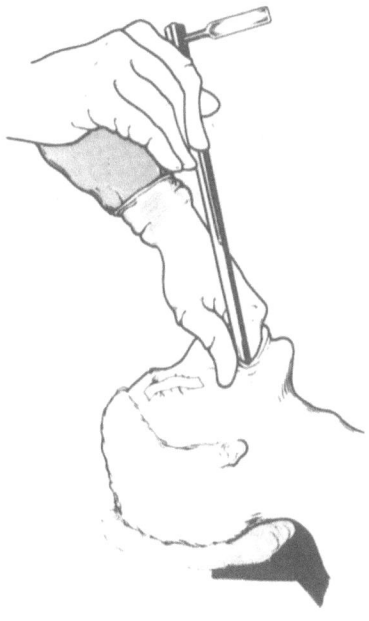

When passed under general anaesthesia the patient will be on his back and unable to assist by swallowing. Passage of the endoscope, therefore may be facilitated by elevating the larynx with a laryngoscope. The cricopharyngeus under full anaesthesia is totally relaxed and should present no resistance. If it is

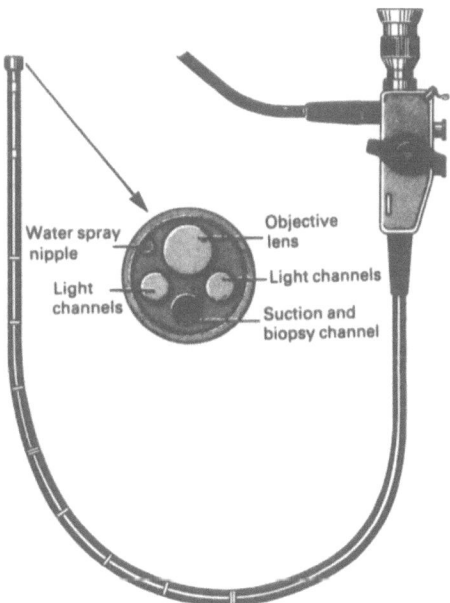

**Fig. 4.4.** The fibreoptic gastroscope. Reproduced, with permission, from Jackson JW, Cooper DKC (eds) (1986) Operative Surgery by Rob and Smith, 4th edn. Butterworths, London.

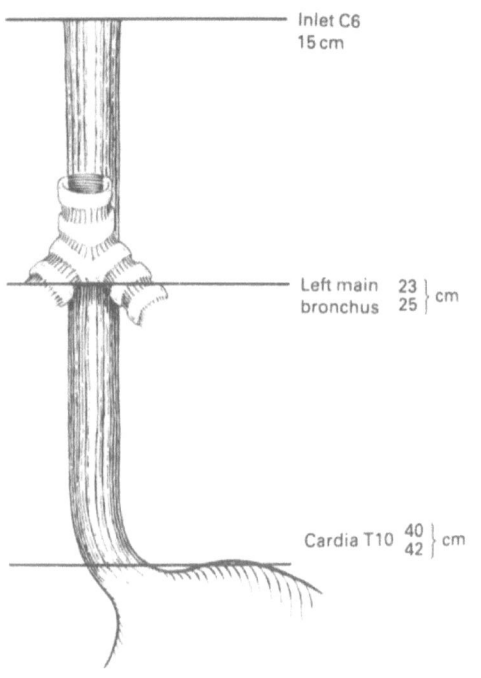

◀ **Fig. 4.5.** Oesophageal lesions should be related to normal landmarks. Reproduced, with permission, from Jackson JW, Cooper DKC (eds) (1986) Operative Surgery by Rob and Smith, 4th edn. Butterworths, London.

Inlet C6
15 cm

Left main    23 } cm
bronchus    25

Cardia T10  40 } cm
            42

**Fig. 4.6.** Lower oesophageal sphincter tone as seen from below. Reproduced, with permission, from Jackson JW, Cooper DKC (eds) (1986) Operative Surgery by Rob and Smith, 4th edn. Butterworths, London.
▼

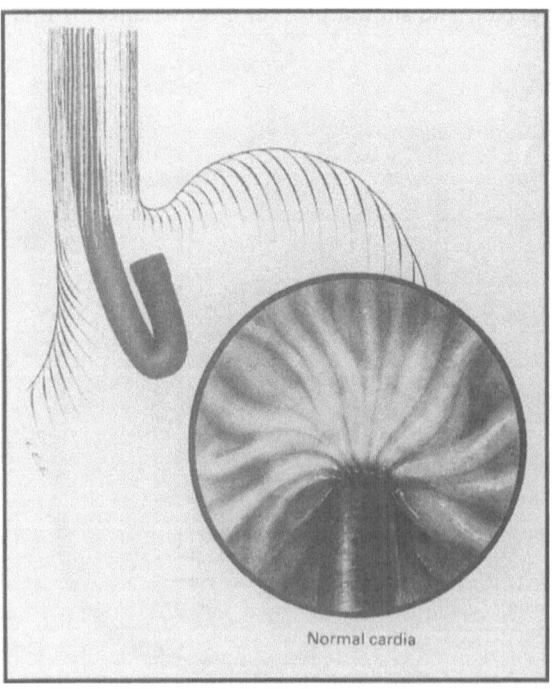

Normal cardia

resistant then it is important to attend to the anaesthesia rather than risk injuring the pharynx while trying to negotiate a contracted sphincter.

# Preoperative Preparation

Many surgeons advise preoperative barium swallow to exclude lesions which might be inadvertently injured by endoscopy, particularly a pharyngeal pouch. In practice, resources both in terms of time and money often dictate otherwise. With care, diagnostic endoscopy very rarely causes complications and the risk of not doing a barium swallow is largely theoretical. More important, perhaps, is to discourage the casual use of the instrument by inexperienced operators who might be unaware of the pitfalls.

# Normal Endoscopic Appearances

The oesophagus is a tube lined by pink, almost magenta, mucosa. It commences at the cricopharyngeal sphincter at usually about 15 cm from the incisor teeth and terminates at 40 cm from the incisor teeth where it joins the stomach. The endoscope can be passed easily as the oesophagus is gently insufflated with air. At the lower end, the lower oesophageal sphincter tone may resist insufflation but will not impede the passage of the endoscope into the stomach. The impression of the left main bronchus may be seen anteriorly at about 25 cm from the incisor teeth (Fig. 4.5).

Just above the oesophagogastric junction, at a variable distance, the "dentate" junction of the magenta-pink squamous epithelium above and the salmon-pink columnar epithelium below will be seen.

Finally, viewed from below by retroflexion, the normal lower oesophageal sphincter will snugly encircle the endoscope even when the stomach is inflated (Fig. 4.6).

# Pathological Appearances

## Inflammation

The most common cause is gastro-oesophageal reflux of acid or bile and inflammation will be seen extending upwards for a variable distance commencing at the squamocolumnar junction. There is a spectrum of changes possible from mild hyperaemia through to confluent mucosal ulceration finally leading to fibrous stricture. The degree of oesophagitis should be recorded on a scale that denotes the severity and allows comparison in the subsequent assessment of therapy. Biopsy can document the findings for scientific purposes but in practice visual appearances suffice.

### Ulceration

Ulceration is more readily diagnosed endoscopically than radiologically. Diagnostic appearances, however, are unreliable and multiple biopsy specimens should be taken around the circumference. A photographic record may facilitate comparison when the results of medication are to be monitored by serial endoscopy.

### Stricture

Stricture is the possible end result of severe gastro-oesophageal reflux. The smooth tapering of the oesophagus into the smoothly narrowed stricture usually differentiates it from an exophytic friable malignant stricture. However, certain malignant strictures, where there is a predominant spread submucosally coupled with external glandular compression, may mimic a peptic stricture. Peptic stricture always occurs at the squamocolumnar junction so that biopsy of the normal mucosa above and below a stricture may provide circumstantial evidence to aid diagnosis. Drug, radiation or corrosive-induced strictures may be suspected from the history.

### Tumour

Carcinoma of the oesophagus is generally easily recognised by the protuberance of friable, haemorrhagic tumour tissue within the lumen. Occult tumour may, however, be missed. It is important when assessing a tumour to remember to look for evidence of submucosal spread which can give a "cobbled" appearance to the mucosa, together with "skip" lesions which can occur in 10% of cases elsewhere in the oesophagus and oropharynx. "Skip" lesions may be highlighted by staining the oesophagus with toluidine blue. Tumours more than 28 cm from the incisor teeth may involve the tracheobronchial tree and bronchoscopy should be included in the assessment.

The benign tumour, leiomyoma, will be recognisable by its protrusion into the oesophageal lumen but with a normal mucosal covering which usually prevents the procurement of a biopsy specimen.

## Therapeutic Procedures

### Biopsy

A variety of biopsy forceps suit different circumstances. Those with the rigid instrument obtain larger specimens but by the same token can do greater damage.

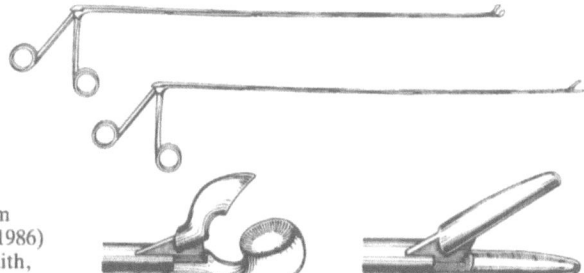

**Fig. 4.7.** Rigid biopsy forceps. Reproduced, with permission, from Jackson JW, Cooper DKC (eds) (1986) Operative Surgery by Rob and Smith, 4th edn. Butterworths, London.

Angled rigid forceps are suitable for sessile lesions which the straight forceps may slide over (Fig. 4.7). The flexible equivalent is a forceps with a central spike that can impale the lesion and prevent the cups skidding across the surface (Fig. 4.8).

It is recommended that several specimens should be taken to assure a representative specimen. It is important to obtain viable rather than necrotic tissue and this is usually assured if a little bleeding is seen at the point from where the specimen has been removed. It is further recommended that a brush biopsy specimen should in addition be sent for cytological examination – two positives are better than none!

## Dilatation

A variety of methods can be used to dilate malignant strictures but these largely fall into three groups.

### Semirigid Bougies

Semirigid bougies are usually gum elastic or, in the case of the Chevalier Jackson bougies, a metal stem with a gum elastic tip (Fig. 4.9). They are used through the rigid endoscope, under direct vision and under general anaesthesia, and are restricted by the internal diameter of the oesophagoscope which is usually around

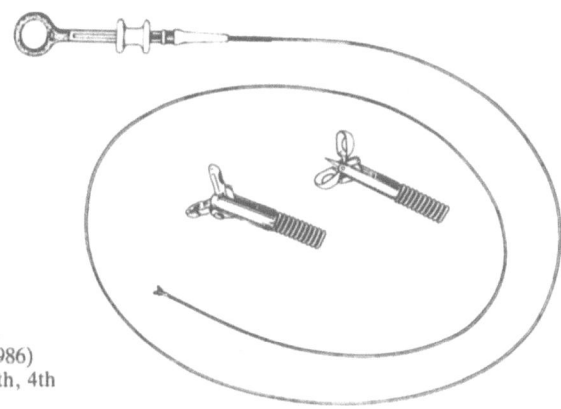

**Fig. 4.8.** Flexible biopsy forceps. Reproduced, with permission, from Jackson JW, Cooper DKC (eds) (1986) Operative Surgery by Rob and Smith, 4th edn. Butterworths, London.

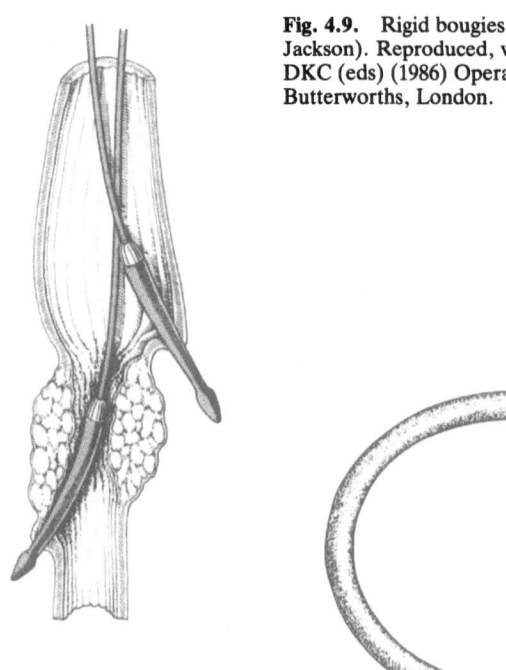

**Fig. 4.9.** Rigid bougies must be used with care (Chevalier Jackson). Reproduced, with permission, from Jackson JW, Cooper DKC (eds) (1986) Operative Surgery by Rob and Smith, 4th edn. Butterworths, London.

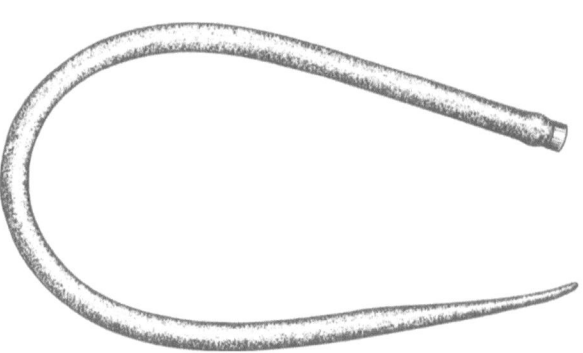

**Fig. 4.10.** Flexible mercury-filled rubber bougies (Maloney). Reproduced, with permission, from Jackson JW, Cooper DKC (eds) (1986) Operative Surgery by Rob and Smith, 4th edn. Butterworths, London.

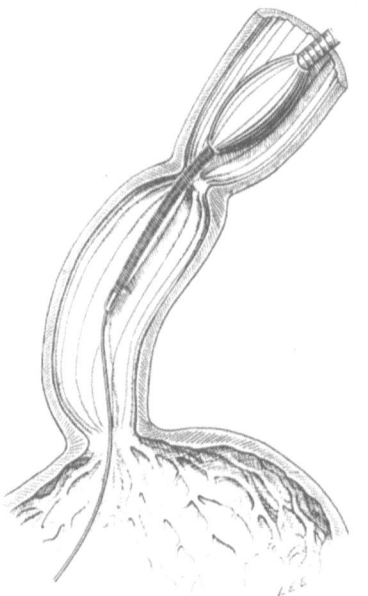

**Fig. 4.11.** Guided bougies (Eder Puestow). Reproduced, with permission, from Jackson JW, Cooper DKC (eds) (1986) Operative Surgery by Rob and Smith, 4th edn. Butterworths, London.

40 French gauge (FG). Because they are semirigid and because once through the stricture the tip cannot be visualised there is a real risk of perforation.

## Flexible Bougies

Flexible bougies are usually mercury-filled such as the blunt-nosed Hurst bougies or the flexible tipped Maloney bougies (Fig. 4.10). They rely more on the weight of the mercury than on forward pressure. Indeed, when resistance is encountered their flexibility prevents undue forward pressure and this makes these bougies extremely safe. They also follow the contour of the oesophagus, taking the line of least resistance. They may be used under local or general anaesthesia – indeed certain patients learn to pass them in their own home without any form of anaesthesia. Many strictures can be taken up to 52–60 FG quite safely as perforation is extremely rare with flexible bougies.

## Guided Bougies

Guided bougies are railroaded down a guide wire placed endoscopically into the stomach, thus discouraging the creation of a false passage. Ideally the wire is introduced while the tip of the endoscope is in the stomach. However, if the stricture is too tight to permit the passage of the endoscope, the wire is passed through the stricture and may be seen fluoroscopically to pass into the stomach. Once positioned, the bougies, such as the Eder Puestow olivary dilators (Fig. 4.11) or the Celestin stepped dilators, are passed at ever-increasing diameters through the stricture. These are somewhat rigid dilators and although the guide wire prevents a false passage it is possible to damage the oesophagus by over forcibly dilating the stricture which can then split. If a stricture is proving rather rigid it may be prudent to achieve dilatation in two or even three separate sessions two days apart.

## Intubation

The early oesophageal stent, a Souttar tube, was inserted endoscopically but has generally been replaced by the larger Celestin or Mousseau–Barbin tubes that could be pulled through via laparotomy. In the last decade it has been possible to pass similar sized tubes entirely through the oesophagus from above, and this has significantly reduced the mortality, morbidity and the length of hospital admission. Having dilated the malignant stricture to about 45 FG the tube can be railroaded over a guide wire through the tumour where it can be accurately positioned radiographically (Fig. 4.12). The Atkinson tube (Fig. 4.13) is used with an introducer which has an expanding flange to grip the tube from within. The Celestin tube (Fig. 4.14) is held from within by an inflatable balloon that is deflated when the tube is correctly positioned.

Tubes come in a variety of sizes. They need to be at least as long as the tumour and perhaps need 2–3 cm extra to allow for tumour growth. On the other hand, the longer the tube the more likely it will get blocked by a bolus. A tube that

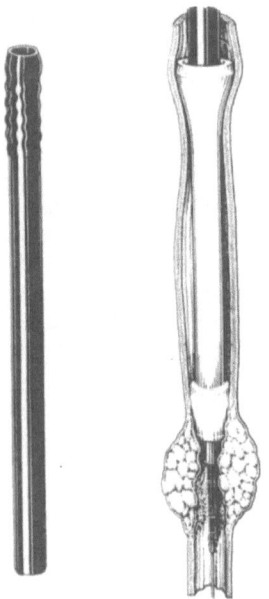

**Fig. 4.12.** Atkinson tube being railroaded through a malignant stricture. Reproduced, with permission, from Jackson JW, Cooper DKC (eds) (1986) Operative Surgery by Rob and Smith, 4th edn. Butterworths, London.

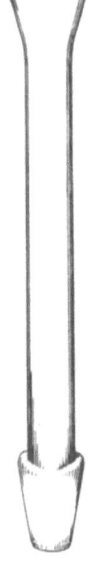

**Fig. 4.13.** Atkinson tube. Reproduced, with permission, from Jackson JW, Cooper DKC (eds) (1986) Operative Surgery by Rob and Smith, 4th edn. Butterworths, London.

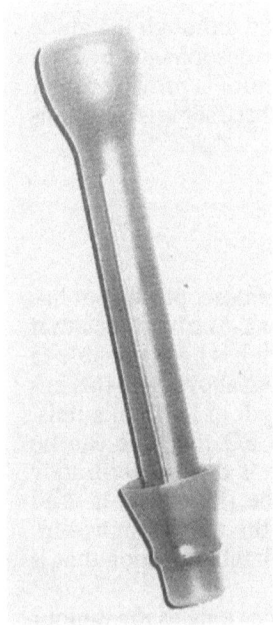

**Fig. 4.14.** The Celestin tube.*

---

*There are two types of Celestin tube, shown in Fig. 4.14 and in Fig. 11.1—Editor

bridges the cardia will encourage gastro-oesophageal reflux and if at all possible a tube that stops short of a normal lower oesophageal sphincter is preferable.

Having placed the tube in position the endoscope should be passed again to ensure that it is well sited, but care must be taken not to dislodge it. Subsequent bolus obstruction is usually amenable to the passage of a nasogastric tube though sometimes it may need to be unblocked endoscopically. A dislocated tube can usually be retrieved endoscopically by passing a guide wire through it and then inserting the Nottingham introducer to effect the extraction.

*Chapter 5*

# Radiological Diagnosis and Assessment

Alison M. McLean and R. H. Reznek

## Introduction

The diagnosis of oesophageal carcinoma is usually made by barium study or endoscopy. Symptoms of dysphagia commonly develop only when the tumour has encompassed the oesophageal lumen or invaded the perioesophageal lymphatics or mediastinal structures (Skinner 1984) and at this stage many tumours are unresectable. The various therapeutic options available have not substantially improved the long-term survival and there is considerable controversy as to the best method of treatment (Moertel 1978; Parker 1978; Earlam and Cunha-Melo 1980). Treatment planning requires assessment of the extent of disease to determine prognosis and resectability. Although conventional radiology can give some indication of tumour extent (Yamada 1979), computerised tomography (CT), by virtue of its cross-sectional imaging ability offers the potential of accurate, non-invasive pretherapy staging of disease. On the basis of the CT findings, potentially curable tumours may be identified, and the need for exploratory surgery obviated in some cases (Halvorsen and Thompson 1987a).

## Diagnosis

### Early Oesophageal Cancer

Early oesophageal cancer is defined as cancer limited to the mucosa or submucosa without lymph node metastases (Japanese Society for Oesophageal Diseases 1976). In contrast to the grave prognosis of patients with advanced disease, true early cancer is a curable lesion (Guojun et al. 1981). However, early carcinoma is often symptomless and population screening offers the only method of diagnosis in these patients. In areas of high incidence such as in China, detection rates of early squamous cell carcinoma as high as 70%–80% are reported using exfoliative balloon cytology, resulting in 5-year survival rates approaching 90% (Coordinating Group for Research on Oesophageal Carcinoma 1976; Guojun et al. 1981; Shu 1983). This does not, however, reflect our experience in the West where detection rates of early cancer are less than 5% (Levine et al. 1986). The terms "early", "small" and "superficial" oesophageal cancer have been used interchangeably but should not be regarded as synonymous as some "small" and seemingly "superficial" lesions have invaded regional lymph nodes and thus carry a prognosis comparable with advanced disease (Zornoza and Lindell 1980). In contrast, "early" cancers are not always small as they may undergo considerable intraluminal growth and still be classified histologically as early oesophageal cancer (Levine et al. 1986).

Many patients in whom superficial oesophageal cancer is detected have some oesophageal symptoms of dysphagia or a sensation of food sticking in the throat

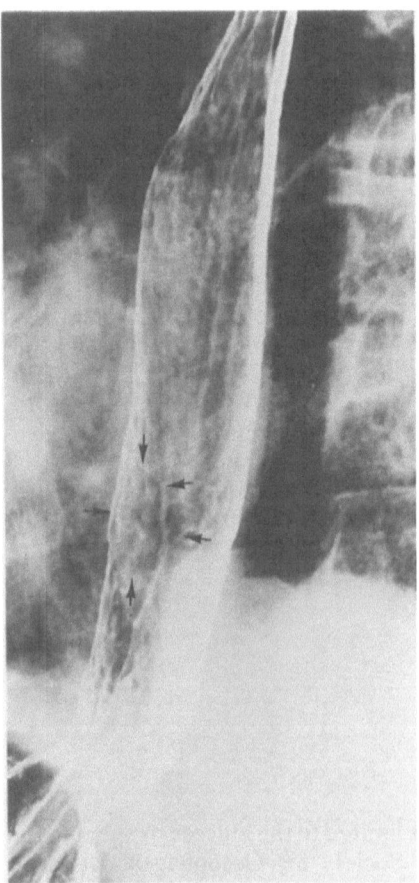

**Fig. 5.1.** Small oesophageal cancer. Double contrast examination demonstrating superficial plaque causing distortion of the mucosal pattern.

(Itai et al. 1978). Detailed double contrast examination of the oesophagus is essential in order to detect small and potentially early lesions, the radiological signs of which can be subtle and may be overlooked (Koehler et al. 1976; Zornoza and Lindell 1980) (Fig. 5.1). Early tumour may be easily confused with benign lesions such as polyps, oesophagitis or peptic stricture, and subtle areas of inelasticity may be overlooked. In one study, 27% of subsequently proven small oesophageal carcinomas were initially misdiagnosed as benign abnormalities or as normal, with the great majority demonstrating some abnormality on the initial study (Moss et al. 1976). It may be necessary to accept an increased proportion of false-positive diagnoses with a high index of radiological suspicion and further evaluation by endoscopy and biopsy.

Most early cancers are elevated lesions appearing as plaques or flat, broad-based sessile polyps ranging in size from 0.8–3.5 cm and extending less than 1 cm into the oesophageal lumen (Zornoza and Lindell 1980) (Fig. 5.2). The contour of the lesion is usually well defined and lobulated and may demonstrate a granular, nodular or smooth surface. Polypoid tumours may become quite large and still remain confined to the submucosa (Levine et al. 1986). Tumours

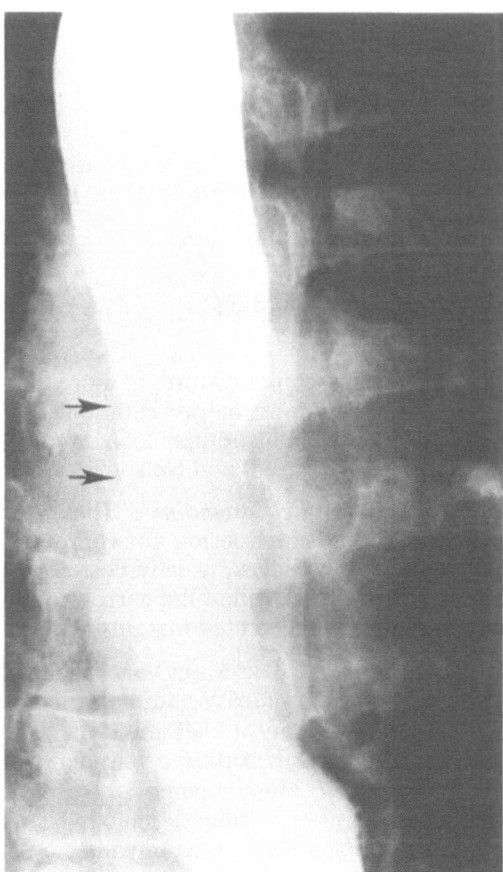

**Fig. 5.2.** Small oesophageal cancer. An irregular plaque-like lesion is demonstrated on the lateral aspect of the oesophagus. Areas of limited distensibility are optimally shown on the contrast-filled single contrast views of the oesophagus.

appearing as shallow ulcers or flat plaques may be very difficult to detect radiologically. Malignant ulcers appear as shallow, irregular barium pools accompanied by various protrusions and a degree of rigidity of the oesophageal wall, requiring multiple projections and different phases of distension to detect the subtle changes (Itai et al. 1978). Rarely, a superficial spreading malignancy may give rise to a fine reticular appearance with diffuse mucosal elevations, simulating oesophagitis, leukoplakia or acanthosis nigricans (Itai et al. 1977).

Most reported cases of early oesophageal cancers are from Chinese or Japanese investigators, and are histologically squamous cell carcinoma (Endo et al. 1971; Suzuki et al. 1972; Itai et al. 1978). In a recent study from the USA, however, five of seven histologically proven early cancers were adenocarcinomas arising in Barrett's oesophagus (Levine et al. 1986). There is strong evidence of the premalignant nature of this condition with a risk of developing carcinoma approximately 40 times greater than the general population (Levine et al. 1984; Agha 1985). The invariable association with reflux oesophagitis which results in columnarisation of the squamous epithelium probably accounts for the earlier symptoms and presentation.

## Advanced Cancer

### Squamous Cell Carcinoma

Four basic radiographic patterns on barium study reflect the gross morphology of advanced carcinoma (Goldstein et al. 1981).

1. Annular constricting
2. Polypoid
3. Infiltrating or stenosing
4. Ulcerating

Many neoplasms exhibit features of more than one pattern. Despite the advanced nature of most tumours on presentation, 8%–10% of carcinomas are missed on the initial study and another 15% are misdiagnosed as a benign condition (Appelqvist 1972; Bruni and Nelson 1975).

*Annular Constricting Carcinomas.* These occur most commonly and resemble a malignant "apple-core" lesion anywhere in the gastrointestinal tract with over-hanging, shelf-like edges, usually best appreciated at the upper margins of the tumour. The mucosa within the narrowed lumen is destroyed with characteristi-cally irregular and ulcerated margins (Fig. 5.3).

*Polypoid Tumours.* These may vary greatly in size, initially arising from one wall of the oesophageal mucosa and with increasing size may eventually spread to encircle the oesophageal wall and create an annular stricture. Small polypoid tumours may be easily confused with benign lesions and histological diagnosis is usually required. Many benign polyps, either fibrovascular, lipomatous or inflammatory, have a smooth mucosal surface and may develop a pedicle. Intramural polyps such as leiomyoma, cysts or haemangioma can usually be recognised by the radiological appearance of a smooth, semicircular lesion arising

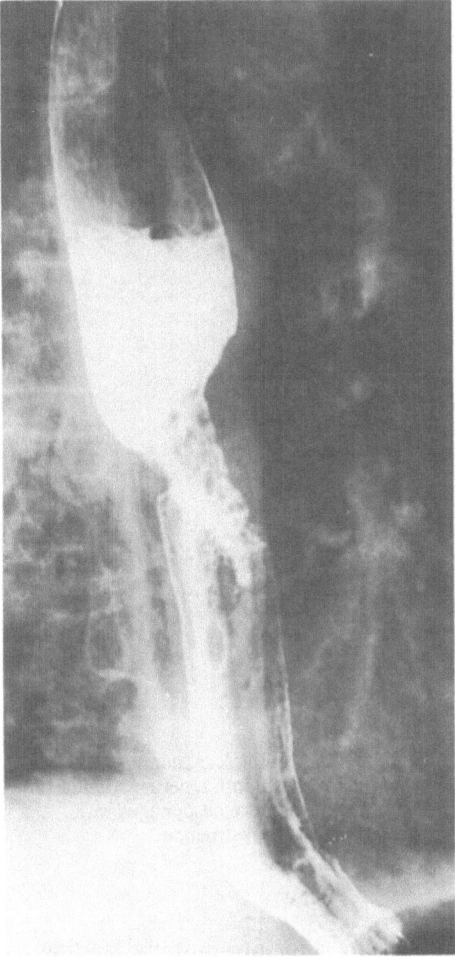

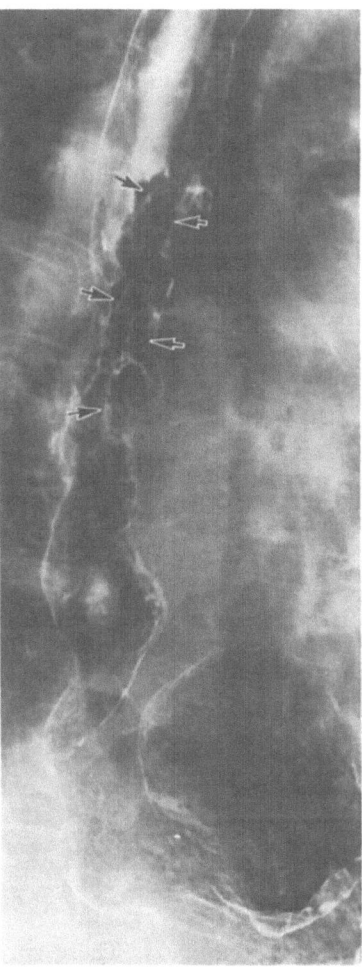

**Fig. 5.3.** Asymmetrical annular constricting carcinoma showing shelf-like edges and mucosal destruction. There is partial oesophageal obstruction.

**Fig. 5.4.** Submucosal spread of a midoesophageal carcinoma resulting in a "varicoid" appearance of the oesophageal folds. There is an associated hiatus hernia.

from the oesophageal wall and indenting the barium column, creating an obtuse angle with the adjacent mucosa.

*Verrucous Carcinoma.* This locally aggressive but non-invasive type of squamous cell carcinoma characteristically presents as a lobulated polypoid mass within the distal oesophagus (Sridhar et al. 1980). Occasionally, spread of a polypoid carcinoma along a considerable length of the oesophagus may simulate the appearance of oesophageal varices (Fig. 5.4). This so-called varicoid carcinoma may be distinguished from varices by the rigidity and unchanging appearance of the enlarged folds (Silver and Goldstein 1974).

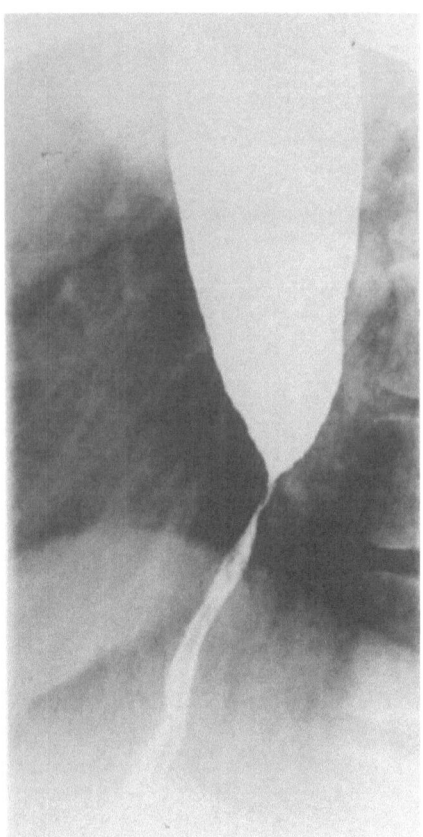

**Fig. 5.5.** Infiltrating carcinoma resulting in a tight, relatively smooth tapering stricture in the lower third of the oesophagus with marked proximal obstruction.

*Infiltrating Tumours.* These spread submucosally and intramurally leading to loss of the normal oesophageal pliability. The resulting stricture may have tapering margins and may be confused with a benign peptic stricture, although the narrowing tends to be more irregular and there is often shallow mucosal ulceration (Fig. 5.5). However, the mucosa may be intact over an area of submucosal infiltration, particularly at the margins, and this may result in negative endoscopic biopsies (Edwards 1974; Goldstein et al. 1981). Although most oesophageal neoplasms are ulcerated in part, a *primarily ulcerative* lesion is unusual (Gloyna et al. 1977). The appearances result from almost complete ulceration of a flat mass on one wall of the oesophagus. In profile, the ulcer demonstrates a meniscoid shape with a raised edge due to a rim of tumour tissue.

## Adenocarcinoma

The true incidence of primary adenocarcinoma of the oesophagus is low, being between 1% and 3% of all carcinomas occurring in the upper and middle third (Bosch et al. 1979). In the lower third, incidence figures of up to 19% are reported but this figure includes upward extension of primary gastric lesions arising at the cardia and invading the lower oesophagus across the gastro-oesophageal junction (Bosch et al. 1979; Faintuch et al. 1984). There have been reports of adenocarcinoma arising in submucosal or deep oesophageal glands (Azzopardi and Menzies 1962) and in heterotopic nests of gastric mucosa (Carrie 1950), but the majority of adenocarcinomas arising away from the gastro-oesophageal junction occur in Barrett-type columnar epithelium, usually in the mid or lower third (Agha 1985).

A small adenocarcinoma may appear as a prominent distal oesophageal fold which develops a polypoid configuration. It may be confused radiologically with an inflammatory oesophagogastric polyp which complicates reflux oesophagitis (Styles et al. 1985). In a patient with reflux, an inflamed gastric fold may evolve gradually into a polyp at or immediately below the squamocolumnar junction and the demonstration of a prominent and straight gastric fold, terminating in a smooth polypoid expansion at this level is characteristic. Any deviation from this easily recognisable entity must be regarded with suspicion. A polyp which is bilobular or multinodular, irregular or sessile, or does not clearly represent the proximal expansion of a gastric fold, must be biopsied to exclude malignancy (Fig. 5.6).

With more advanced adenocarcinoma, the distal oesophageal folds become more distorted and ulcerated and in such cases careful examination of the gastric fundus may reveal a carcinoma with retrograde spread. The presence of normal gastric folds within a collapsed hiatus hernia may occasionally cause diagnostic difficulty and adequate distension of the distal oesophagus is essential.


## Other Unusual Oesophageal Malignancies

Other neoplasms occurring less frequently than squamous or adenocarcinoma may be confused with them, but some have characteristic radiological features which may suggest the correct diagnosis.

*Carcinosarcoma* is a rare tumour composed of both epithelial and connective tissue elements, and presents radiologically as a bulky polypoid mass which, unlike most squamous cell carcinomas, tends to expand the lumen, although infiltrative forms occur (McCort 1972) (Fig. 5.7). Rarely, *primary melanosarcoma* may present a similar large polypoid appearance, although metastatic melanoma is more usually seen, presenting the typical "bullseye" appearance of an ulcerated polypoid mass (Burnett and Toffler 1951). *Oesophageal lymphoma* accounts for less than 1% of gastrointestinal lymphoma and is most commonly non-Hodgkin's lymphoma. Like lymphoma elsewhere in the gastrointestinal tract, a wide spectrum of radiological appearances has been described. It most frequently presents as nodularity and occasional narrowing of the distal oesophageal lumen. This may extend into the stomach, but infiltration of any segment of the oesophagus may occur (Carnovale et al. 1977). *Secondary oesophageal carcinoma* occurs in approximately 3% of autopsy series of patients dying from malignant disease, most commonly originating from a primary site in either stomach, lung or breast (Anderson and Harell 1980). Other infradiaphragmatic primary tumours may metastasise to lymph nodes in the mediastinum and secondarily invade the oesophagus, but mediastinal involvement is usually obvious on the chest X-ray film.

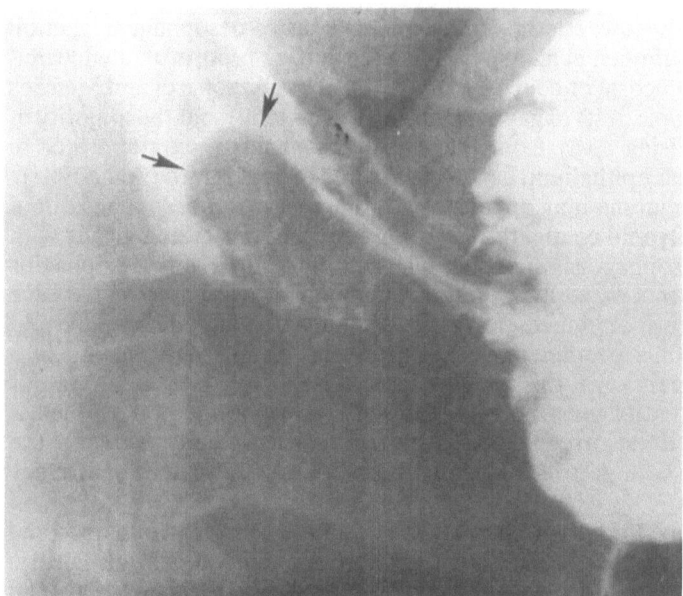

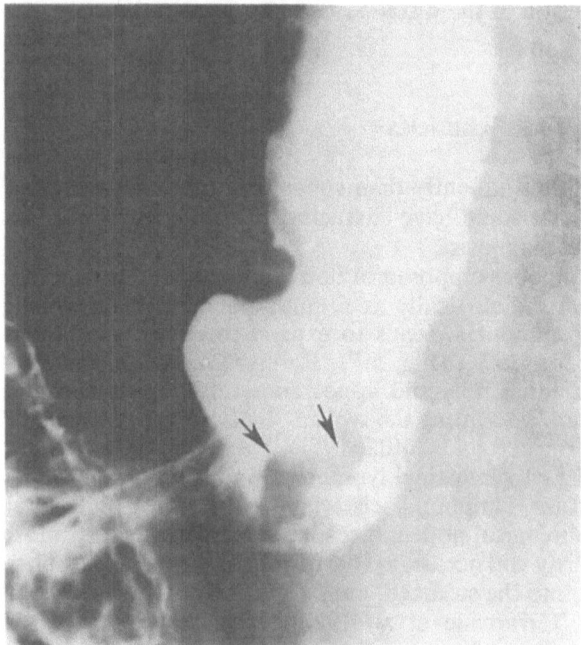

**Fig. 5.6a,b.** Polypoid lesions of the distal oesophagus. **a** Inflammatory thickening of a mucosal fold within a hiatus hernia has given rise to a smoothly marginated polyp in a patient with gross reflux. The irregular margins of the polyp demonstrated in **b** raise the diagnosis of distal oesophageal tumour which was confirmed to be adenocarcinoma.

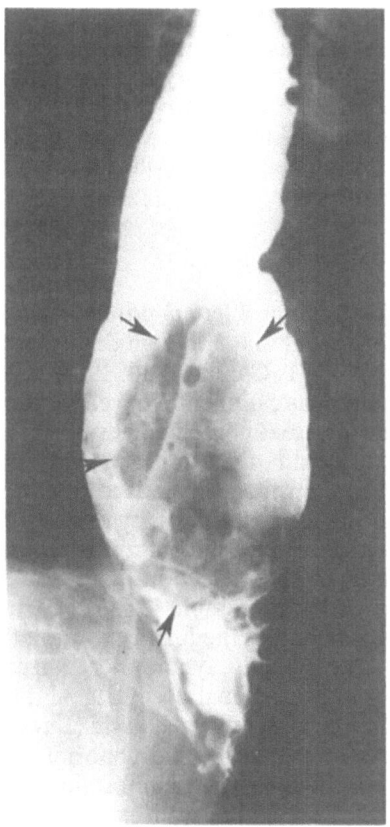

**Fig. 5.7.** Bulky polypoid mass with expansion of the oesophageal lumen – typical appearance of a carcinosarcoma.

Haematogenous metastases from lung or breast appear as short, segmental narrowings, although occasionally may present with longer tapering strictures, usually affecting the middle third of the oesophagus, which may be difficult to differentiate radiologically from a benign stricture. Lymphatic metastases spread through the subepithelial lymphatic plexus and usually originate in the stomach or elsewhere in the oesophagus (Steiner et al. 1984). They appear as smooth-surfaced polypoid masses and with progression of disease the submucosal lymphatic vessels may become filled with tumour and varicoid filling defects may result. Metastatic disease may resemble primary oesophageal tumour but the mucosa is usually preserved and smooth resulting in negative endoscopic biopsy.

## Predisposing Conditions

Occasionally the radiological appearances are dominated by the features of an underlying condition, predisposing to the development of oesophageal carcinoma. Such predisposing factors include achalasia, caustic stricture, Barrett's oesophagus and the presence of a cervical web in the Plummer–Vinson syndrome. A history of alcohol and smoking, carcinoma of the head and neck (Goldstein and Zornoza 1978), adult coeliac disease (O'Brien et al, 1985) and tylosis (Shine and Allison 1966) also have a strong association with the development of oesophageal carcinoma.

## Achalasia

A special problem is posed by the increased incidence of carcinoma in patients with achalasia, although this association has recently been questioned (Wychulis et al. 1971; Chuong et al. 1984). Characteristically, the tumour, a bulky polypoid squamous carcinoma, develops in the middle third of the oesophagus at the site of the pretreatment fluid level in an area of chronic oesophagitis. Diagnosis is usually late, the symptoms of dysphagia being attributed to advancing achalasia. Partial obstruction leads to retention of fluid and food residue in the oesophagus and hinders detection by endoscopy or barium swallow. Preceding oesophageal lavage or the use of fizzy drinks prior to barium examination may improve the radiographic detection. Some have advocated routine surveillance for the early detection of curable lesions (Carter and Brewer 1975), although in the light of recent studies the justification for this approach is in doubt (Chuong et al. 1984).

Occasionally, symmetrical constriction caused by an infiltrating carcinoma may result in proximal oesophageal dilatation and simulate the "bird-beak" appearance of idiopathic achalasia (Lawson and Dodds 1978). There may be associated loss of peristalsis and abnormal response to Mecholyl which in some patients appears to be due to infiltration of the myenteric plexus. Careful attention to the radiological appearances may discriminate, particularly in patients with a short duration of symptoms. Any suggestion of mucosal nodularity or ulceration, fold thickening or gastric fundal distortion may provide the correct diagnosis (Fig. 5.8). The absence of a "jet effect" as the oesophagus empties in the erect position may also be a helpful clue in suggesting malignancy.

## Caustic Stricture

The incidence of squamous carcinoma developing in prior caustic strictures is high. Stricturing usually occurs in the midthoracic region at the bronchial bifurcation. Nodularity of the mucosa within the narrowed segment may be demonstrated and obstructive symptoms occur early as the lumen is already compromised. It has been suggested that the presence of perioesophageal scar tissue may limit extraoesophageal spread and this, together with the early presentation, may account for the improved prognosis in this group of patients (Applequist and Salmo 1980).

## Barrett's Oesophagus

The strong association between columnarisation of the squamous epithelium and the development of oesophageal adenocarcinoma has been discussed (*vide*

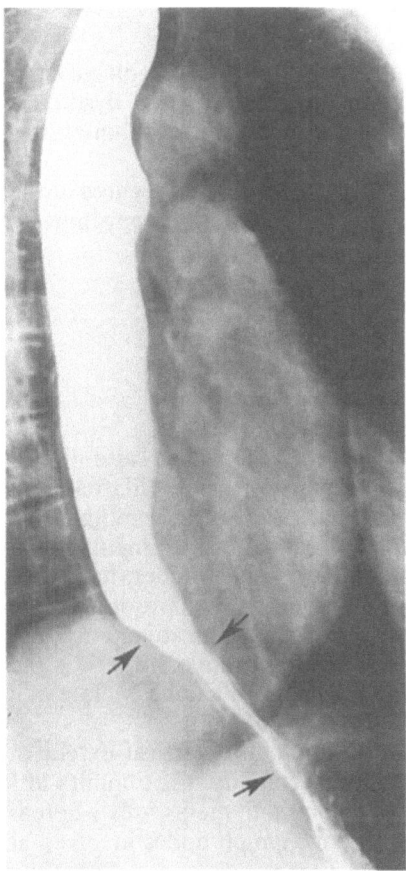 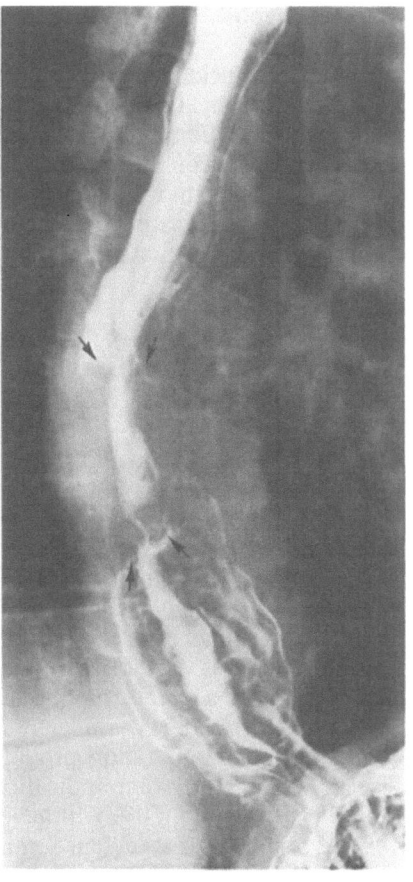

**Fig. 5.8.** Narrowed oesophagus at the level of the gastro-oesophageal junction, with proximal oesophageal dilatation simulating achalasia. The slight nodularity of the mucosal folds gives the clue to the biopsy-proven diagnosis of adenocarcinoma.

**Fig. 5.9.** The development of a carcinoma in a patient with gross reflux and Barrett's oesophagus is shown as an apple-core lesion in the lower third of the oesophagus. (The thickened distal oesophageal folds were due to reflux.)

*supra*). Certain radiological features may distinguish this lesion from conventional squamous cell or gastric cardia carcinoma (Agha 1985).

In established Barrett's oesophagus, adenocarcinoma develops at the level of the stricture or ulceration, but tends to infiltrate submucosally creating a relatively long stricture (Fig. 5.9). This may be confused with a benign stricture or occasionally with varices as the extensive submucosal tumour may create a varicoid appearance of the oesophageal folds. The overlying mucosa is frequently preserved or shows changes only of chronic oesophagitis and negative endoscopic biopsies may result. When the radiological appearances suggest a Barrett's carcinoma, a negative biopsy must be regarded with suspicion and adequate tissue samples obtained (Agha 1985).

## Cervical Webs

An increased incidence of carcinoma in the upper third of the oesophagus and hypopharynx has been reported in association with sideropenic dysphagia (Paterson–Kelly/Plummer–Vinson syndrome) and cervical webs, although this association has been questioned (Jacobsson 1961).

When a malignant lesion occurs in a patient with a web, it is not located at the site of the web, indicating that the web itself is not precancerous but may indicate the presence of a concomitant malignancy (Ekberg 1981).

# Staging of Oesophageal Carcinoma

Once the diagnosis of oesophageal carcinoma has been established, attention is directed towards the therapeutic options. Despite reports of successful treatment with radiotherapy and chemotherapy (Leichman et al. 1984), surgery remains the primary treatment *in most centres*. Accurate pretreatment assessment of the extent of disease may identify patients with potentially curable tumours and those in whom only palliative surgery or conservative management is appropriate. The avoidance of unnecessary surgery together with the lower operative morbidity and mortality associated with palliative as opposed to curative surgery is the justification for accurate preoperative staging (Earlam and Cunha-Melo 1980; Heck and Rossi 1980; Orringer 1984).

The barium examination provides information about the vertical extent of disease which gives some indication of potential resectability. Of tumours less than 5 cm in length, 50% will have developed lymph node metastases whereas 90% of tumours greater than 5 cm in length will have lymph nodes involved at surgery (Earlam and Cunha-Melo 1980).

However, the major factors influencing the prognosis and choice of therapy are the extent of invasion of vital mediastinal structures by extraoesophageal spread of disease and the presence of distant metastases. Retrotracheal abnormalities with displacement of the trachea on the lateral film have been suggested as signs of tracheo-bronchial invasion (Daffner et al. 1978) and occasionally the presence of a malignant tracheo-bronchial fistula may be inferred from a chest X-ray film which demonstrates recurrent pneumonia or pulmonary abscess. In general, however, conventional radiological assessment of resectability by barium studies (Yamada 1979), azygos venography (Mori et al. 1979) or gallium scanning (Kondo et al. 1982) has been disappointing. The value of bronchoscopy and mediastinoscopy has also been limited in the assessment of spread (Murray et al. 1971) and resectability has, until recently, only been reliably assessed by surgical exploration.

### Computed Tomography

CT enables visualisation of the cross-sectional relationships in the mediastinum and has become an increasingly valuable tool in the pretherapy staging of squamous cell oesophageal carcinoma.

## CT Technique

Careful attention to technique is important to avoid errors of interpretation. Scans of the entire oesophagus and upper abdomen should be obtained at 1-cm intervals with the patient maintaining deep inspiration which results in full distension of the airways. Standard dilute oral contrast media is given and patients are instructed not to swallow during scanning. For the detection of subtle areas of wall thickening we have found the use of hyoscine-N-butyl bromide (Buscopan) with effervescent tablets to be helpful in obtaining maximal distension of the oesophageal wall (Fig. 5.10). This technique is also helpful in assessing the gastro-oesophageal junction where the oblique course of the oesophagus as it

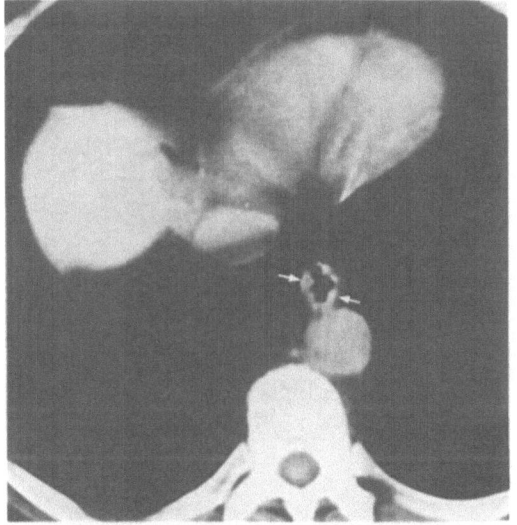

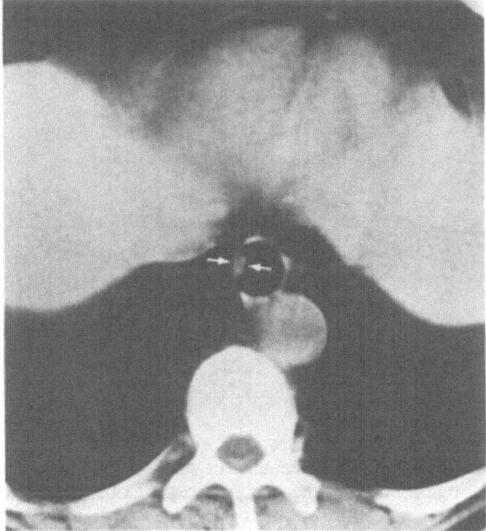

**Fig. 5.10a.** The distal oesophagus is partially collapsed resulting in apparent irregular circumferential thickening (arrow heads). **b.** After administration of gas-producing tablets and a relaxant, the resulting distension accurately shows a small plaque of mural thickening indicating a small oesophageal cancer. (Same patient as demonstrated in Fig. 5.1.)

enters the stomach may result in the appearance of a "pseudo mass" which may be misinterpreted as tumour. It may also be necessary to scan in the left lateral decubitus position which allows gas to rise and distend the gastro-oesophageal junction.

Rapid sequential "dynamic" scanning after a bolus of i.v. contrast medium may be of value to delineate more clearly the vascular structures in the mediastinum and may be particularly useful in cachectic patients in whom the fat

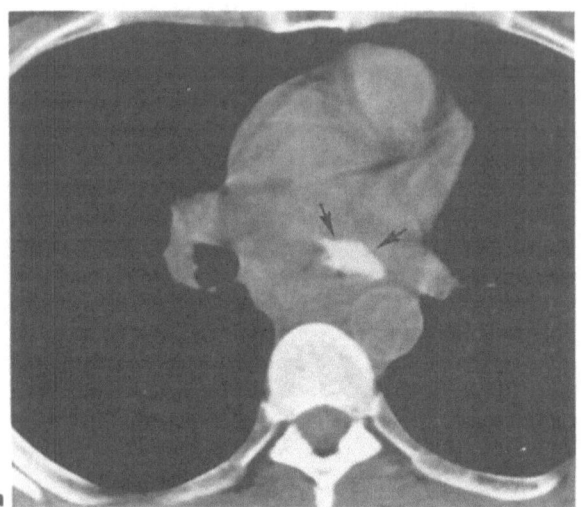

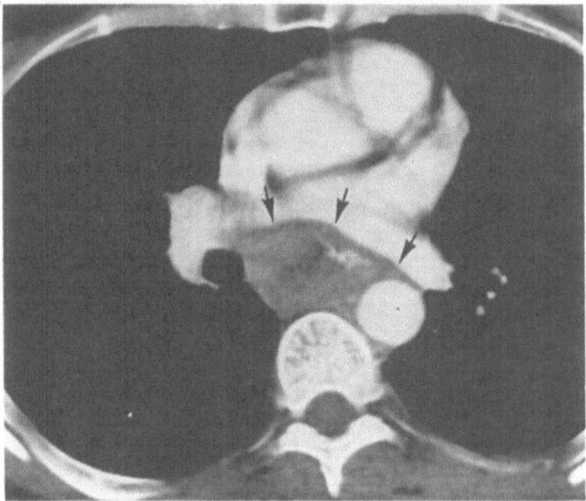

**Fig. 5.11a.** On a precontrast scan, a large tumour of the midoesophagus is demonstrated with distension and displacement of the oesophageal lumen. The margins of the tumour cannot be distinguished from the posterior aspect of the heart and great vessels. **b.** A scan during dynamic intravenous contrast enhancement clearly delineates the tumour mass (arrowheads) and shows the distortion of the left atrium and encasement of the aorta. The tumour is almost certainly unresectable.

planes cannot be distinguished (Fig.5.11). Its use may also elucidate equivocal liver metastases but routine use is not advocated.

## Normal Appearances

On CT, the oesophageal wall is defined by intraluminal air, perioesophageal fat and the adjacent airways. Oesophageal wall thickness depends on the degree of distension and ranges between 3 and 5 mm (Halber *et al.* 1979). The cervical oesophagus extends from the cricopharyngeus muscle to the thoracic inlet. There is virtually no perioesophageal fat in this region, which makes CT assessment of oesophageal abnormalities very difficult. The thoracic oesophagus is surrounded by a variable amount of fat which may be markedly reduced in the cachectic patient. It is loss or encroachment on this normal fat which enables an assessment of extraoesophageal spread of malignant disease.

In the lower thorax, the oesophagus lies directly posterior to the pericardium covering the left atrium and moves to the left of the midline as it enters the diaphragmatic hiatus anterior to the descending aorta. At the level of the hiatus, the diaphragmatic crura surround the oesophagus on both sides and then come to lie posterior to the intra-abdominal segment. The anatomical level of the gastro-oesophageal junction is easily identified on CT by the most cranial portion of the fissure for the gastro-hepatic ligament (Marks et al. 1981).

## Staging Systems

The TNM system of staging has been widely adopted (Beahrs and Myers 1983) (Table 5.1). T1 and T2 represent limited disease and the presence of extra-oesophageal spread places the tumour in a T3 category. Lymph node involve-

**Table 5.1.**  TNM staging system for oesophageal carcinoma (American Joint Committee)

*Clinical diagnostic primary tumour (T)*

| | |
|---|---|
| T1 | A tumour that involves 5 cm or less of oesophageal length, that produces no obstruction and that has no circumferential involvement and no extraoesophageal spread |
| T2 | A tumour that involves more than 5 cm of oesophageal length without extraoesophageal spread or a tumour of any size that produces obstruction or that involves the entire circumference but without extraoesophageal spread |
| T3 | Any tumour with evidence of extraoesophageal spread |

*Regional lymph node involvement (N)*

| | |
|---|---|
| N0 | Regional nodes not involved |
| N1 | Unilateral regional nodes involved |
| N2 | Bilateral regional nodes involved |
| N3 | Extensive multiple regional nodes involved |

*Distant metastasis (M)*

| | |
|---|---|
| M0 | No distant metastasis |
| M1 | Distant metastasis present |

*Clinical-diagnostic classification*

| | |
|---|---|
| Stage I | T1, N0, M0 |
| Stage II | T1, N1–N2, M0 or T2, N0–N2, M0 |
| Stage III | T2, any N, M0 or any T, N3, M0 |
| Stage IV | Any T, any N, M1 |

ment below the diaphragm is considered as distant metastases. Stage groups have been defined with Stage I and II corresponding to T1 and T2, without evidence of metastatic disease, and are therefore considered potentially resectable for cure. Stage III includes tumours with extraoesophageal spread and/or regional lymph node involvement, and the presence of distant metastases leads to a Stage IV categorisation. Palliative therapy is generally considered appropriate for Stage III and IV disease.

A separate and somewhat simpler staging system has been devised based on CT criteria which has been applied generally to all tumours of the gastrointestinal tract (Moss et al. 1981) (Table 5.2). This closely parallels the TNM staging system in that Stages I and II are considered potentially resectable for cure.

**Table 5.2.**   CT staging of oesophageal carcinoma (Moss 1981)

| | |
|---|---|
| Stage I | Intraluminal polypoid mass without thickening of the oesophageal wall, no mediastinal extension or metastasis |
| Stage II | Thickened oesophageal wall (greater than 5 mm) without invasion of adjacent organs or distant metastasis |
| Stage III | Thickened oesophageal wall with direct extension into surrounding tissue: local or regional mediastinal metastases |
| Stage IV | Any tumour stage with distant metastatic disease |

## Staging Criteria for Squamous Cell Oesophageal Carcinoma

### The Tumour

The earliest indication of oesophageal tumour on CT is eccentric thickening of the wall (Figs. 5.10, 5.12) which, with more advanced disease, may become circumferential. The presence of obstruction can be inferred by increased diameter of the oesophageal lumen above the strictured segment, with reduced distension below. The length of tumour on CT shows moderately good correlation with barium studies and oesophagoscopy (Moss et al. 1981; Thompson et al. 1983). Discrepancies do occur, particularly in more distal tumours where concomitant reflux oesophagitis may result in diffuse wall thickening, which may be indistinguishable from tumour infiltration (Schneekloth et al. 1983). The longest measurement obtained from CT, barium examination or endoscopy should be taken to avoid understaging, and most studies show tumour measurements to correlate within 2–3 cm of the pathological specimen.

### Extraoesophageal Extension

Increase in size of an oesophageal carcinoma frequently results in transmural invasion and the lack of a defined serosa facilitates extension into the perioesophageal fat. On CT, blurring or obliteration of the fat surrounding the oesophagus has been found to be a reliable criterion for perioesophageal spread (Coulomb et al. 1981) (Fig. 5.13) and immediately places the tumour in Stage III category. Minor degrees of perioesophageal spread do not, however, preclude

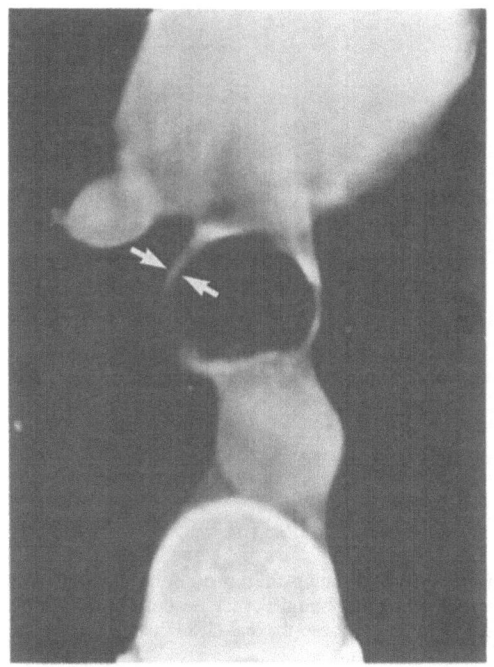

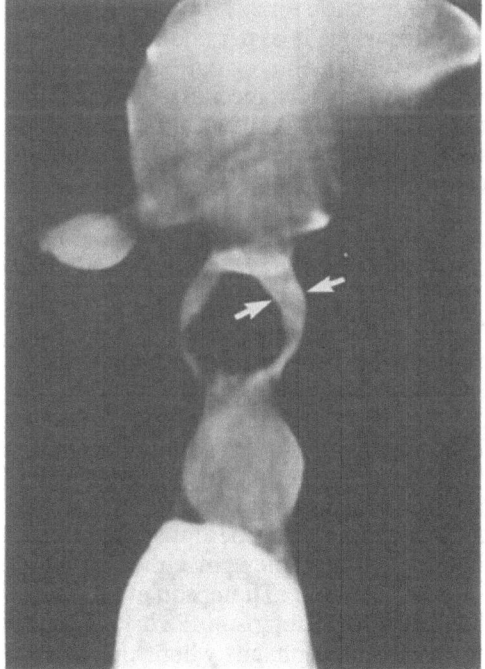

**Fig. 5.12a.** The normal oesophageal wall measures less than 3 mm in the distended state (arrowheads). **b.** Irregular thickening of the wall indicates the presence of tumour (arrowheads), although inflammatory change may give a similar appearance.

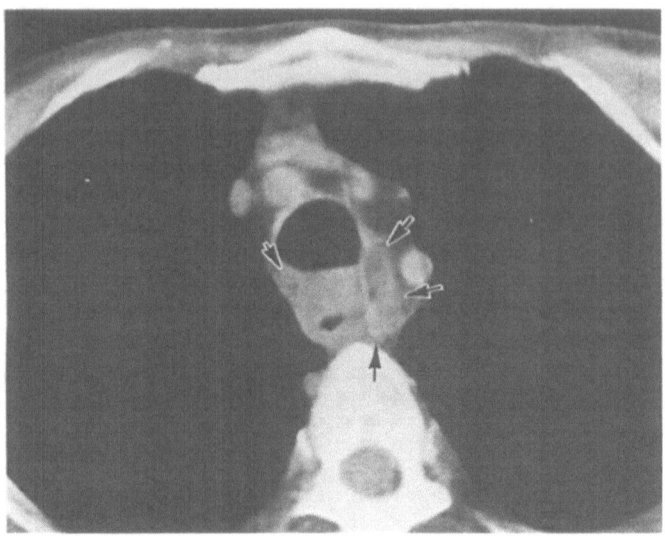

**Fig. 5.13.** Thickening of the oesophageal wall is demonstrated in an upper-third oesophageal tumour. The outer margin of the oesophagus is poorly defined (arrows) and the increased soft tissue density in the perioesophageal fat indicates extraoesophageal spread.

surgical resection for cure and it is invasion into the surrounding vital mediastinal structures which is of paramount importance. Fat planes may be completely lost in cachectic patients or patients who have undergone prior radiotherapy, and under these circumstances assessment of mediastinal invasion is difficult (Daffner et al. 1979). Contiguity of structures does not necessarily imply invasion and other well-defined criteria are required before invasion can be predicted accurately by CT.

*Tracheobronchial Invasion*

There is normally an absence of fat between the oesophagus and the trachea and loss of the fat plane can therefore not be used as an indication of invasion. Specific criteria of invasion have been described, namely displacement and indentation of the trachea or left main bronchus by the tumour mass (Fig. 5.14). Although on expiration the posterior membranous part of the trachea may normally be bowed inwards, on inspiration the posterior wall of the normal trachea is flat or bowed outwards (Gamsu and Webb 1982) and under these circumstances any indentation by an adjacent oesophageal carcinoma is indicative of tumour invasion. Similarly, displacement of either of these structures by the mass will reliably predict infiltration (Thompson et al. 1983; Picus et al. 1983; Daffner et al. 1979; Halvorsen and Thompson 1987b). These criteria cannot be accurately applied in the cervical oesophagus where the narrow AP diameter may result in normal indentation of the cervical trachea by the cervical oesophagus. It should be appreciated that these criteria apply only to squamous cell carcinoma of the oesophagus, as some benign oesophageal conditions and oesophageal sarcoma

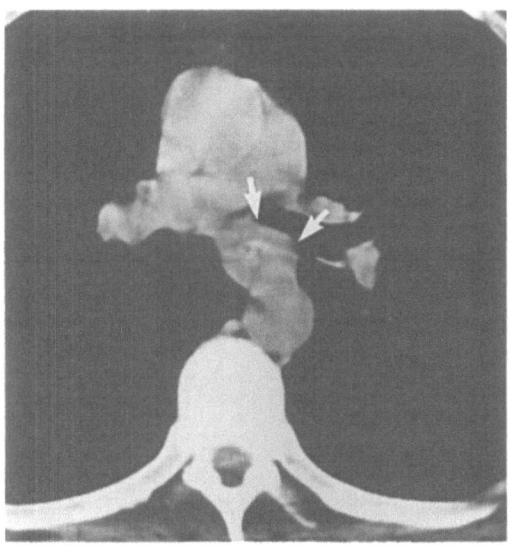

**Fig. 5.14.** The posterior wall of the left main bronchus is bowed inwards by an oesophageal mass (arrowheads). The appearances indicate bronchial wall invasion.

and lymphoma can cause tracheal indentation without implying tumour invasion (Thompson et al. 1983). Using the above criteria, the sensitivity of invasion predicted by CT is high at approximately 98% (Halvorsen and Thompson 1987b). False-positive results occur, but specificity is still as high as 95% (Coulomb et al. 1981; Picus et al. 1983; Thompson et al. 1983). Occasional spontaneous malignant oesophagotracheal fistulas can be demonstrated with a reported incidence of 7% (Little et al. 1984).

*Aortic Invasion*

Tumours lying in the middle third of the oesophagus are closely related to the descending aorta. A discernible fat plane is usually seen separating these structures and, if visualised, excludes aortic invasion by tumour. Cachexia and radiotherapy may both result in loss of the fat planes but if a clear fat plane is visible above and below the tumour, then obliteration at the tumour level suggests malignant invasion. The CT criteria for aortic invasion are based on the degree of contact between the tumour and aortic circumference (Picus et al. 1983). If the tumour is in contact with less than 45° of the aortic circumference, then the aorta is considered normal with no evidence of invasion. However, contact over an arc greater than 90° predicts invasion with an accuracy of 80% or more (Picus et al. 1983; Thompson et al. 1983). An arc of contact of between 45° and 90° is considered indeterminate (Fig. 5.15). A recent study assessing accuracy of CT staging quoted an accuracy of only 55% for aortic invasion (Quint et al. 1985b). These investigators, however, included 11 indeterminate scans as false-positives which may be inappropriate, and if these patients are excluded from

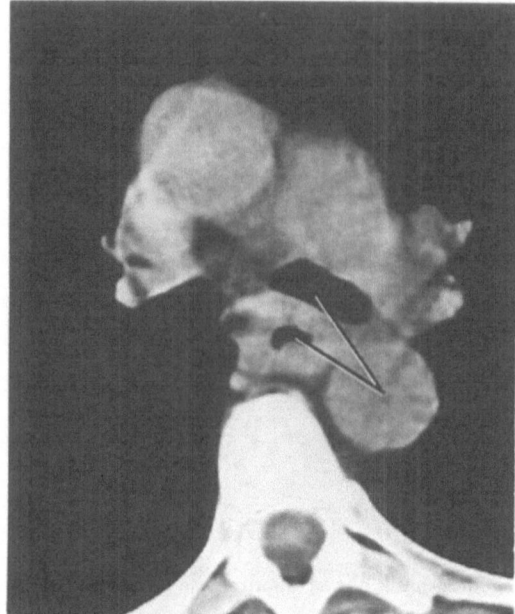

a

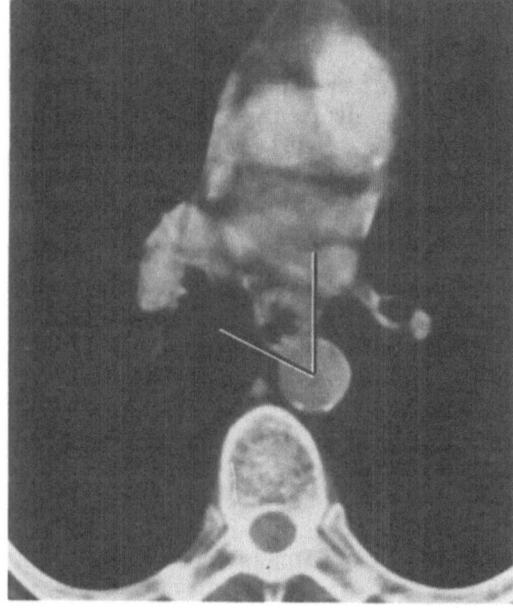

b

**Fig. 5.15a.**   A midoesophageal tumour with marked concentric wall thickening is in contact with the aorta over an arc of less than 45°. This is negative for aortic invasion. There is, however, slight indentation of the posterior aspect of the left main bronchus suggesting invasion. **b.** There is eccentric thickening of the oesophageal wall subtending an angle between 45° and 90° with the aorta and therefore indeterminate for aortic invasion. **c.** The aortic circumference is in contact with a large irregular tumour and over greater than 90°. There is associated pleural thickening and a left pleural effusion (arrowheads).

Fig 5.15 (*continued*)

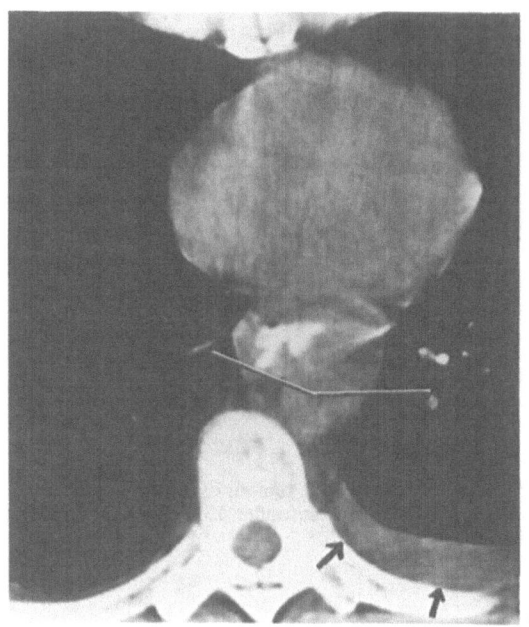

c

their results, the accuracy of assessment of aortic invasion rises to 82%
(Halvorsen and Thompson 1987a).


## Invasion of Other Mediastinal Structures

Involvement of the pericardium at the level of the left atrium may be difficult to
determine, in part because of artefact from cardiac motion and partly as a result
of the frequent absence of an intervening fat plane. Strict criteria for invasion
have not been clearly defined. If direct contact between the tumour and
pericardium is visualised, invasion is suspected but only regarded as positive if
clear fat planes are visualised on contiguous CT sections above and below the
level of the lesion (Halvorsen and Thompson 1987b). In the presence of cachexia,
scans are commonly indeterminate.

Pleural invasion may be very difficult to assess accurately by CT. Rarely
invasion of the vertebral bodies may be demonstrated.


## Lymph Node Staging

CT is limited in its ability to detect tumour in lymph nodes. On CT, 95% of
normal mediastinal nodes measure less than 11 mm (Genereux and Howie 1984)
and 1 cm is a generally accepted upper limit of normal size. However, metastatic
foci in nodes of less than 1 cm cannot be differentiated on CT. Conversely, lymph
node enlargement may be due to benign causes rather than malignant infiltration,
particularly if there is an inflammatory component to the tumour (Lackner et al.

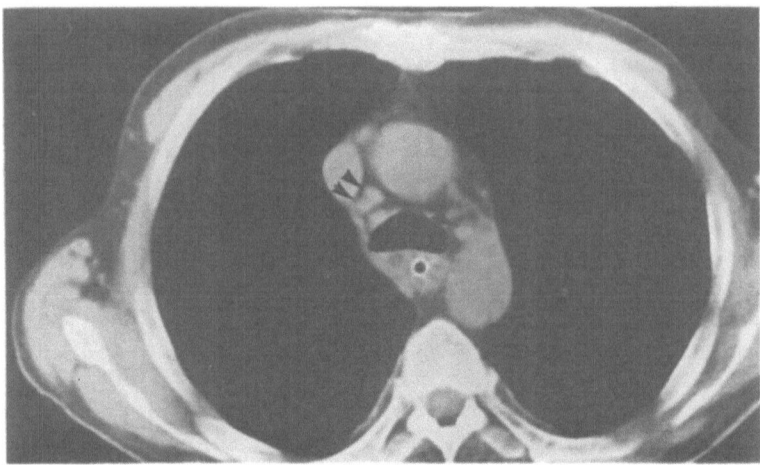

**Fig. 5.16.** An inoperable tumour of the upper third of the oesophagus has spread to involve lymph nodes in the middle mediastinum. Enlarged right pretracheal and subaortic nodes are demonstrated (arrowheads).

1981). However, in general, the larger the lymph node the greater the probability of tumour involvement.

It is almost impossible to distinguish local para-aortic lymph node involvement from extraoesophageal spread. The distinction is academic with no influence on resectability or prognosis as both would be considered as Stage III disease. The abundant lymphatic drainage of the oesophagus which is orientated in a longitudinal plane allows rapid and often non-segmental and skipping involvement of perioesophageal lymph nodes (Becker and Fuchs 1986) (Fig. 5.16). The accuracy of regional nodal staging has been variably reported as between 55% (Picus et al. 1983) and 96% (Samuelsson et al. 1984), with differences in part due to the different upper limit of normal lymph node size adopted. In one series with surgical confirmation, almost all perioesophageal nodes containing tumour were less than 7 mm (Picus et al. 1983).

## Subdiaphragmatic Metastases

### Lymph Nodes

Subdiaphragmatic lymph node spread is common, occurring with similar incidence to mediastinal lymphadenopathy. The prevalence of abdominal lymph node involvement at diagnosis varies widely. A surgical series with careful lymph node dissection reported an incidence of 59% (Akiyama et al. 1981). Some authors have considered coeliac axis and left gastric nodes as regional lymph nodes for distal oesophageal tumours (Quint et al. 1986) and this also influences prevalence figures. The upper limit of normal size for gastrohepatic ligament nodes has been established as 8 mm (Balfe et al. 1984). It is, however, common in this region for metastatic foci to exist in normal-sized nodes which reduces the sensitivity of CT diagnosis. This can be a difficult area for CT interpretation as normal structures may be confused with lymphadenopathy. The accuracy of CT diagnosis varies between 39% (Lee et al. 1984) and 85% (Quint et al. 1986; Samuelsson et al. 1984). In general, CT is less accurate in the detection of subdiaphragmatic nodal metastases than in the detection of direct mediastinal invasion.

*Liver*

A recent review of CT staging of oesophageal carcinoma, comparing results of several investigators, quotes a sensitivity rate of 78% for the detection of liver metastases. Small deposits may go undetected, although the use of dynamic intravenous contrast enhancement may improve delineation. The specificity approaches 100% (Halvorsen, 1987b).

# Gastro-oesophageal Junction Tumours

CT is considered to be less accurate in preoperative staging of tumours in this region, with an accuracy between 50% and 68% (Thompson et al. 1983; Terrier et al. 1984). Deep intramural tumour growth cannot be accurately differentiated from early infiltration of the perioesophageal and perigastric soft tissue planes (Fig. 5.17). Almost all tumours arising in this region appear to be in close contact with the pleura and diaphragmatic crura, whether or not they are directly involved (Picus et al. 1983). Assessment of the extent of gastric invasion may be further complicated by the presence of a hiatus hernia or collapsed gastric folds. However, in advanced carcinoma, CT accurately predicts unresectability by showing extensive local infiltration (Terrier et al. 1984).

The value of preoperative staging of gastro-oesophageal junction tumours depends largely upon local surgical policy (Freeny and Marks 1982). If unresectable, tumours are invariably treated by palliative surgery, and there is little indication for preoperative CT staging. If, however, other palliative methods such as peroral endoscopic intubation or chemotherapy are considered as alternative palliative procedures, then the preoperative CT diagnosis of unresectability may guide management.

# Ultrasound

Although CT provides the greatest accuracy in the assessment of liver metastases (Snow et al. 1979), a technically satisfactory ultrasound examination images most metastatic disease to the liver. In addition, hepatic ultrasound is occasionally abnormal in patients who have completely normal CT examinations (Mayes and Bernadino 1982).

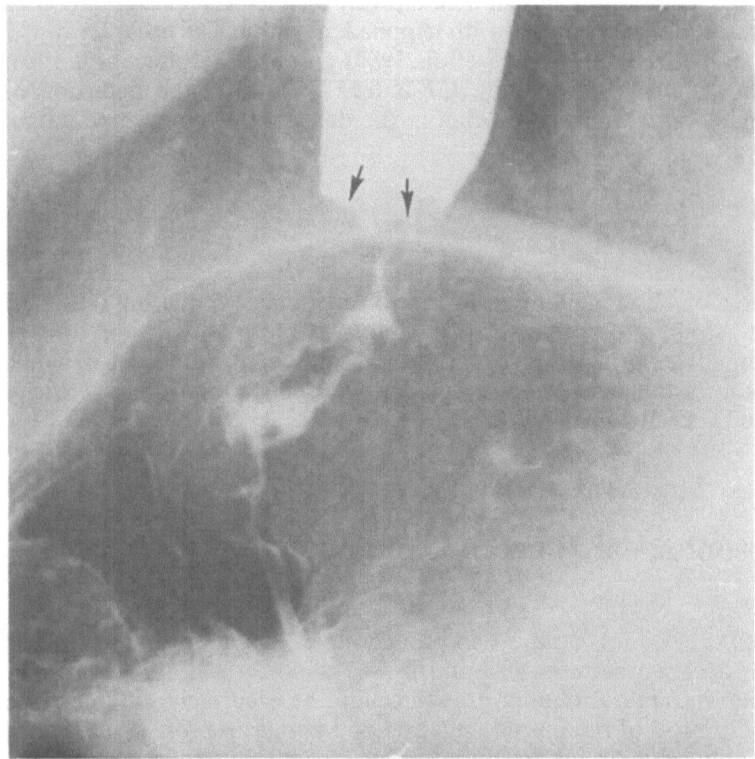

a

**Fig. 5.17a–c.** A gastro-oesophageal adenocarcinoma diagnosed on barium examination, **a**, is demonstrated on CT as an irregular soft tissue mass, **b**, indenting the medial aspect of the gastric fundus. The outer margin of the mass is poorly defined (arrowheads) which probably represents perioesophageal spread. **c**, Enlarged coeliac axis and left gastric nodes are demonstrated (white arrows).

Endoscopic ultrasound is a new technique which produces high resolution real-time ultrasound images from within the gastrointestinal tract by means of an ultrasound probe mounted at the tip of a fibreoptic endoscope (Fig. 5.18). This technique is currently under evaluation in several centres with some promising results in the oesophagus (Shorvon et al. 1987; Tio and Tytgat 1984). The layers of the oesophageal wall can be clearly visualised and it is possible to differentiate between localised tumour (T1) and tumour which has spread beyond the muscularis propria and therefore represents T3. Although early degrees of transmural spread do not render a tumour unresectable, it is likely to be incurable. Perioesophageal and mediastinal lymph nodes are clearly seen and there is evidence to suggest that metastatic and hyperplastic lymphadenopathy may be distinguished by the shape and internal ultrasonic structure of the nodes (Murata et al. 1987), giving an accuracy of nodal staging of 89%. The technique has limitations, particularly where the presence of a tight stricture limits the passing of the endoscope (Shorvon 1987). However, there is clearly a future role for this technique if accurate preoperative staging is required.

**Fig 5.17** (*continued*)

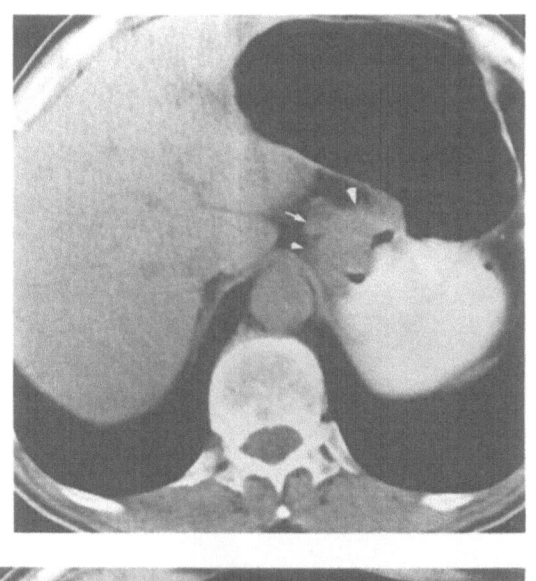

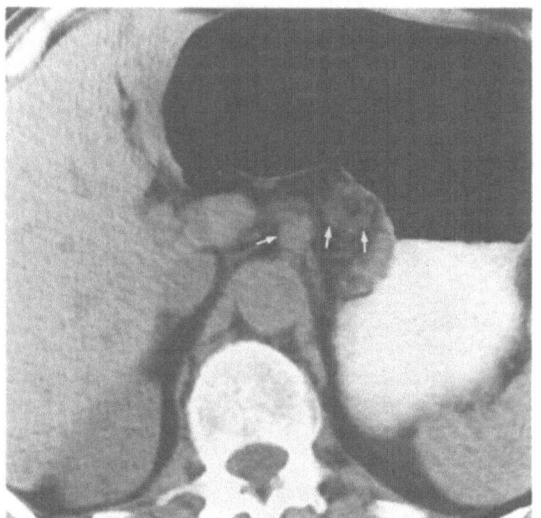

# Magnetic Resonance Imaging (MRI)

The technical development of MRI is evolving rapidly but its exact role in clinical practice has not yet been defined. There are major limitations to its use in the thorax. Cardiac gating is necessary to eliminate cardiac motion artefact; respiratory movement artefact is less readily dealt with. Despite these shortcomings, the cross-sectional images provided by MRI may be compared with CT.

There have been few reports of the MRI appearances of oesophageal carcinoma (Smith et al. 1981; Alfidi et al. 1982; Quint et al. 1985a). Available

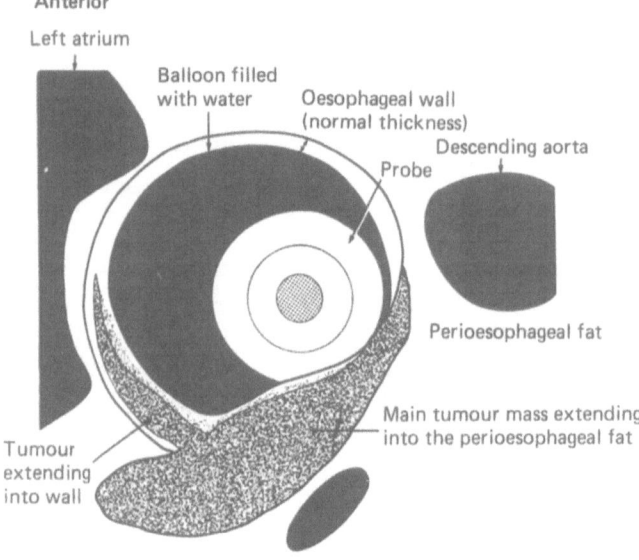

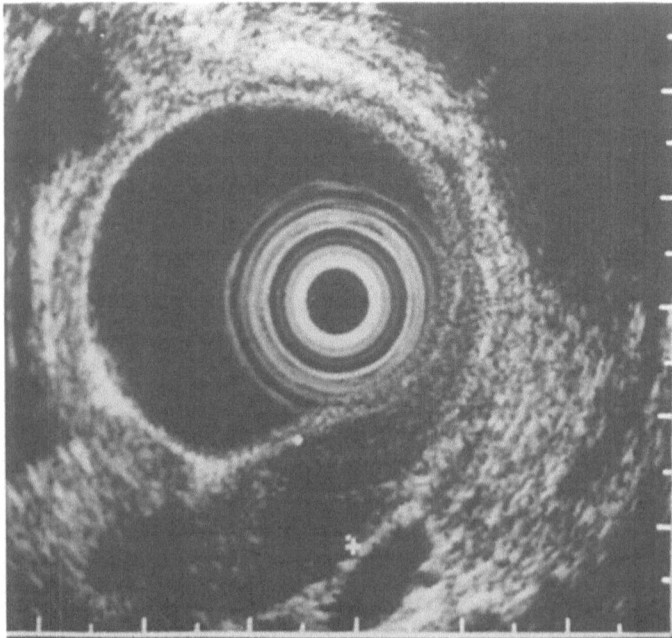

**Fig. 5.18.** Transverse scan of the lower one-third of the oesophagus obtained by endoscopic ultrasonography. The tumour is arising from the posterior aspect of the oesophagus and extending into the mediastinum. The tumour is not circumferential at this point and the oesophageal wall anterolaterally on the left is of normal thickness. The wall is seen as three lines: an echodense line at the junction of the mucosa with the water-filled balloon, an echolucent line representing submucosa and muscularis and a rather poorly defined echodense line representing the adventitia. Illustration kindly provided by Dr P. Shorvon, Central Middlesex Hospital, London, NW10.

data suggest that non-respiratory gated MRI is inaccurate in preoperative staging of oesophageal cancer, tending to understage the primary tumour more frequently than CT (Quint et al. 1985a). In part, this reflects a well-recognised difficulty in imaging the tracheo-bronchial tree with MRI (Webb et al. 1984; Ross et al. 1984).

The two major weaknesses of CT in lymph node imaging are also inherent in MRI: inability to detect metastases in normal-sized nodes, and an inability to distinguish the causes of node enlargement. In evaluating the mediastinal and hilar nodes, MRI has some theoretical advantages in that no contrast medium is required and normal vascular structures are easily differentiated from masses. The main disadvantages in comparison with CT are a lack of spatial resolution, an inability to show calcium reliably and confusion between the oesophagus and subcarinal nodes (Levitt et al. 1985). The absence of a suitable bowel contrast medium creates a major diagnostic difficulty in the abdomen in that loops of bowel can simulate lymph node enlargement.

Most investigators suggest roughly comparable results for MRI and CT in the detection of focal liver disease (Moss et al. 1984; Heiken et al. 1984). It may be that with advancing technology, MRI will surpass CT in the detection of liver metastases. This assumption is supported by a recent preliminary report of patients with liver metastases studied with both modalities (Lee et al. 1985).

# Postoperative Assessment and Tumour Recurrence

## Early Complications

Technical improvements in surgery including the introduction of transhiatal oesophagectomy and of an end-to-end anastomotic stapler have considerably decreased the morbidity and mortality associated with oesophageal resection (Steichen and Ravitch 1980; Orringer and Orringer 1983). Most deaths are related to anastomotic dehiscence (Postlethwaite 1983) and the early demonstration of this is essential as the morbidity and mortality of oesophageal perforation are directly related to the interval between diagnosis and the instigation of appropriate therapy (Agha et al. 1985). The radiological diagnosis of anastomotic leakage depends on the demonstration of extravasation of contrast material into the mediastinum or pleural space. A suggestive plain film finding may be the sudden marked increase in pleural effusion after removal of the chest drain around the third postoperative day (Owen et al. 1983). Contrast examination requires fluoroscopy in two oblique projections after ingestion of water-soluble contrast medium (Gastrografin) followed, if negative, with dilute barium. Blind sinus tracks at the anastomotic sites may indicate walled-off leaks and warrant repeat contrast examinations to ensure adequate healing. Many such tracks will resolve without specific therapy (Owen et al. 1983). In the presence of a negative barium study, CT examination may reveal the development of mediastinal or subphrenic abscess in patients with persistent symptoms (Heiken et al. 1984) (Fig. 5.19).

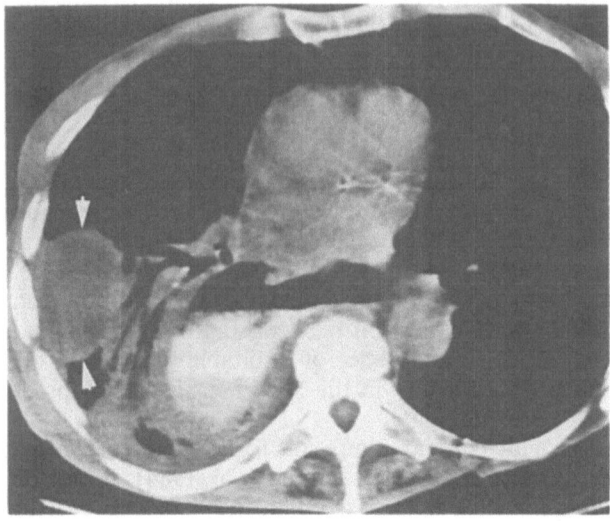

**Fig. 5.19.** CT examination following oesophageal resection with the stomach having been mobilised into the chest. Anastomotic leakage into the pleura has resulted in the development of a loculated abscess (arrowheads). There is associated consolidation of the right lower lobe with a clearly demonstrated air bronchogram.

Twenty to twenty-five per cent of patients develop cricopharyngeal inco-ordination and a tendency to aspirate into the tracheo-bronchial tree following transhiatal oesophagectomy (Agha et al. 1985). Extreme caution is required when using water-soluble contrast agents in these patients as aspiration into the lungs may result in pulmonary oedema. Gastric outlet obstruction may occur at the level of the diaphragmatic hiatus if not accompanied by an appropriate drainage procedure. Radiographically, the intrathoracic stomach appears distended and contains an excessive amount of secretions with marked delay in emptying in the upright position (Agha et al. 1985). Gastric necrosis may result from impairment to the blood supply of the mobilised stomach and present as perforation of the gastric wall away from the level of the sutures, with extravasation of contrast medium into the mediastinum.

## Late Complications

The development of symptoms of dysphagia occurring several months after oesophago-gastrectomy may indicate the development of a benign stricture, or recurrence of disease. Barium examination may reveal anastomotic stenosis, often due to fibrosis. This appears as a smoothly tapered narrowing of variable length, terminating inferiorly at the oesophago-gastric anastomosis and is often associated with mucosal ulceration (Owen et al. 1983). The absence of any significant mass effect favours benign disease. Malignancy may however coexist with oesophagitis. Tumour recurrence often occurs at the level of the primary tumour, suggesting recurrent growth from residual tumour or adjacent lymph-

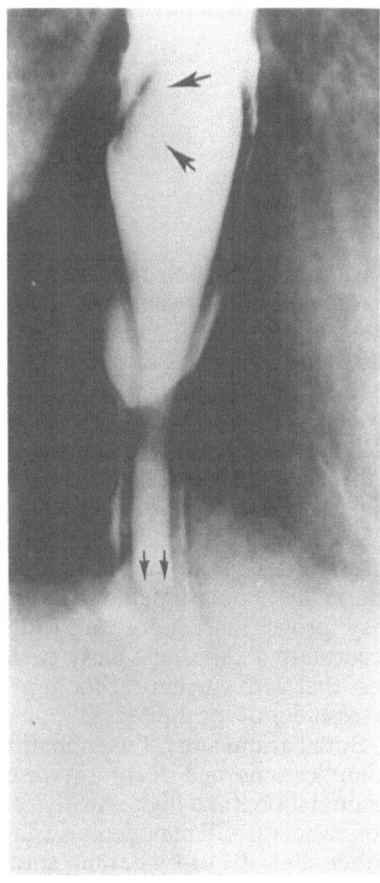

**Fig. 5.20.** Following insertion of an
endoprosthesis for unresectable tumour, this
patient presented with dysphagia. There is tumour
growth over the rim of the prosthesis (arrowheads)
and the distal lumen is completely blocked.

node metastases (Becker et al. 1987) (Fig. 5.20). Disease may also recur above or
below the primary tumour level or anywhere along the intrathoracic course of the
resected oesophagus. In one series 50% of patients were demonstrated to have
distant metastases at the time of recurrence (Becker et al. 1987). CT is more
sensitive than barium examination in the assessment of extramucosal tumour
recurrence and distant metastases, and may detect disease before it is symptomatic. Following gastric interposition the prevertebral region may contain increased
fat, as part of the omentum is brought into the chest with the stomach, and the
right crus may also be displaced laterally by surgical enlargement of the
diaphragmatic hiatus (Heiken et al. 1984). The mediastinal fat planes may be
absent or distorted, or may demonstrate increased density as a result of scar
formation or radiotherapy (Gross et al. 1985). The azygos vein may also impress
the gastric wall and simulate recurrence, as may underdistension of the inter-
posed stomach (Becker et al. 1987). However, the demonstration of an abnormal
soft tissue mediastinal mass is likely to represent recurrent carcinoma. Although
there is currently no general agreement regarding treatment of patients with
recurrent disease, the early detection may enable the instigation of further

palliative treatment or the discontinuation of chemotherapy with its attendant side-effects.

# Conclusions

Barium examination remains the primary method of diagnosis of oesophageal carcinoma and presents a wide variety of radiological appearances. Careful attention to subtle mucosal abnormalities in patients with dysphagia may enable the earlier diagnosis of potentially curable lesions.

In established disease, CT has emerged as an acceptable method of preoperative staging. Although there has been controversy over the accuracy and value of CT, most recent studies indicate that a high staging accuracy can be achieved by adherence to strict CT criteria in squamous cell tumours of the oesophagus. CT may therefore be recommended in routine preoperative staging of such lesions. Oesophago-gastric junction tumours, which are more commonly adenocarcinomas, are less accurately staged and CT may be of value only in selected cases where the tumour is demonstrated to be clearly unresectable. Further experience may prove that endoscopic ultrasound is a valuable additional technique, accurately determining early perioesophageal spread. Preliminary reports suggest that with current technology MRI is less accurate than CT in preoperative assessment of local disease.

Both barium and CT examination are of value in the detection of postoperative complications and recurrent disease and are often complementary. Barium examination has a high sensitivity for benign and malignant mucosal abnormalities, whereas CT may demonstrate mediastinal recurrence before it is apparent either clinically or by barium study.

*Acknowledgements.* Our grateful thanks go to Julie Jessop for typing the manuscript and to Dr PJ Shorvon for kindly providing Fig. 5.18.

# References

Agha FP (1985) Barrett carcinoma of the esophagus: clinical and radiographic analysis of 34 cases. AJR 145:41–46

Agha FP, Orringer MB, Amendola MA (1985) Gastric interposition following transhiatal esophagectomy: radiographic evaluation. Gastrointest Radiol 10:17–24

Akiyama H, Tsuramaru M, Kawanura T, Ono Y (1981) Principles of surgical treatment for carcinoma of the esophagus. Analysis of lymph node involvement. Ann Surg 194:438–446

Alfidi RJ, Hagga JR, El Yousef SJ et al. (1982) Preliminary experimental results in humans and animals with a superconducting whole body nuclear magnetic resonance scanner. Radiology 143:175–187

Anderson MF, Harell GS (1980) Secondary esophageal tumors. AJR 135:1243–1246

Applequist P (1972) Carcinoma of the esophagus and gastric cardia: a retrospective study based on statistical and clinical material from Finland. Acta Chir Scand [Suppl] 430:1

Applequist P, Salmo M (1980) Lye corrosion carcinoma of the oesophagus. Cancer 45:2655–2658

Azzopardi JG, Menzies T (1962) Primary oesophageal adenocarcinoma: confirmation of its existence by the finding of mucous gland tumours. Br J Surg 49:497–506

Balfe DM, Mauro MA, Koehler RE et al. (1984) Gastrohepatic ligament: normal and pathologic CT anatomy. Radiology 150:485–490

Beahrs OH, Myers MH (1983) Digestive system sites: oesophagus. In: American Joint Committee on Cancer, Beahrs OH, Myers MH (eds) Manual for staging of cancer, 2nd edn. Lippincott, Philadelphia, pp 61–66

Becker CD, Fuchs WA (1986) Carcinoma of the esophagus and gastroesophageal junction. In: Meyers Morton A (ed) Computed tomography of the gastrointestinal tract. Springer-Verlag, Berlin Heidelberg New York pp 1–20

Becker CD, Barbier PA, Terrier F, Porcellini B (1987) Patterns of recurrence of oesophageal carcinoma after transhiatal esophagectomy and gastric interposition AJR 148:273–277

Bosch A, Frias Z, Caldwell WL (1979) Adenocarcinoma of the esophagus. Cancer 43:1557–1561

Bruni HC, Nelson RS (1975) Carcinoma of the esophagus and cardia: diagnostic evaluation in 113 cases. J Thorac Cardiovasc Surg 70:367

Burnett M, Toffler R (1951) Primary melanosarcoma of the esophagus. Radiology 57:868–870

Carnovale RL, Goldstein HM, Zornoza J, Dodd GD (1977) Radiologic manifestations of esophageal lymphoma. AJR 128:751–754

Carrie A (1950) Adenocarcinoma of the upper end of the oesophagus arising from ectopic gastric epithelium. Br J Surg 37:474

Carter R, Brewer L (1975) Achalasia and esophageal carcinoma: studies in early diagnosis for improved surgical management. Am J Surg 130:114

Chuong J. DuBovik S, McCallum RW (1984) Achalasia as a risk factor for esophageal carcinoma: a reappraisal. Dig Dis Sci 29:1105–1108

Coordinating group for research on esophageal cancer, Linhsien County, Honan (1976) Early diagnosis and surgical treatment of esophageal cancer under rural conditions. Chin Med J (Engl) 2:113–116

Coulomb M, Leas JF, Sarrazin R, Geindre M (1981) Computed tomography and esophageal carcinoma. J Radiol 62:475–487

Daffner RH, Postlethwait RW, Putman CE (1978) Retrotracheal abnormalities in esophageal carcinoma: prognostic implications. AJR 130:719–723

Daffner RH, Halber MD, Postlethwait RW et al. (1979) CT of the esophagus. II. Carcinoma. AJR 133:1051–1055

Earlam R, Cunha-Melo JR (1980) Oesophageal squamous carcinoma. I. A critical review of surgery. Br J Surg 67:381–390

Edwards DAW (1974) Carcinoma of the esophagus and fundus. Postgrad Med J 50:223

Ekberg O (1981) Cervical oesophageal webs in patients with dysphagia. Clin Radiol 32:633–641

Endo M, Kobayashi S, Suzuki H, Takemoto T, Nakayama K (1971) Diagnosis of early esophageal cancer. Endoscopy 2:61–66

Faintuch J, Shepard KV, Levin B (1984) Adenocarcinoma and other unusual variants of esophageal cancer. Semin Oncol 11:192–202

Freeny PC, Marks WM (1982) Adenocarcinoma of the gastrooesophageal junction: barium and CT examination. AJR 138:1077–1084

Gamsu G, Webb NR (1982) Computed tomography of the trachea: normal and abnormal. AJR 139:321–326

Genereux GP, Howie JL (1984) Normal mediastinal lymph node size and number: CT and anatomic study. AJR 142:1095–1100

Gloyna RE, Zornoza J, Goldstein HM (1977) Primary ulcerative carcinoma of the oesophagus. AJR 129:599–600

Goldstein HM, Zornoza J (1978) Association of squamous cell carcinoma of the head and neck with cancer of the esophagus. AJR 131:791–794

Goldstein HM, Zornoza J, Hopens T (1981) Intrinsic disease of the adult esophagus: benign and malignant tumors. Semin Roentgenol XVI(3):183–197

Gross BH, Agha FP, Glazer GM, Oringer MB (1985) Gastric interposition following transhiatal esophagectomy: CT evaluation. Radiology 155:177–179

Guojun H, Lingfang S, Davies Z et al. (1981) Diagnosis and surgical treatment of early esophageal carcinoma. Chin Med J (Engl) 94:229–232

Halber MD, Daffner RH, Thompson WM (1979) CT of the esophagus: I. Normal appearance. AJR 133:321–326

Halvorsen RA Jr, Thompson WM (1987) Critical review: esophageal carcinoma, CT findings. Invest Radiol 22(1):84–87

Halvorsen RA, Thompson WM (1987) Computed tomographic staging of gastrointestinal tract malignancies. Part I. Esophagus and stomach. Invest Radiol 22:2–16

Heck HA, Rossi NP (1980) Esophageal and gastroesophageal junction carcinoma: an evolved philosophy of management. Cancer 46:1873–1878

Heiken JP, Balfe DM, Roper CL (1984) CT evaluation after esophagogastrectomy. AJR 143:555–560

Itai Y, Kogure T, Okuyama Y et al. (1977) Diffuse finely nodular lesion of the oesophagus. AJR 128:563

Itai Y, Kogure T, Okuyama Y, Akiyama H (1978) Superficial esophageal carcinoma. Radiology 126:597–601

Jacobsson F (1961) The Paterson–Kelly (Plummer–Vinson) syndrome and carcinoma of the esophagus. In: Tanner NC, Smithers DW (eds) Tumours of the oesophagus. Churchill Livingstone, London

Japanese Society for Oesophageal Diseases (1976) Guidelines for the clinical and pathological studies on carcinoma of the esophagus. Jap J Surg 6:69–78

Koehler RE, Moss AA, Margulis AR (1976) Early radiographic manifestations of carcinoma of the esophagus. Radiology 119:1–5

Kondo M, Ando N, Kosuda S et al. (1982) GA-67 scan in patients with intrathoracic esophageal carcinoma planned for surgery. Cancer 49:1031–1034

Lackner K, Weiand G, Koster O, Engel K (1981) Computed tomography for tumours of the oesophagus and stomach. Fortschr Geb Roentgenstr 134(4):364–370

Lawson TL, Dodds WJ (1976) Infiltrating carcinoma simulating achalasia. Gastrointestinal Radiol 1:245–248

Lee JKT, Heiken JP, Dixon WT (1985) Detection of hepatic metastases by proton spectroscopic imaging. Work in progress. Radiology 156:429–432

Lee JW IV, Prager RL, Bender HW Jr (1984) The questionable role of computed tomography in preoperative staging of esophageal cancer. Ann Thorac Surg 38:479–481

Leichman L, Steingar Z, Segel HG, Vaitkeviius VK (1984) Combined preoperative chemotherapy and radiation therapy for cancer of the esophagus. The Wayne State University, South-West Oncology Group and Radiation Therapy Oncology Group Experience. Semin Oncol 11:178–185

Levine MS, Caroline D, Thompson JJ, Kressel HY, Laufer I, Herlinger H (1984) Adenocarcinoma of the esophagus: relationship to Barrett mucosa. Radiology 150:305–309

Levine MS, Dillon EC, Saul SH, Lauter I (1986) Early esophageal cancer. AJR 146:507–512

Levitt RG, Glazer HS, Roper CL et al. (1985) Magnetic resonance imaging of mediastinal and hilar mases: comparison with CT. AJR 145:9–14

Little AG, Ferguson MK, DeMeester TR, Hoffman PC, Skinner DB (1984) Esophageal carcinoma with respiratory tract fistula. Cancer 53:1322–1328

Marks WM, Callen PW, Moss AA (1981) Gastroesophageal region: source of confusion on CT. AJR 136:359–362

Mayes GB, Bernadino ME (1981) The role of ultrasound in the evaluation of hepatic neoplasms. Semin Ultrasound II(3)

McCort JJ (1972) Esophageal carcinosarcoma and pseudosarcoma. Radiology 102–519–524

Moertel CG (1978) Carcinoma of the oesophagus: is there a role for surgery? Am J Dig Dis 23:735–736

Mori S, Kasai M, Watanabe I, Shibuya I (1979) Preoperative assessment of resectability for carcinoma of the thoracic esophagus. Part I. Esophagogram and azygogram. Ann Surg 190:100–105

Moss AA, Koehler RE, Margulis AR (1976) Initial accuracy of esophagograms in detection of small esophageal carcinoma. AJR 127:909–913

Moss AA, Schnyder P, Thoeni R, Margulis AR (1981) Esophageal carcinoma: pretherapy staging by computed tomography. AJR 136:1051–1056

Moss AA, Goldberg HI, Stark DB et al. (1984) Hepatic tumours: magnetic resonance and CT appearance. Radiology 150:141–147

Murata Y, Muroi M, Yoshida M, Ide H, Hanyu F (1987) Endoscopic ultrasonography in the diagnosis of oesophageal carcinoma. Surg Endosc 1:11–16

Murray GF, Wilcox BR, Stare KPJK (1977) The assessment of operability of esophageal carcinoma. Ann Thorac Surg 23:393–399

O'Brien CJ, Saverymuttu S, Hodgson HJF, Evans DJ (1985) Coeliac disease, adenocarcinoma of the jejunum and in-situ carcinoma of the esophagus. J Clin Pathol 36:62–67

Orringer MB, Orringer S (1983) Esophagectomy without thoracotomy: a dangerous operation? J Thorac Cardiovasc Surg 85:72–80

Orringer MB (1984) Transhiatal esophagectomy without thoracotomy for carcinoma of the thoracic esophagus. Ann Surg 200:282–288

Owen JW, Balfe DM, Koehler RE, Roper CL, Weyman PJ (1983) Radiologic evaluation of complications after esophagogastrectomy. AJR 140:1163–1169

Parker EF (1978) Carcinoma of the oesophagus: is there a role for surgery? The case for surgery. Am J Dig Dis 23: 730–734

Picus D, Balfe DM, Koehler RE, Roper CL, Owen JW (1983) Computed tomography in the staging of esophageal carcinoma. Radiology 146:433–438

Postlethwait RW (1983) Carcinoma of the thoracic esophagus. Surg Clin North Am 64(4):933–939

Quint LE, Glazer GM, Orringer MB (1985a) Esophageal imaging by MR and CT: study of normal anatomy and neoplasms. Radiology 156:727–731

Quint LE, Glazer GM, Orringer MB, Gross BH (1985b) Esophageal carcinoma: CT findings. Radiology 155:171–175

Quint LE, Glazer GM, Orringer MB (1986) CT staging of esophageal carcinoma. In: Siegelman S (ed) Staging of neoplasms. Churchill Livingstone, New York, pp 79–99 (Contemporary issues in computed tomography, vol 7)

Ross JS, O'Donovan DB, Novoa R et al. (1984) Magnetic resonance of the chest: initial experience with imaging and in vivo T1 and T2 calculations. Radiology 152:95–101

Samuelsson L, Hambraeus GM, Mercke CE, Tyler U. (1984) CT staging of oesophageal carcinoma. Acta Radiol Diagn [Stockh] 25:7–11

Schneekloth G, Terrier F, Fuchs WA (1983) CT in carcinoma of the oesophagus and cardia. Gastrointest Radiol 8:97–101

Shine I, Allison PR (1966) Carcinoma of the oesophagus with tylosis (keratosis palmaris et plantaris). Lancet I: 951–953

Shorvon PJ, Lees WR, Frost RA, Cotton PB (1987) Upper gastrointestinal endoscopic ultrasonography in gastroenterology. Br J Radiol 60:429–438

Shu YJ (1983) Cytopathology of the oesophagus. An overview of cytopathology in China. Acta Cytol 27:7–16

Silver TM, Goldstein HM (1974) Varicoid carcinoma of the esophagus. Am J Dig Dis 19:56

Skinner DB (1984) Surgical treatment for esophageal carcinoma. Semin Oncol 11(2):136–143

Smith FW, Hutchinson JMS, Mallard JR et al. (1981) Oesophageal carcinoma demonstrated by whole-body nuclear magnetic resonance imaging. Br Med J 282:510–512

Snow JH, Goldstein HM, Wallace S (1979) Comparison of scintigraphy, sonography and computed tomography in the evaluation of hepatic neoplasms. AJR 132:915–918

Sridhar C, Zeskind J, Rising JA (1980) Verrucous squamous cell carcinoma. An unusual tumour of the esophagus. Radiology 136:614

Steichen FM, Ravitch MM (1980) Mechanical sutures in esophageal surgery. Ann Surg 191:373–381

Steiner H, Lanimer J, Hackl A (1984) Lymphatic metastases to the esophagus. Gastrointest Radiol 9:1–4

Styles RA, Gibb SP, Tarshis A, Silverman ML, Scholz FJ (1985) Esophago-gastric polyps: radiographic and endoscopic findings. Radiology 154:307–311

Suzuki H, Kobayashi S, Endo M, Nakayama K (1972) Diagnosis of early esophageal cancer. Surgery 71:99–103

Terrier F, Schapira G, Fuchs WA (1984) CT assessment of operability in carcinoma of the oesophagogastric junction. Eur J Radiol 4:114–117

Thompson WM, Halvorsen RA Jr, Foster WL et al. (1983) Computed tomography for staging esophageal and gastroesophageal cancer: re-evaluation. AJR 141:951–958

Tio TL, Tytgat GN (1984) Endoscopic ultrasonography in the assessment of intra- and transmural infiltration of tumours in the oesophagus, stomach and papilla of Vater and in the detection of extraoesophageal lesions. Endoscopy 16:203–210

Webb WR, Gamsu G, Stark DD, Moore EH (1984) Magnetic resonance imaging of the normal and abnormal pulmonary hila. Radiology 152:89–94

Wychulis AR, Woolam GL, Anderesen HA, Ellis FH (1971) Achalasia and carcinoma of the esophagus. JAMA 215:1638–1641

Yamada A (1979) Radiologic assessment of resectability and prognosis in esophageal carcinoma. Gastrointest Radiol 4:213–218

Zornoza J, Lindell MM (1980) Radiologic evaluation of small esophageal carcinoma. Gastrointest Radiol 5:197–111

# Chapter 6

# Pathology

J.R. Salisbury and W.F. Whimster

## Introduction

The microscopical confirmation of the diagnosis of carcinoma of the oesophagus, together with its history and pathogenesis, are discussed in this chapter. Rational management also requires assessment of the extent of the disease (staging) and prediction of its behaviour (cell typing and grading), which also come within the purview of the pathologist.

## Pathological Diagnosis

The pathological diagnosis of oesophageal carcinoma requires the identification of malignant epithelial cells of oesophageal origin in cytological or histological material (see Chap. 4).

In cytological specimens the pathologist's task is to distinguish malignant from non-malignant cells. Cytological screening of asymptomatic people, using the Chinese balloon technique, has been particularly applied in high risk areas, with endoscopy and biopsy to confirm positives. Western pathologists generally have little experience of interpreting cytological specimens from the oesophagus because it is usual to proceed directly to endoscopy and biopsy in patients with symptoms. It is, however, the practice of some endoscopists to pass a brush through an obstructed lumen to obtain cells for cytology when the lumen is too

**Table 6.1.**   Histological types of oesophageal carcinoma

1. *Squamous cell carcinoma*
   *In situ*
   Invasive
   Spindle cell variant (Stout et al. 1949)
   Verrucous variant (Oota & Sabin 1977)
   Paget's disease (Yates and Ross 1968)

2. *Adenocarcinoma*
   *In situ*
   Invasive

3. *Tumours showing mixed differentiation*
   Adenosquamous carcinoma
   Mucoepidermoid carcinoma (Woodard et al. 1978)
   Other mixtures (Dodge 1961; McKechnie and Fechner 1971; Cook et al. 1976)

4. *Adenoid cystic carcinoma* (Marcial Rojas and Vallecillo 1959)

5. *Oat cell carcinoma* (McKeown 1952; Cook et al. 1976)

6. *Carcinoid tumour* (Brenner et al. 1969)

7. *Melanocytic tumours*
   Malignant melanoma (DiCostanzo and Urmacher 1987)

8. *Metastatic carcinoma*
   Lung and stomach are the commonest primary sites (Rosai 1981)

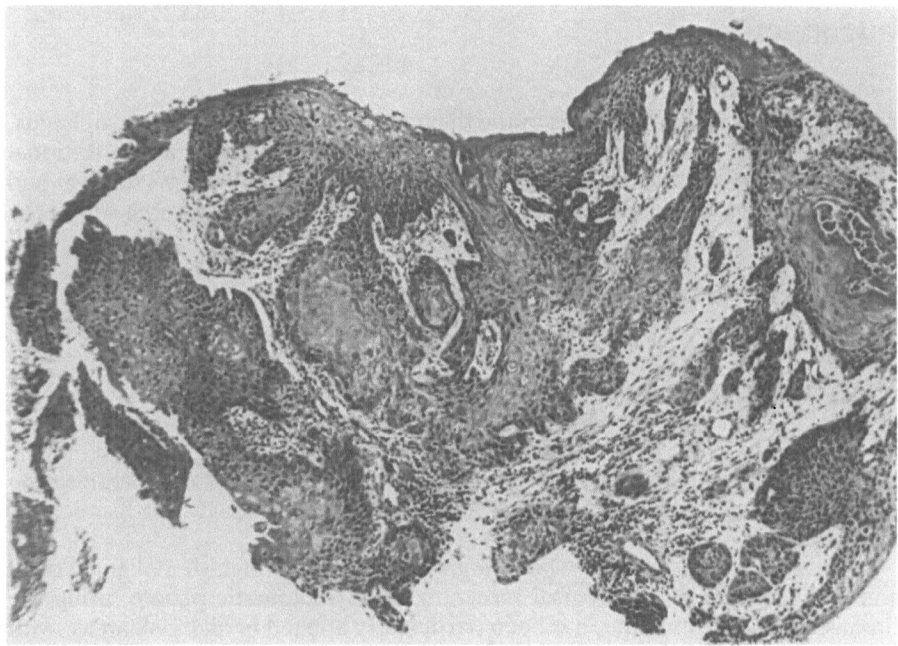

**Fig. 6.1.**   An endoscopic biopsy of a well-differentiated squamous cell carcinoma of the oesophagus. There are dysplastic changes in the overlying epithelium and tongues of abnormal epithelium are dipping downwards into the connective tissue. Distinguishing between *in situ* and invasive carcinoma can be almost impossible in this type of material. ×35.

**Table 6.2.**  Staging of carcinoma of the oesophagus (Hermanek et al. 1987 and American Joint Committee on Cancer 1987)

*TNM Clinical Classification (pretreatment)*

| | |
|---|---|
| *T –* | *Primary tumour* |
| TX | Primary tumour cannot be assessed |
| T0 | No evidence of primary tumour |
| Tis | Pre-invasive carcinoma (carcinoma *in situ*) |
| T1 | Tumour invades lamina propria or submucosa |
| T2 | Tumour invades muscularis propria |
| T3 | Tumour invades adventitia |
| T4 | Tumour invades adjacent structures |

| | |
|---|---|
| *N –* | *Regional lymph nodes* |
| NX | Regional lymph nodes cannot be assessed |
| N0 | No regional lymph node metastasis |
| N1 | Regional lymph node metastasis |

| | |
|---|---|
| *M –* | *Distant metastasis* |
| MX | Presence of distant metastasis cannot be assessed |
| M0 | No distant metastasis |
| M1 | Distant metastasis |

| | |
|---|---|
| *G – Histopathological grading* | |
| GX | Grade of differentiation cannot be assessed |
| G1 | Well differentiated |
| G2 | Moderately differentiated |
| G3 | Poorly differentiated |
| G4 | Undifferentiated |

*pTNM Pathological Classification (postsurgical histopathological)*
The pT, pN, pM categories correspond to the T, N, M categories.

| | |
|---|---|
| *R – Residual tumour after treatment* | |
| RX | Presence of residual tumour cannot be assessed |
| R0 | No residual tumour |
| R1 | Microscopic residual tumour |
| R2 | Macroscopic residual tumour |

*Stage grouping*

| | | | |
|---|---|---|---|
| Stage 0 | Tis | N0 | M0 |
| Stage I | T1 | N0 | M0 |
| Stage IIA | T2 | N0 | M0 |
| | T3 | N0 | M0 |
| Stage IIB | T1 | N1 | M0 |
| | T2 | N1 | M0 |
| Stage III | T3 | N1 | M0 |
| | T4 | Any N | M0 |
| Stage IV | Any T | Any N | M1 |

narrow for adequate biopsy (e.g., Kasugi et al. 1978). In biopsies, the task is to recognise dysplastic or malignant cells. If present, an attempt should be made to type the carcinoma (Table 6.1) and grade it according to whether it is *in situ* or invasive, and, if the latter, its degree of differentiation (Table 6.2). This requires good judgement and experience in assessing the minute tissue samples obtained through the modern fibreoptic oesophagoscope (Fig. 6.1). On the false-positive side, crushing of the fragments by the biopsy forceps can easily make non-malignant epithelial cells more haematoxyphil and malignant looking. On the false-negative side, it is possible to miss malignant cells by examining too few sections through the tissue block. Furthermore, the absence of malignant cells does not necessarily mean that the patient does not have a carcinoma. A false-negative result can arise because of swelling and inflammation of the mucosa proximal to the carcinoma or because the malignant cells have proliferated intramurally rather than intraluminally. Further biopsy, upsetting for the patient, calls for good liaison between the diagnostic parties.

## Normal Histology

To identify malignancy in the oesophagus one must have a clear idea about its normal structure. The luminal squamous mucosa is normally longitudinally ridged and has a matt grey opaque appearance. The transition from the squamous mucosa of the oesophagus to the glandular mucosa of the stomach is usually clearcut, especially after fixation (Fig. 6.2).

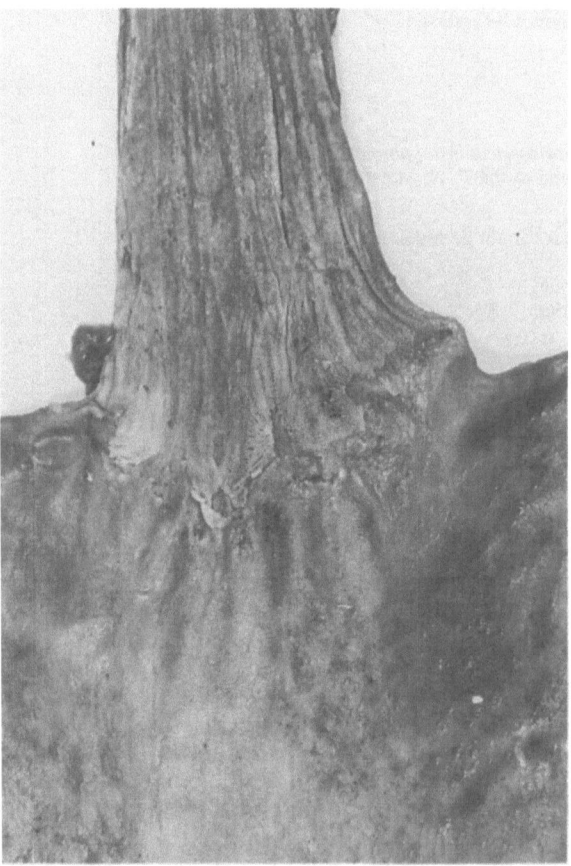

**Fig. 6.2.** The squamocolumnar junction of the lower oesophagus after fixation shows an abrupt transition. The longitudinal ridges of the oesophageal mucosa are evident.

Histologically, the structure of the oesophagus conforms to the pattern for the rest of the gut. The oesophageal lumen is lined by a mucous membrane which is continuous with the hypopharynx (muscle behaviour makes the transition visible to the endoscopist but it is not obvious to the pathologist in the resected specimen or at autopsy). The mucous membrane consists of a layer of stratified squamous epithelium overlying lamina propria and muscularis mucosae, submucosa, mucularis propria (three layers: circular, longitudinal, circular), and adventitia (Fig. 6.3). Keratinisation of the stratified squamous epithelium is abnormal in man although found in mammals with coarser diets. Focal thickening of the epithelium with an increase in the glycogen content is common (Rywlin and Orteya 1970). Scanty melanocytes (De la Pava et al. 1963), a small neuroendocrine cell population (Tateishi et al. 1974) and some Langerhans' cells are present

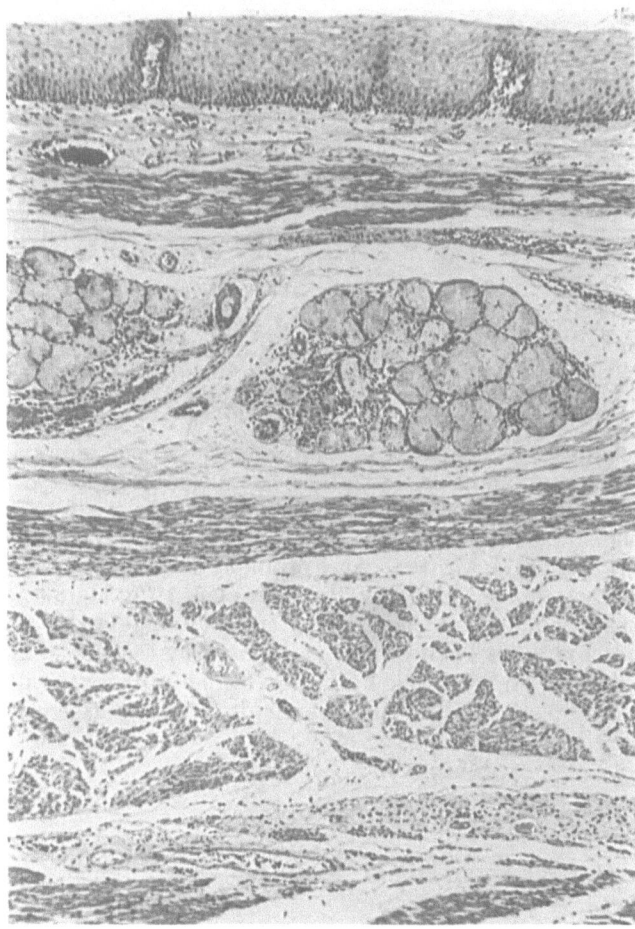

**Fig. 6.3.** Normal appearance of a longitudinal section through the oesophageal wall. Stratified squamous epithelium (SE) overlies lamina propria (LP), muscularis mucosae (MM), submucosa (SM) and muscularis propria (MP). Oesophageal glands (OG) are present in the submucosa with some of their secretory ducts (SD) in transverse section.

in the basal layers of the stratified squamous epithelium. At the squamo-columnar junction of the lower oesophagus, the stratified squamous epithelium usually shows an abrupt transition to the simple mucin-secreting epithelium of the gastric cardia.

Small mucous-secreting compound racemose glands, which discharge their secretions via ducts, are present in the submucosa of the oesophagus (Johns 1952). These secretions are thought to lubricate the oesophageal mucosa and aid the passage of food. Melanocytes are absent from these oesophageal glands and ducts (Tateishi et al. 1974). Sectioning the whole oesophagus at 5 mm intervals in a Japanese series of 250 adults revealed between six and 620 gland ducts, with an average of 227 (Takubo et al. 1981).

Islands of heterotopic gastric mucosa can occur throughout the oesophagus (Schmidt 1805). In an autopsy study of 1000 infants and children, Rector and Connerley (1941) found gastric mucosa in 7.8% of oesophagi. Of the heterotopic mucosal islands 51% were in the upper third of oesophagus, 41% in the middle third and 8% in the lower third. In a Japanese series of 264 adults heterotopic islands of gastric mucosa were found in 20% (Takubo et al. 1981). Macroscopi-cally, heterotopic gastric mucosa appears sharply delineated and the border with the normal stratified squamous epithelium is abrupt. Microscopically, the gastric mucosa is composed of typical mucin-secreting gastric glands. There is often an extensive inflammatory reaction with both acute and chronic inflammatory cells. Parietal cells were present in one-third of Rector and Connerley's cases (1941) but others have found them to be rare (Rosai 1981). Chief cells are uncommon, but ulceration does occur.

## Barrett's Oesophagus (Columnar-lined Lower Oesophagus)

In some people a significant part of the lower oesophagus is lined by columnar secretory epithelium – a condition known as Barrett's oesophagus (Barrett 1957; Mossberg 1966). Histologically, three different epithelial patterns are found: atrophic gastric fundal, intestinal and junctional. A neuroendocrine cell popula-tion is also present (Rindi et al. 1987). Most cases are probably due to gastric cells colonising areas ulcerated by reflux oesophagitis (Bremner et al. 1970; Hamilton and Yardley 1977) although metaplastic change is presumably responsible for those where a total gastrectomy has been performed previously (Meyer et al. 1979). *Campylobacter pyloridis*, an anaerobic bacterium found in patients with chronic active gastritis, can be observed over the gastric mucous cells in Barrett's oesophagus (Yardley 1987).

## Squamous Cell Dysplasia and Carcinoma *in situ*

In biopsy specimens, as in the resected specimen (see below) dysplasia is the term used to describe cells that have undergone irregular, atypical proliferative changes in response to chronic irritation or inflammation (Robbins et al. 1984). Dysplasia is strongly implicated in the causation of cancer but does not

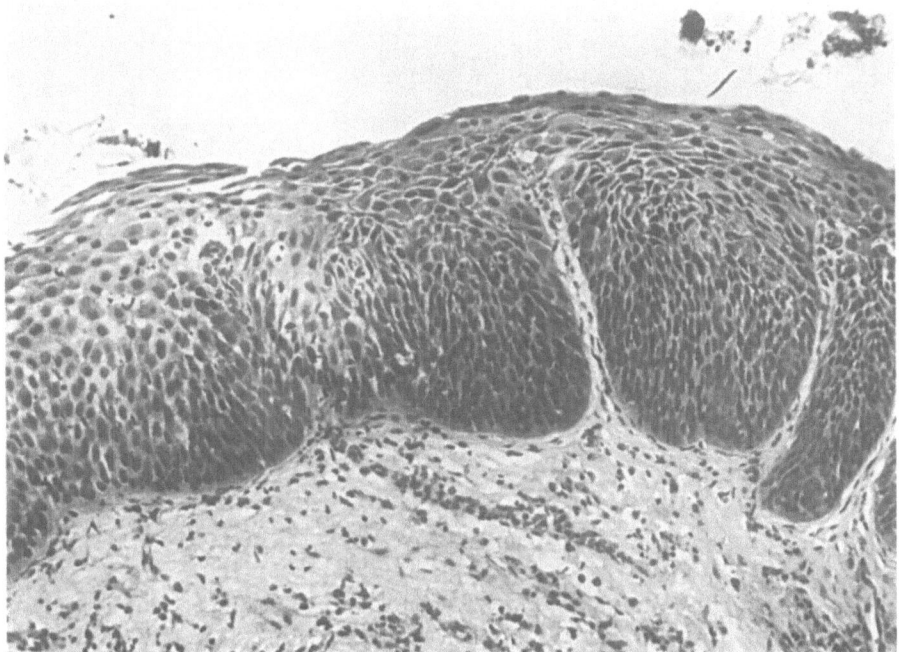

**Fig. 6.4.** An endoscopic biopsy showing focal severe dysplasia of the squamous epithelium, in which there is loss of polarity with abnormally large cells with hyperchromatic nuclei throughout the epithelium. ×90.

necessarily progress to cancer in all cases. The changes in lesser grades of dysplasia may be reversible. By light microscopy, dysplastic oesophageal epithelium shows both architectural and cytological abnormalities, well illustrated by Morson and Jass (1985). Enlarged immature cells are present at higher than usual levels in the epithelium and these cells may show loss of polarity. The nuclei may vary in size, shape and staining (Fig. 6.4). Mitoses are no longer restricted to the basal layers. The degree of dysplasia can be graded as mild, moderate or severe, with severe dysplasia merging into carcinoma *in situ*, but these gradings are obviously subjective as the disease is a spectrum of abnormality and they are not reliably reproducible. It is often possible to find all grades of dysplasia in different areas of one specimen. Distinction between severe dysplasia/carcinoma *in situ* and early invasive carcinoma may be difficult, if not impossible, especially on small biopsies. Takubo et al. (1981), using 5 mm histological sections, have mapped dysplasia and carcinoma *in situ* throughout the oesophagus and shown great variability.

Dysplasia may, in present usage, represent either preneoplastic changes or regenerative changes associated with inflammation and injury. Arguments against describing regenerative change in the gut as dysplastic and for reserving dysplasia for changes thought to represent intraepithelial neoplasia have been made but the histological distinction may not be straightforward and long-standing regenerative efforts might themselves lead in time to neoplastic

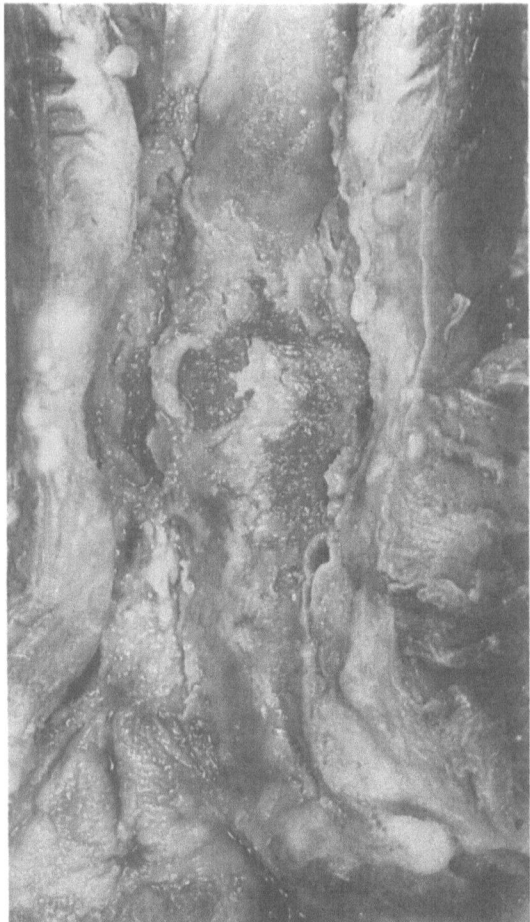

**Fig. 6.5.** Fixed surgical resection specimen with the distal oesophagus opened longitudinally to show a 4-cm diameter ulcerated squamous cell carcinoma. Nodules of carcinoma are seen infiltrating through the muscular wall and on the external surface. Lymph node metastases were present.

transformation (Robbins et al. 1984). Clearly the finding of dysplasia in an oesophageal biopsy is an indication for follow-up and further biopsies. Close co-operation with regular meetings between clinicians and histopathologists allows discussion of these problem cases.

## Squamous Cell Carcinoma

This is the common epithelial malignant tumour of the oesophagus and numerous studies worldwide confirm that it accounts for over 90% of primary oesophageal malignancies (Fig. 6.5). It is composed of cells resembling those of squamous epithelium and is usually graded as well, moderately or poorly differentiated (Table 6.2). The World Health Organization defines well differentiated tumours as those with abundant keratin, easily demonstrable intercellular bridges and minimal nuclear and cellular pleomorphism. Poorly differentiated tumours are those with no or virtually no keratin and intercellular bridges or with marked cellular and nuclear pleomorphism. Moderately differentiated carcinomas are those intermediate between well and poorly differentiated (Oota and Sobin 1977). Grading has not, however, been found to be of prognostic value in carcinoma of the oesophagus (Broders and Vinson 1928; Takahashi 1961; Ming 1971). Figure 6.1 shows an example of a well-differentiated carcinoma and also illustrates the difficulty in deciding whether the abnormal epithelium dipping into the deeper layers is truly invasive or whether the carcinoma is still *in situ*.

Tumour cells at the periphery of invasive islands may show a palisaded arrangement reminiscent of the peripheral palisading seen in basal cell carcinoma of the skin.

Variants of squamous cell carcinoma include the spindle cell and verrucous forms (Stout et al. 1949; Oota and Sobin 1977). The spindle cell carcinomas are often polypoid and contain squamous cell and sarcomatous elements intermingled together, with both possessing metastatic capability. Battifora (1976) demonstrated desmosomes, tonofilaments and collagen production by the spindle cells and suggested that the sarcomatous elements arose from metaplastic squamous cells. It has been possible to show a transition from squamous carcinoma *in situ* through invasive squamous carcinoma to the spindle cell elements in some cases (Matsusaka et al. 1976). Adenocarcinomatous elements may also be present (Du Boulay and Isaacson 1981).

The verrucous variant is exophytic, warty and cauliflower-like, and thus easily biopsied. It invades locally in a relentless fashion yet rarely metastasises (Agha et al. 1984). Microscopically, it is well-differentiated with hyperkeratotic and markedly acanthotic epithelium invading with a pushing margin rather than as individual or small groups of cells.

Strangely, Paget's disease of the oesophageal epithelium has been described in association with primary squamous cell carcinoma (Yates and Koss 1968) but not with adenocarcinoma of the oesophagus.

The tissues deep to the submucosa are seldom included in the diagnostic biopsy (see Fig. 6.1), so it is usually not possible to tell whether the muscularis propria is invaded but it is sometimes possible to see malignant cells in the submucosal lymphatics.

## Adenocarcinoma

Primary adenocarcinomas of the oesophagus are very rare tumours if all adenocarcinomas involving both sides of the oesophagogastric junction are considered as primary gastric carcinomas with oesophageal spread (Figs. 6.6 and 6.7). The only unquestionable cases are then those with normal epithelium in the proximal as well as in the distal margin.

The epithelium of the columnar-lined (Barrett's) oesophagus may show dysplastic changes. These have been well described by Morson and Jass (1985) and by Day (1986). Mitoses are often seen within the surface epithelium or in the

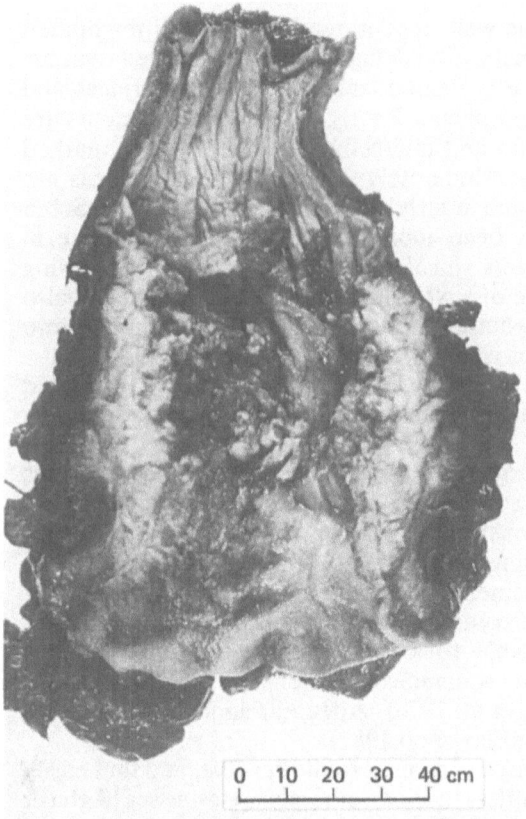

0    10   20   30   40 cm

**Fig. 6.6.** Fixed surgical resection specimen of lower oesophagus and upper part of stomach. A 6-cm diameter ulcerated adenocarcinoma has destroyed the gastro-oesophageal junction. White tumour tissue can be seen thickening the wall.

upper parts of glands and there may be mucin depletion. The dysplasia can be superficial giving rise to papillary or villous configurations or can affect entire glands. In severe dysplasia the glands may appear "back to back" without intervening stroma and the distinction between severe dysplasia and intramucosal carcinoma can be difficult.

## Other Carcinomas

Carcinomas showing mixed squamous and glandular differentiation are known as adenosquamous carcinomas when poorly differentiated and as mucoepidermoid carcinomas (as in the salivary glands) when well differentiated (Woodard et al. 1978; Matsufuji et al. 1985). Adenoid cystic carcinomas also showing histological features identical with those seen in the salivary glands are seen very rarely (Marcial Rojas and Vallecillo 1959; Azzopardi and Menzies 1962). Primary oat cell carcinomas (McKeown 1952) and primary carcinoid tumours of the oesopha-

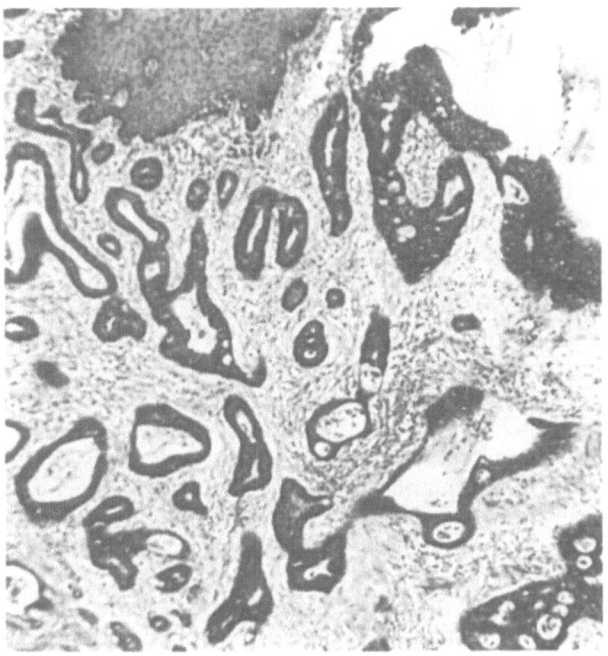

**Fig. 6.7.** Section of the squamocolumnar junction and underlying connective tissue infiltrated by a moderately differentiated adenocarcinoma. ×40.

gus occur (Brenner et al. 1969) and histologically resemble their counterparts elsewhere in the body. A case of a mixed carcinoid and mucin-producing adenocarcinoma has been reported (Chong et al. 1979). Case reports of primary oesophageal choriocarcinomas exist; some of the tumours were admixed with adenocarcinoma (McKechnie and Fechner 1971).

## Carcinomas Metastatic to the Oesophagus

The pathologist does not usually have to consider the possibility of an endo-oesophageal metastasis from a carcinoma elsewhere when trying to interpret an oesophageal biopsy but such metastases do occur. Invasion by tumours of nearby structures (carcinoma of stomach, carcinoma of lung, primary and secondary tumours of mediastinal lymph nodes) is quite common as is leukaemic infiltration. Within the gastrointestinal tract, the oesophagus is the most common site for metastases from primary carcinoma of the lung and is frequently involved by direct extension (Antler et al. 1982). Dysphagia may be caused by metastatic carcinoma of the breast which shows a tendency to infiltrate the submucosal lymphatics in the middle third of the oesophagus and the adjacent mediastinal lymph nodes (Polk et al. 1967). Cases of malignant melanoma (Butler et al. 1975; Wood and Wood 1975) and hepatocellular carcinoma (Sohn et al. 1965) metastasising to the oesophagus have been reported.

# Natural History

## The Early Phase

The current hypothesis is that the carcinoma starts with a normal epithelial cell becoming transformed into a malignant cell which then divides to form a clone of malignant cells. The malignant cells proliferate initially within the epithelium (carcinoma *in situ*, Tis, see Table 6.2) but have the capacity to invade through the epithelial basement membrane into the mucosa and through the muscularis mucosae into submucosal tissues and ultimately beyond.

In this hypothesis it is not entirely clear how epithelial dysplasia (see p. 108) fits in. In practice, most pathologists regard themselves as capable of recognising mild, moderate and severe dysplasia. The latter is now usually regarded as a form of intraepithelial carcinoma (carcinoma *in situ*), although there is the possibility of reversibility, with Yang (1980), for example, quoting Chinese experience to the effect that of 79 patients with severe dysplasia 40% regressed to mild dysplasia or normality over a four-year period while 27% became cancerous, and 33% remained unchanged.

Mild and moderate dysplastic changes in epithelia are usually regarded as of little significance, often secondary to inflammation and/or healing of ulcerated epithelium, and unrelated to the development of neoplasia. But recent work on the uterine cervix has caused this opinion to be revised for that site (Fox 1987). Similarly Yang (1980) quoted Chinese experience to the effect that of 105 patients with mild dysplasia 15% progressed to severe dysplasia over a four-year period while 40% remained unchanged and 45% returned to normal.

Nevertheless, oesophageal squamous cell carcinoma can arise from areas of preceding squamous dysplasia, and various stages of dysplasia and carcinoma *in situ* can be found adjacent to the primary invasive carcinoma in resected surgical specimens (O'Gara and Horn 1955). Follow-up of Northern Chinese in whom screening cytology had revealed dysplastic oesophageal squamous cells showed some to progress to carcinoma (Ackerman et al. 1978). The latent period from the cytological detection of dysplasia to the development of clinical cancer was between 3 and 12 years. How long it may take carcinoma *in situ* to become invasive is unknown but there are estimates of between 3 and 7 years (Ackerman et al. 1978; Rajindranath et al. 1984).

Carcinoma *in situ* can also be found apart from the primary tumour; evidence for the concept of multiple foci of origin (Ushigome et al. 1967). The finding by Takubo et al. (1987) of 175 primary carcinomas in oesophagi resected from 165 patients must also mean that more than one malignant clone can develop at around the same time, although this aspect has not received much attention.

Areas of carcinoma *in situ* are not easily recognisable macroscopically, but may be picked up by exfoliative cytology (Ackerman et al. 1978). Microscopically, areas of carcinoma *in situ* are often separated from each other by normal epithelium. The change may be abrupt or gradual through increasing grades of dysplasia. The host–tumour junctions in intraepithelial oesophageal carcinomas have been studied ultrastructurally (Takubo et al. 1984) and shown to consist of mesenchymal cells, degenerated epithelial cells and amorphous material. Occasionally, however, tumour cells are attached directly to normal cells by well-developed desmosomes suggesting a stable state at some parts of the junction. It is not clear whether carcinoma *in situ* can regress in the same way as dysplasia.

Early oesophageal carcinoma, which is limited by definition (Japanese Society for Oesophageal Diseases 1976) to the mucosa or submucosa without lymph node metastases, was seldom seen before screening programmes for oesophageal carcinoma were initiated in areas of high incidence, particularly in the Henan Province in China, where in one series cytological screening of 28 139 people revealed 115 cases of early carcinoma (Guanrei et al. 1982). Endoscopically, 52 had an erosive appearance with a slightly depressed greyish mucosa, 39 were plaque-like with a slightly raised granular mucosa, 21 were congestive, and 3 were polypoid. In 91 cases of early carcinoma followed up without treatment for 19–42 months Guanrei et al. (1982) found that only 6 became advanced. This finding gives some idea of the rate of progression of early carcinoma. Barge et al. (1981) found that their 10 French cases could also be classified as erosive, plaque-like, papillary, and occult.

From Japan, Endo et al. (1986) have recently illustrated five types of endoscopic appearance: polypoid; plateau-like; flat, red, coarse, greyish-white; erosive; and ulcerated. Both groups also noted that if the oesophageal surface is sprayed with aniline blue or 2% toluidine blue, the carcinomatous area stains blue but the normal mucosa does not, and if sprayed with 3% Lugol's iodine, the normal mucosa stains black-grey (due to the glycogen content of the normal epithelial cells) while the carcinomatous area is brown. Such staining can also be applied to the resected or postmortem oesophagus.

The Chinese and Japanese series of early oesophageal carcinomas have nearly all been squamous but 5 of the 7 cases described by Levine et al. (1986) were adenocarcinomas, all arising in Barrett's mucosa. They concluded that this must reflect a higher prevalence of Barrett's oesophagus in the West. In the series of Barge et al. (1981), to which more than 40 more have now been added (Bogomoletz 1987, personal communication), the carcinomas are all squamous, with none in Barrett's mucosa.

### The Late Advanced, Invasive Phase

Extension beyond the submucosa, either more deeply or to lymph nodes, even if still superficial or small (less than 3.5 cm diameter), takes the carcinoma into the advanced phase, which has a dramatically reduced 5-year survival rate (Levine et al. 1986). Takagi and Karasawa (1982) reported a mean increase in tumour length of 0.51 cm/month in seven patients followed up with serial barium swallow examinations. The tumour doubling time was five months which compares with three months for squamous carcinoma of the lung (Geddes 1979).

Takubo et al. (1987) have recently drawn attention to the extension of intraepithelial carcinoma along the ducts of the submucosal glands and suggest that this route of invasion into the deeper tissues may be important. Further direct invasion is possible in three directions: through the muscularis propria into the adventitia, and thence into adjacent structures, particularly the tracheo-bronchial tree and the aorta; circumferentially, around the oesophagus; and longitudinally, up and/or down the oesophagus. These possibilities of invasion give rise to the three types of advanced lesion usually described (illustrated by

Mannell 1982), in order of frequency: ulcerative and stenotic; infiltrative, with thickening and narrowing; and fungating or exophytic, including verrucous and papillary variants. The ulcers in the first group frequently exceed 5 cm in diameter (43% of 105 in Sons' and Borchard's (1984) series). Features of all these types may be seen together. The adenocarcinomas of the cardia tend to be larger, more florid, and less infiltrative than the squamous carcinomas of the oesophagus.

It is customary to identify the site of origin of the carcinomas within the middle third of the oesophagus (commonest), the lower third (25%–40%, including most adenocarcinomas), and the upper third (less than 20%). This distribution applies in the West (see Mannell 1982) and in the East (Yang 1980). Thirds are easily measured by the pathologist at postmortem, but Miller (1962) pointed out that to him, as a surgeon, the upper "third", above the aortic arch, is about a quarter, and the lower "third", below the inferior pulmonary vein, is also about a quarter. The UICC (1987) and the American Joint Committee on Cancer (1987), which are now harmonised (Table 6.2), use four unequal distances, as measured on the oesophagoscope, i.e., the cervical oesophagus, beginning at the pharyngeal–oesophageal junction, ends approximately 18 cm from the upper incisor teeth, the upper thoracic portion ends 26 cm, the lower thoracic portion 32 cm, and the lower oesophagus at the cardiac orifice approximately 40 cm from the upper incisor teeth. The Japanese Society for Oesophageal Diseases (1976), on the other hand, using radiological anatomy, had five divisions: cervical (to upper sternum), upper thoracic (to tracheal bifurcation), middle thoracic (half way to oesophago-gastric junction), lower thoracic (to diaphragm), and abdominal (to oesophago-gastric junction). These differences make comparisons between series and assessment of the possible aetiological contributions of risk factors more difficult. At one time it was thought that, like strictures due to swallowing caustic substances, carcinomas arose preferentially at sites of physiological narrowing of the oesophagus i.e., the cricoid cartilage, the tracheal bifurcation, and the diaphragmatic foramen, or of anatomical (radiological) indentation by the arch of the aorta, the left bronchus and the left atrium, but there seems to be no supporting evidence.

## The Resected Specimen

Whether the carcinomatous oesophagus is resectable depends on surgical judgement which includes the clinical state of the patient and the extent of the tumour as determined by imaging, to which the Clinical Classification (pretreatment clinical classification, TNM or cTNM) (UICC 1987) may be thought to contribute. On receipt of a resected oesophagus, however, the pathologist's main task is to try to determine by macroscopic observation and microscopic sampling whether the carcinoma extends to the external surface of the specimen or to the upper or lower resection margins, and whether any lymph nodes included are invaded. Miller (1962) reported microscopic spread, after fixation, proximal to the visible tumour to be less than 1 cm in 46 of 72 cases, but just under 3.5 cm in 2 cases. Fixation experiments showed that 1 cm of oesophagus after fixation was equivalent to 3 cm *in situ*. In no case of adenocarcinoma at the cardia, however, were malignant cells seen more than 1.5 cm above the visible tumour after fixation. On this basis, the Pathological Classification (postsurgical histopathological classification (pTNM) (UICC 1987) can be carried out, according to Table 6.2. Neither of these include assessment of the resection margins, although the Japanese Society for Oesophageal Diseases (1976) guidelines for pathological studies do.

The use of the rapid frozen section technique to show that the resection margins are clear of tumour at the time of operation has been advocated (Kay 1963; Cliffton 1970) but it is generally impractical to sample the resection margins adequately, although small areas of particular concern to the surgeon may be usefully examined in this way.

It has been suggested (Takahashi 1961; Younghusband and Aluwihare 1970) that the patient may mount an immune response to the carcinoma and that this may be a favourable prognostic feature, but the data given are difficult to assess.

## Allegedly Predisposing Pathological Conditions

### Oesophageal Webs and the Paterson–Brown-Kelly (Plummer–Vinson) Syndrome

Oesophageal shadows resembling rings and webs, not only in the postcricoid region, are sometimes demonstrated radiologically in patients complaining of dysphagia. These are either folds of mucosa or localised annular thickening of the muscle (Clements et al. 1974), as are the lower oesophageal rings (Goyal et al. 1971; Tedesco and Morton 1975).

Vinson (1921) reported 69 cases of dysphagia without radiological or oesophagoscopic abnormalities of whom 37 were anaemic and 12 had splenomegaly, and also stated that Plummer had first noted this association (no date or reference given). In May 1919, however, at the Laryngological Section of the Royal Society of Medicine, Paterson (1919) had read a paper on dysphagia and glossitis and mentioned that "malignant disease at the mouth of the gullet" happened too often in these cases to be a coincidence; Brown-Kelly (1919) had also read a paper on patients with dysphagia, preceded by a long period of anaemia, dyspepsia or impaired general health, in whom oesophageal webs might be found oesophagoscopically. Waldenstrom (1938) and Waldenstrom and Kjellberg (1939) later confirmed the association with iron-deficiency anaemia and a beneficial response to iron therapy in patients who were not anaemic, and demonstrated webs radiologically in the postcricoid region in both female and male patients.

Postcricoid webs in the Paterson–Brown-Kelly syndrome have been variously reported as showing hyperkeratosis and chronic inflammation (Chisholm et al. 1971) together with atrophy (McNab Jones 1961), normal epithelium with mild submucosal inflammation (Shamma'a and Benedict 1958; Entwistle and Jacobs 1965; Chisholm et al. 1971) or no histological abnormality (Entwistle and Jacobs 1965; Chisholm et al. 1971). Entwistle and Jacobs (1965) also reported chronic inflammation and carcinoma *in situ* in biopsies of associated upper oesophageal strictures, but their illustration of carcinoma *in situ* would be regarded as dysplasia today. It thus seems unlikely that the webs or rings themselves are premalignant.

McNab Jones (1961) noted that in many cases of postcricoid carcinoma a history of the Paterson–Brown-Kelly syndrome could be elicited (up to 66% of his, 90% of Ahlbom's (1936)), and the sex ratio of the carcinoma was similar to that of the syndrome, i.e., the reverse of that of carcinoma of the upper alimentary tract, and her series and review of the literature showed that between 10% and 50% of patients with the syndrome developed carcinoma. Of Chisholm et al.'s (1971) 72 patients, 4 developed carcinomas.

## Achalasia of the Cardia

Just-Viera and Haight (1969), reviewing the literature since 1872, found 167 examples of squamous carcinoma at all levels, but mainly in the middle and lower thirds, in oesophagi affected by achalasia of the cardia. The incidence varied from 0% to 20% of cases of achalasia of the cardia, usually of longstanding. Since then Wychulis et al. (1971) have reported 7 out of 1318 cases and Hankins and McLaughlin (1975) 3 out of 156 cases.

## Chronic Oesophagitis

In 430 people screened in Northern Iran oesophagoscopy revealed chronic oesophagitis in 344, with dysplasia in 16 and invasive carcinoma in 11 (Crespi et al. 1979); and in 527 people screened in Henan Province in China the same group found chronic oesophagitis in 84%, with dysplasia in 10% and carcinoma of the oesophagus in 4 patients and of the cardia in 5 (Muñoz et al. 1982). The oesophagitis affected the middle and lower thirds of the oesophagus in both series but differed from that seen in the West by a lack of association with reflux or ulceration. Smithers (1955) reported four primary squamous and five primary adenocarcinomas of the oesophagus associated with sliding hiatus hernias.

## Barrett's Oesophagus

Dysplasia may be seen in the columnar epithelium (Day 1986). Morson and Belcher (1952) reported the first case of adenocarcinoma arising within Barrett's oesophagus. Normal columnar epithelium separated the carcinoma from the anatomic cardia. Agha (1985) recently reported 34 cases and reviewed the literature, concluding that a Barrett oesophagus had a 10% chance of developing "Barrett's carcinoma" and that 20% of true oesophageal adenocarcinomas occur in Barrett's oesophagi.

## Lye Strictures

Bigelow (1953) reported a case of squamous carcinoma occurring in the oesophagus of a 43-year-old female who developed a stricture 20 cm from the incisor teeth after swallowing lye at the age of one year, and reviewed 9 previously reported cases. The carcinoma had developed in the narrowed segment and not in the proximal dilated oesophagus as happens in achalasia. Lansing et al. (1969) reported another example in a 54-year-old female who had swallowed lye 22 years previously and whose stricture was at the level of the bifurcation of the trachea. The carcinoma was confined to the area of the stricture and was successfully resected.


## Oesophageal Diverticula

Garlock and Richter (1961) reported a case of squamous carcinoma arising in a pharyngo-oesophageal diverticulum of about 15 years' standing, and reviewed 12 previously reported cases.


## Tylosis

In keratosis palmaris et plantaris (tylosis), one of many forms of dyskeratosis, there is marked hyperkeratosis of the palms and soles. Howel-Evans et al. (1958) reported carcinoma of the oesophagus in association with tylosis in 17 members of two Liverpool families but in none of those who did not have tylosis. The families were reviewed and two new cases added by Harper et al. (1970). Shine and Allison (1966) reported a further example.

It should be noted that only a few patients with these conditions develop oesophageal carcinomas. Nevertheless, the pathologist should be on the look out for carcinomas in patients known to have these conditions, and should search for evidence of these conditions in patients with carcinomas of the oesophagus.


## The Autopsy

The aims of the autopsy on an individual case are to complete the natural history by identifying residual local and metastatic carcinoma, identifying effects of treatment (surgery, radiotherapy (see Oota and Sobin 1977, and Fig. 6.8), chemotherapy), determining the cause of death, in particular whether it was due to the disease or to some other cause, and by recording some measure of prognosis, of which the interval between onset of symptoms or diagnosis and death is the simplest, especially if different forms of treatment are being studied. In this way, they may be studied in relation to the overall natural history of the disease as reported in the literature. For example, of Miller's (1962) 60 radical resections, at 5 years 32 had died of recurrent carcinoma and 9 from unrelated disease. The extent of residual tumour may be recorded by the TNM system (see Table 6.2). This presumably includes tumour present at autopsy, which was mentioned in previous American Joint Committee on Cancer versions but not by UICC (1987).

The obstacles to getting a clear overall picture of the natural history of the disease from other people's experience are illustrated by the three most recently published autopsy series (Mandard et al. 1981; Anderson and Lad 1982; Sons and Borchard 1984; there seems to be no autopsy series reported from eastern high incidence areas such as northern Iran or the Henan Province in China or from Japan), which may be compared with the outcome as reported by surgeons. For

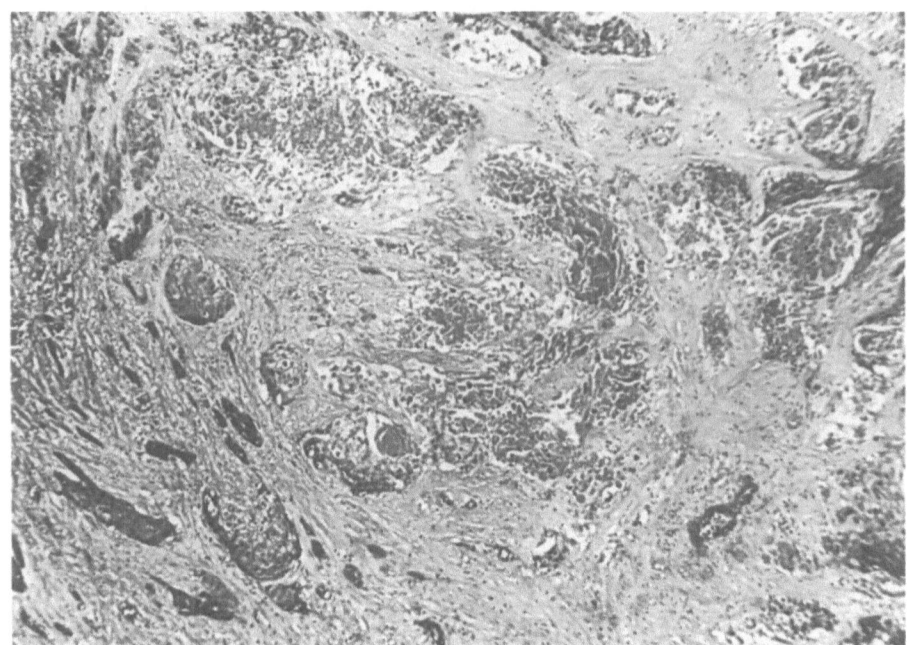

**Fig. 6.8.** A squamous cell carcinoma of the oesophagus which has been treated by radiotherapy. Many of the islands of tumour have undergone necrosis. ×40.

example, Mannell (1982), with a large surgical experience of the disease in South Africa, summarised the picture in untreated patients as death within a few months (Miller's (1962) inoperable cases survived for a mean of 5 months) from cachexia and aspiration pneumonia secondary to oesophageal obstruction, and quotes Roberts (1980) in maintaining that at autopsy in untreated cases, cancer was confined to the perioesophageal tissues in one third. She also quotes Mandard (1981, see below) who had lymph node metastases in 74% and visceral metastases in 50%, the lungs and liver being the most frequent sites. Roberts' (1980) argument was that, as lymph node metastases were invariably present in patients dying of disseminated disease, absence of disseminated disease could be inferred from the absence of lymph node metastases – at diagnosis as well as at autopsy.

Mandard et al. (1981) found no residual carcinoma in 25% of 111 autopsies performed between 1975 and 1977 in Caen, France, but 60% had spread to neighbouring structures (trachea and bronchi 48%, aorta 18%, pericardium 13%, pleura 10%), with fistula formation in 28%. In 77 cases, extension of the carcinoma within the oesophagus was greater than estimated clinically in 16% and less in 10%; histological comparisons revealed some discrepancy in 3%. *In situ* or invasive carcinoma distant (2–10 cm) from the original tumour was found in 13.5%. In 11 autopsies performed within days of surgical resection residual tumour was found in the oesophagus in 3. Lymph node and distant metastases were studied in 98 cases, and the well-tabulated data show metastases in lymph nodes in 74.5% (cervical 37%, mediastinal 64%, abdominal 47%), and in viscera in 50% (lungs 31%, liver 23%, pleura 17%, bone 13%). Alcoholic liver disease, atherosclerosis, chronic pancreatitis and other malignancies (oropharyngeal cancer in 16 cases and unrelated cancers in 14 cases) were frequent. No clear distinction was made between deaths attributable directly or indirectly to the disease and deaths due to unrelated causes. Only 17 had been treated surgically. Mean survival from the onset of symptoms was 10.6 months.

Anderson and Lad (1982) reviewed 79 autopsies performed in Chicago between 1965 and 1979. Five were free of disease, 7 had disease localised to the oesophagus and mediastinal structures, 2 had distant metastatic disease alone, and 65 had persistent or recurrent local disease and distant metastases in up to 10 sites (lymph nodes 73%, lung 52%, liver 47%). There were 20 fistulae (17 tracheobronchial, one aortic, pleural and mediastinal). Only 5 had had surgery. Survival (presumably from diagnosis) ranged up to 84 months with a mean of 6 months and median of 4 months. Other conditions found at autopsy are not mentioned. The authors argue, on the basis of tumour doubling times (Charbit et al. 1971), that many of the metastatic lesions found at autopsy would have been present at the time of diagnosis.

In Sons' and Borchard's (1984) German autopsy series of 169 carcinomas dating from 1950 to 1982 oesophagectomy had been performed in 56 cases. The time from onset of symptoms or diagnosis to death was not given. At autopsy, oesophageal submucosal metastases were seen in 12 patients. Carcinomas of the upper third of the oesophagus had the greatest tendency to extend into adjacent structures (13/16, 81%) as compared with the middle (67/87, 77%) and lower thirds (46/68, 68%). In the whole series, 29% had no metastases, 67% had lymph node metastases (a nice graphic presentation of the distribution), and 30% had visceral metastases. Pneumonia (40%), fatty change and cirrhosis of the liver (20%), deep femoral vein thrombosis (8%), pancreatitis (6%), and other neoplastic disease (6%) were also found, but whether the prosector attributed death to the disease or to other causes is not recorded.

Thus the surgeons appear to be more concerned about the timing and cause of death, whereas the autopsy pathologists concentrate on the details of the residual carcinoma. Surely both approaches are needed? It is interesting that in the total of 359 autopsy cases reported above the allegedly predisposing pathological conditions (see p. 117) are not mentioned even to note their absence, while Miller (1962) reports treating oesophageal carcinomas in 7 members of the two families with tylosis reported by Howel-Evans et al. (1958), and 4 adenocarcinomas in an oesophagus extensively lined by columnar epithelium. He also records hiatus hernias in 14 out of 57 radical resections for adenocarcinoma of the cardia but none in 83 radical resections for squamous carcinoma of the oesophagus.

## Staging

The factors that determine the natural history of oesophageal cancer are largely unknown but, as with other neoplasms, the anatomical extent of the carcinoma or tumour burden appears to be important. Schemes for staging have been developed independently, and therefore not uniformly, by the Japanese Society for Oesophageal Diseases (1976), the American Joint Committee on Cancer and the UICC (1987) (see Table 6.2) to categorise the anatomical extent of oesophageal carcinoma, at various times between diagnosis and death, to help assess prognosis in individuals, and for research and therapeutic trials in groups of comparable patients. Staging is appropriate, firstly, after histological diagnosis but before any treatment is undertaken. At this stage (cTNM) the pathologist's role is confined to diagnosing histologically any tissue obtained from the primary tumour or local or distant sites. The extent of the disease at this point in the natural history is more the domain of the imaging specialists than of the pathologist, being assessed on the results of plain X-ray films, tomography, CT scanning, NMR scanning, ultrasonography, etc.

After resection of the carcinomatous oesophagus the pathologist can do no more than attempt to assess whether the tumour is confined to the resected specimen and whether any lymph nodes submitted are involved. The pathologist is not involved in assessing responses to radiotherapy and/or chemotherapy in life, but he clearly has an important part to play in postmortem staging, as already described.

As discussed by Jass and Morson (1987) in relation to colorectal cancer, the TNM system is not itself a research tool, merely a method of encoding pathological and clinical data at successive points in the natural history of the disease. What is needed now is the statistical analysis of prospective prognostic factors by modern techniques, as has been done for example for inoperable lung cancer (Stanley 1980); in 4840 patients, of 50 prognostic factors the three most important were the initial performance status, the extent of disease (i.e., simplified TNM staging), and weight loss in the previous 6 months. Histological type came 20th. Thus the pathologist's only contribution at the time of diagnosis was to confirm it histologically. With carcinoma of the oesophagus, also, efforts must be directed to clarifying further the information required from each of the specialties at each stage in the natural history and ensuring that it is obtained, recorded and used meticulously to assess individual prognosis and treatment.

# Pathogenesis

## Histogenesis

It seems probable that the different types of oesophageal carcinoma recognised histologically arise from different stem cell populations. It is thought that the oesophageal squamous carcinomas arise from the basal cells of the surface epithelium and that oesophageal adenocarcinomas arise from undifferentiated isthmus or neck cells in the gastric glands of gastric heterotopias. These cells are the stem cell populations at these sites (Leblond et al. 1967; Hunt and Hunt 1962). The rare adenoid cystic and mucoepidermoid carcinomas probably arise from the oesophageal glands, but the adenosquamous carcinomas are thought to develop from the surface epithelium (Rosai 1981). The oesophageal oat cell carcinomas are presumed to arise from neuroendocrine cells in the basal epithelium (Tateishi et al. 1974).

Some tumours show evidence of multiple forms of differentiation. The adenosquamous and mucoepidermoid carcinomas have both squamous and

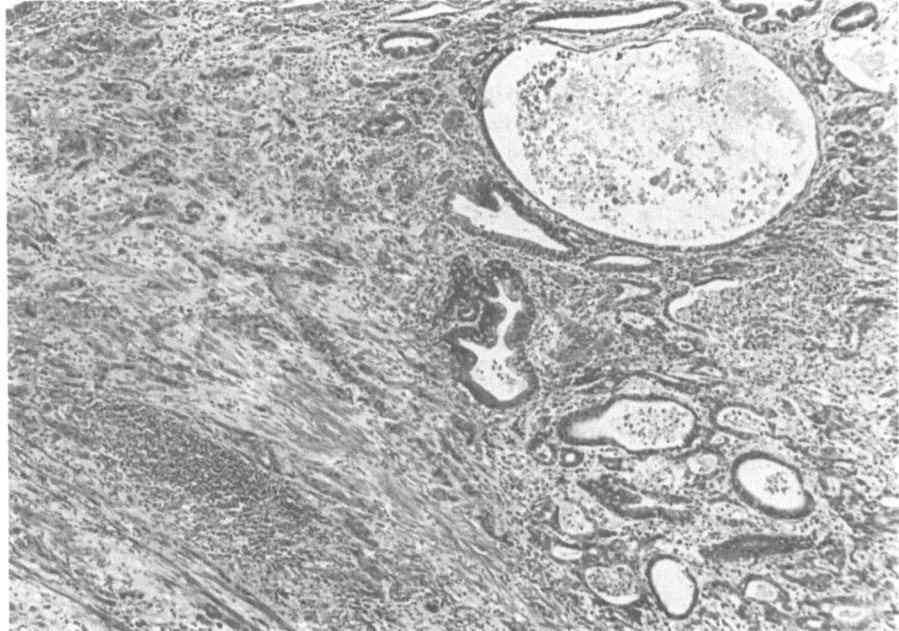

**Fig. 6.9.** "Collision" tumour formed by a primary oesophageal squamous cell carcinoma on the left of the photograph abutting onto a primary gastric adenocarcinoma on the right. ×40.

glandular components. Mixed oat cell and squamous cell carcinomas occur (Cook et al. 1976), as they do in the lung. The spindle cell carcinoma histologically resembles a mixed carcinoma and sarcoma but there is ultrastructural evidence that both components are of epithelial origin (Battifora 1976; Du Boulay and Isaacson 1980).

"Collision" tumours, where an oesophageal squamous carcinoma meets a gastric adenocarcinoma, are seen occasionally (Majmudar et al. 1978) (Fig. 6.9).

## Chemical Carcinogens

Chemicals may act as initiators or promoters of oesophageal carcinoma but much is speculative. Oesophageal carcinoma arising after long-term exposure to benzene has been reported and a direct activation of cellular oncogenes by benzene proposed (Boewer 1986). Tumour promoters of the phorbol ester type can be isolated from the roots of *Croton flavens* which are eaten in Curaçao (Netherlands Antilles) and may be causally related to the high rate of oesophageal carcinoma in that area (Weber and Hecker 1978). Phorbol esters act directly on protein kinase C leading to DNA synthesis and increased mitotic activity and also reduce the metabolic co-operation between cells.

N-nitrosamine compounds are thought to be relevant to oesophageal cancer in China. Both nitrosamines and precursor secondary amines are present in food in high-incidence areas (Singer et al. 1986) and several N-nitrosamines have been detected in gastric juice and urine (Lu et al. 1986a, b). A correlation between the amount of nitrosamines ingested and oesophageal epithelial lesions has been reported (Lu et al. 1986a).

Mycotoxins have also been suggested as playing a role in inducing oseophageal carcinoma (Lu and Lin 1982) as have polycyclic aromatic hydrocarbons, smoking and chewing tobacco and excessive consumption of alcoholic beverages (Mahboubi 1977). A link between nitrosamines and alcohol consumption has been proposed as ethanol prevents the first pass hepatic clearance of dimethylnitrosamine in rats and increases the amount of dimethylnitrosamine activated in the oesophagus (Swann 1984).

## Tissue Culture Studies

Nitrosamines have been reported to cause hyperplasia of human foetal oesophageal epithelium in tissue culture (Lu et al. 1986a). The cell kinetics of a cell line derived from an oesophageal squamous carcinoma have been compared with those of cell lines from a pulmonary oat cell carcinoma and from squamous carcinomas at other sites in an experimental nude mouse system (Ikeuchi 1983). All squamous carcinoma cell lines showed similar cell kinetics with a shorter time lag before visible growth, longer $G_1$ and higher growth fractions than the oat cell line. The theoretical volume doubling time was shown to be a reliable estimate of radiosensitivity whilst the labelling index by pulse administration of $^3$H-thymidine was not.

## Human Papillomavirus

Infection of the oesophagus by human papillomavirus (HPV) has been reported and proposed as being responsible for benign proliferation of the squamous epithelium of the oesophagus (Winkler, quoted by Goldsmith 1984). Changes fulfilling the histological criteria for HPV infection have been found in about one-third of cases of oesophageal squamous carcinomas (Syrjanen 1982; Hille et al. 1985) and HPV antigens can be demonstrated by immunohistochemical techniques (Hille et al. 1986). HPV DNA has been reported in five out of ten cases of oesophageal carcinoma studied using a filter *in situ* hybridisation method (Kulski et al. 1986). HPV has been linked to the development of intraepithelial neoplasia and invasive squamous carcinoma in other parts of the body and HPV may prove to be an aetiological factor in human oesophageal carcinoma. A bovine papillomavirus (type 4) is known to cause oesophageal papillomas that become malignant after cattle eat bracken that contains a co-carcinogen and an immunosuppressant (Olson et al. 1969). A hypothesis linking the concept of mucosal immune surveillance with HPV infection of the oesophagus in a sequence of events which leads to squamous dysplasia and oesophageal carcinoma has been presented and involves an aberration of the Langerhans' cell/lymphocyte network and its symbiotic relationship with squamous cells as a result of persistent HPV infection in the epithelium. Neoplastic transformation may occur when this "at-risk" mucosa is exposed to one or several co-carcinogenic factors present in the environment (Morris and Price 1986).

## Cachexia and Tumour Necrosis Factors

The mode of death in most patients with oesophageal carcinoma is cachexia, a symptom complex with wasting of body fat and lean body mass. Obviously, local effects of the oesophageal carcinoma may contribute to the malnutrition. In cancer patients generally, the precise cause of the weight loss is obscure and prospective estimations of energy intake and energy expenditure for reasonable periods are lacking (Editorial 1984). Many patients with malignant disease are anorexic and have metabolic abnormalities such as increased glucose production rates (Heber et al. 1985). These effects remote from the tumour are believed to be mediated by cachexia factors. A similar factor or factors, termed cachectin, produced by endotoxin-stimulated macrophages, is known to inhibit adipocyte gene expression and the activity of lipogenic enzymes in culture (Torti et al. 1985). Structural studies have revealed a marked homology between cachectin and human tumour necrosis factor (Beutler and Cerami 1986).

## DNA Analysis

Analysis of the DNA content of tumour cells of various types has shown an association between high ploidy and poor prognosis, which might be causal. Carcinomas of the oesophagus have been subjected to cytophotometric DNA analysis by Sugimachi and his colleages (Sugimachi et al. 1984; Matsuura et al. 1986; Sugimachi et al. 1987) in both resection and biopsy specimens. In the latter report, on carcinomas from both Chinese and Japanese patients, high ploidy was associated with reduced survival. Further studies, possibly using flow cytometry to study many more cells, are needed to define the value of this approach in assessing prognosis and guiding therapy in individual patients.

## Experimental Carcinoma of the Oesophagus

The successful induction of specific malignancies in experimental animals is an important step in testing theories of aetiology, pathogenesis and therapy. Convincing carcinomas of the oesophagus have been induced experimentally in monkeys (Adamson et al. 1977), dogs (Sasajima et al. 1977), rats (Napalkov and Pozharisski 1969), mice (Nakamura et al. 1974), and hamsters (Herrold 1966). Little use has, however, been made of these models in recent years to unravel the aetiology or pathogenesis of carcinoma of the oesophagus.

# Conclusions

We have shown that the pathologist should have little difficulty in performing the practical tasks for the individual patient with carcinoma of the oesophagus, namely, diagnosing the carcinoma in cytological or biopsy material, in reporting the extent of spread and any lymph node involvement to be found in the resected specimen, or in carrying out an autopsy with attention to the details mentioned above. Nevertheless, these tasks play an essential part in the management of this distressing and lethal disease.

Pathologists may also be expected to contribute to the research into how the oesophageal epithelium becomes malignant, what dysplasia is and whether it is reversible. But possibly the most useful step forward now would be to refine the assessment of prognosis for the individual patient. This calls for multivariate analysis of all the factors thought to contribute to the behaviour of the disease in a large series of patients, as has been done for lung cancer (Stanley 1980). Data about some of these factors will be required from the pathologist and may include quantitative aspects, such as assessment of nuclear or nucleolar size or shape, mitotic indices, or oncogene expression, which have not so far apparently been addressed for this malignancy, or ploidy (see above). It may also be valuable to compare such data with those obtained from experimental animal models under controlled conditions. One may also look out for spin-offs from research into the numerous squamous carcinomas at other sites.

*Acknowledgements.* We are indebted to Gregor Wenning, Shaun Greer and Kate Parker, medical students, for sifting the literature while writing essays for us on this subject; and to Nitu Patel and Jane Codd for photography.

# References

*Notations in parentheses indicate the number of illustrations included. Abbreviations are:* XR, *radiographs including CT scans;* Macro, *macroscopic pictures;* LM, *light microscopic pictures;* EM, *transmission electron micrographs;* Autorad, *autoradiographs.*

Ackerman LV, Weinstein IB, Kaplan HS et al. (1978) Cancer of the esophagus. In: Kaplan HS, Tsuchitani PJ (eds) Cancer in China. Alan R Liss, New York, pp 111–136
Adamson RH, Krolikowski FJ, Correa P, Sieber SM, Dalgard DW (1977) Carcinogenicity of 1-methyl-1-nitrosourea in nonhuman primates. J Natl Cancer Inst 59:415–422 (XR 1, LM 1)
Agha FP (1985) Barrett carcinoma of the esophagus: clinical and radiographic analysis of 34 cases. AJR 145:41–46 (XR 6, Macro 1)
Agha FP, Weatherbee L, Sams JS (1984) Verrucous carcinoma of the esophagus. Am J Gastroenterol 79:844–849 (XR 3, LM 2)
Ahlbom HE (1936) Simple achlorhydric anaemia, Plummer–Vinson syndrome, and carcinoma of the mouth, pharynx, and oesophagus in women. Br Med J ii:331–333.
American Joint Committee on Cancer (1987) Manual for staging cancer, 3rd edn. Lippincott, Philadelphia
Anderson LL, Lad TE (1982) Autopsy findings in squamous-cell carcinoma of the esophagus. Cancer 50:1587–1590
Antler AS, Ough Y, Pitchumoni CS, Davidian M, Thelmo W (1982) Gastrointestinal metastases from malignant tumours of the lung. Cancer 49:170–172
Azzopardi JG, Menzies T (1962) Primary oesophageal adenocarcinoma. Confirmation of its existence by the finding of mucous gland tumours. Br J Surg 49:497–506 (XR 2, Macro 2, LM 12)
Barge J, Molas G, Maillard JN, Fekete F, Bogomoletz WV, Potet F (1981) Superficial oesophageal carcinoma: an oesophageal counterpart of early gastric cancer. Histopathology 5:499–510 (Macro 3, LM 5)
Barrett NR (1957) The lower esophagus lined by columnar epithelium. Surgery 41:881–894
Battifora H (1976) Spindle cell carcinoma. Ultrastructural evidence of squamous origin and collagen production by the tumour cells. Cancer 37:2275–2282 (LM 2, EM 5)
Beutler B, Cerami A (1986) Cachectin and tumour necrosis factor as two sides of the same biological coin. Nature 320:584–588 (Autorad 1)
Bigelow NH (1953) Carcinoma of the esophagus developing at the site of lye stricture. Cancer 6:1159–1164 (Macro 1, LM 1)

Boewer C (1986) Zur Kanzerogenen Wirkung langjahriger Benzenexposition. Auftreten eines Plasmozytoms und zweier solider Malignome an ein und demselben Arbeitsplatz. Folia Haematol 113:615–632

Bremner CG, Lynch VP, Ellis FH (1970) Barrett's esophagus: congenital or acquired? An experimental study of esophageal mucosal regeneration in the dog. Surgery 68:209–216 (Macro 3, LM 12)

Brenner S, Heimlich H, Widman M (1969) Carcinoid of esophagus. N Y State J Med 69:1337–1339 (XR 1, LM 1)

Broders AC, Vinson PP (1928) The degree of malignancy of carcinoma of the esophagus. Arch Otolaryngol 8:79–80

Brown-Kelly A (1919) Spasm at the entrance to the oesophagus. J Laryngol 34:285–289

Butler ML, Van Heertum RL, Teplick SK (1975) Metastatic malignant melanoma of the esophagus: a case report. Gastroenterology 69:1334–1337 (XR 2, LM 2)

Charbit A, Malaise EP, Tubiana M (1971) Relation between the pathological nature and the growth rate of human tumors. Eur J Cancer 7:307–315

Chisholm M, Ardran GM, Callender ST, Wright R (1971) A follow-up study of patients with post-cricoid webs. Q J Med 40:409–420 (XR 3)

Chong FK, Graham JH, Madoff IM (1979) Mucin-producing carcinoid ("composite tumor") of upper third of esophagus. A variant of carcinoid tumor. Cancer 44:1853–1859 (Macro 1, LM 6)

Clements JL, Cox GW, Torres WE, Weens HS (1974) Cervical esophageal webs – a roentgen–anatomic correlation. Observations on the pharyngoesophagus. Am J Roentgenol Rad Ther Nucl Med 121:221–231 (XR 10, Macro 4, LM 4)

Cliffton EE (1970) Treatment of cancer of the esophagus. Mod Treatment 7:1261–1283 (XR 16, Macro 3)

Cook MG, Eusebi V, Betts CM (1976) Oat-cell carcinoma of the esophagus: a recently recognized entity. J Clin Pathol 29:1068–1073 (Macro 1, LM 3, EM 2)

Correa P (1982) Precursors of gastric and esophageal cancer. Cancer 50:2554–2565 (LM 8)

Crespi M, Muñoz N, Grassi A et al. (1979) Oesophageal lesions in Northern Iran: A premalignant condition? Lancet II:217–221

Day DW (1986) Biopsy pathology of the oesophagus, stomach and duodenum. Chapman and Hall, London, pp 21–29 (LM 4)

De la Pava S, Nigogosyan G, Pickren JW, Cabrera A (1963) Melanosis of the esophagus. Cancer 16:48–50 (LM 2)

DiCostanzo DP, Urmacher C (1987) Primary malignant melanoma of the esophagus. Am J Surg Pathol 11:46–52 (XR 1, Macro 1, LM 4, EM 1)

Dodge OG (1961) Gastro-oesophageal carcinoma of mixed histological type. J Pathol Bacteriol 81:459–471 (LM 9)

Du Boulay CEH, Isaacson PG (1981) Carcinoma of the oesophagus with spindle cell features. Histopathology 5:403–414 (Macro 2, LM 13, EM 1)

Editorial (1984) Cancer cachexia. Lancet I:833–834

Endo M, Takeshita K, Yoshida M (1986) How can we diagnose the early stages of esophageal cancer? Endoscopic diagnosis. Endoscopy 18 [Suppl 3]:11–18 (Macro 19, LM 1)

Entwistle CC, Jacobs A (1965) Histological findings in the Paterson–Kelly syndrome. J Clin Pathol 18:408–413 (LM 7)

Fox H (1987) Cervical smears: new terminology and new demands. Br Med J 294:1307–1308

Garlock JH, Richter R (1961) Carcinoma in a pharyngo-esophageal diverticulum: a case report. Ann Surg 154:259–262 (XR 4)

Geddes DM (1979) The natural history of lung cancer: a review based on rates of tumour growth. Br J Dis Chest 73:1–17

Goyal RK, Bauer JL, Spiro HM (1971) The nature and location of lower esophageal ring. N Engl J Med 284:1175–1180 (XR 1, Macro 2, LM 3)

Guanrei Y, He H, Sungliang Q, Yuming C (1982) Endoscopic diagnosis of 115 cases of early esophageal carcinoma. Endoscopy 14:157–161 (Macro 11, LM 3)

Hamilton SR, Yardley JH (1977) Regeneration of cardiac type mucosa and acquisition of Barrett mucosa after esophagogastrostomy. Gastroenterology 72:669–675 (Macro 1, LM 8)

Hankins JR, McLaughlin JS (1975) The association of carcinoma of the esophagus with achalasia. J Thorac Cardiovasc Surg 69:355–360 (XR 2, Macro 1)

Harper PS, Harper RMJ, Howel-Evans AW (1970) Carcinoma of the oesophagus with tylosis. Q J Med 39:317–333 (Macro 3)

Heber D, Byerly LO, Chlebowski RT (1985) Metabolic abnormalities in the cancer patient. Cancer 55:225–229

Hermanek P, Sobin P, Leslie H (eds) (1987) TNM classification of malignant tumours, 4th edn. (UICC) Springer-Verlag, Berlin Heidelberg New York

Herrold KM (1966) Epidermoid carcinomas of esophagus and forestomach induced in Syrian hamsters by N-nitroso-N-methylurethan. J Natl Cancer Inst 37:389–394 (LM8)

Hille JJ, Markowitz S, Margolius KA, Isaacson C (1985) Human papillomavirus and carcinoma of the esophagus. N Engl J Med 312:1707 (letter)

Hille JJ, Margolius KA, Markowitz S, Isaacson C (1986) Human papillomavirus infection related to oesophageal carcinoma in black South Africans. A preliminary study. S Afr Med J 69:417–420 (LM 5)

Howel-Evans W, McConnell RB, Clarke CA, Sheppard PM (1958) Carcinoma of the oesophagus with keratosis palmaris et plantaris (tylosis). A study of two families. Q J Med 27:413–429 (Macro 2, LM 2)

Hunt TE, Hunt EA (1962) Radioautographic study of proliferation in the stomach of the rat using thymidine-$H^3$ and compound 48/80. Anat Rec 142:505–517 (Macro 1, LM 1, Autorad 10)

Ikeuchi S (1983) Radiosensitivity and cell kinetics of the human solid cancer transplanted to nude mouse. Nippon Geka Gakkai Zasshi 84:655–666 (LM 8)

Japanese Society for Oesophageal Diseases (1976) Guide lines for the clinical and pathologic studies on carcinoma of the esophagus. Jap J Surg 6:69–86 (XR 7, Macro 4, LM 6)

Jass JR, Morson BC (1987) Reporting colorectal cancer. J Clin Pathol 40:1016–1023

Johns BAE (1952) Developmental changes in the oesophageal epithelium in man. J Anat 86:431–442 (LM 26)

Just-Viera JO, Haight C (1969) Achalasia and carcinoma of the esophagus. Surg Gynecol Obstet 128:1081–1095

Kasugai T, Kobayashi S, Kuno N (1978) Endoscopic cytology of the esophagus, stomach and pancreas. Acta Cytol 22:327–330

Kay S (1963) A ten-year appraisal of the treatment of squamous cell carcinoma of the esophagus. Surg Gynecol Obstet 117:167–171

Kulski J, Demeter T, Sterrett GF, Shilkin KB (1986) Human papilloma virus DNA in oesophageal carcinoma. Lancet II:683–684 (letter) (Autorad 6)

Lansing PB, Ferrante WA, Oschsner JL (1969) Carcinoma of the esophagus at the site of lye stricture. Am J Surg 118:108–111 (XR 3, Macro 1, LM 2)

Leblond CP, Clermont Y, Nadler NJ (1967) The pattern of stem renewal in three epithelia (esophagus, intestine and testis). Can Cancer Conf 7:3–30 (LM 3, Autorad 5)

Levine MS, Dillon EC, Saul SH, Laufer I (1986) Early esophageal cancer. AJR 146:507–512 (XR 5, LM 1)

Lu SH, Lin P (1982) Recent research on the etiology of esophageal cancer in China. Z Gastroenterol 20:361–367

Lu SH, Montesano R, Zhang MS et al. (1986a) Relevance of N-nitrosamines to esophageal cancer in China. J Cell Physiol [Suppl] 4:51–58

Lu SH, Ohshima H, Fu HM et al. (1986b) Urinary excretion of N-nitrosamino acids and nitrate by inhabitants of high- and low-risk areas for esophageal cancer in Northern China: Endogenous formation of nitrosoproline and its inhibition by vitamin C. Cancer Res 46: 1485–1491

Mahboubi E (1977) The epidemiology of oral cavity, pharyngeal and esophageal cancer outside of North America and Western Europe. Cancer 40:1879–1886

Majmudar B, Dillard R, Susann PW (1978) Collision carcinoma of the gastric cardia. Hum Pathol 9:471–473 (Macro 1, LM 1)

Mandard AM, Chasle J, Marnay J et al. (1981) Autopsy findings in 111 cases of esophageal cancer. Cancer 48:329–335

Mannell A (1982) Carcinoma of the esophagus. Curr Prob Surg 19:553–647 (XR 23, Macro 5)

Marcial Rojas RA, Vallecillo LA (1959) Primary adenoidcystic carcinoma of the esophagus. Report of one case and review of the literature. Arch Otolaryngol 70:197–201 (XR 1, Macro 1, LM 4)

Matsufuji H, Kuwano H, Ueo H, Sugimachi K, Inokuchi K (1985) Mucoepidermoid carcinoma of the esophagus: a case report. Jap J Surg 15:55–59 (Macro 1, LM 4)

Matsusaka T, Watanabe H, Enjoji M (1976) Pseudosarcoma and carcinosarcoma of the esophagus. Cancer 37:1546–1555 (Macro 3, LM 9)

Matsuura H, Sugimachi K, Ueo H, Kuwano H, Koga Y, Okamura T (1986) Malignant potentiality of squamous cell carcinoma of the esophagus predictable by DNA analysis. Cancer 57:1810–1814

McKechnie JC, Fechner RE (1971) Choriocarcinoma and adenocarcinoma of the esophagus with gonadotrophin secretion. Cancer 27:694–702 (XR 6, LM 3)

McKeown F (1952) Oat-cell carcinoma of the oesophagus. J Pathol Bacteriol 64:889–891 (LM 4)

McNab Jones RF (1961) The Paterson–Brown–Kelly syndrome. Its relationship to iron deficiency and postcricoid carcinoma. J Laryngol Otol 75:529–561 (XR 7)

Meyer W, Vollmar F, Bar W (1979) Barrett-esophagus following total gastrectomy. A contribution to its pathogenesis. Endoscopy 11:121–126 (Macro 2, LM 1)

Miller C (1962) Carcinoma of thoracic oesophagus and cardia. A review of 405 cases. Br J Surg 49:507–522 (LM 1)

Ming S-C (1971) Tumors of the esophagus and stomach. Atlas of tumor pathology, second series, fasc 7. Armed Forces Institute of Pathology, Washington

Morris H, Price S (1986) Langerhans' cells, papillomaviruses and oesophageal carcinoma. A hypothesis. S Afr Med J 69:413–417 (LM 5)

Morson BC, Belcher JR (1952) Adenocarcinoma of the oesophagus and ectopic gastric mucosa. Br J Surg 6:127–130 (XR 3, Macro 1, LM 4)

Morson BC, Jass JR (1985) Precancerous conditions of the gastrointestinal tract. A histological classification. Baillière Tindall, London (LM 29)

Mossberg SM (1966) The columnar-lined esophagus (Barrett syndrome) – an acquired condition? Gastroenterology 50:671–676 (XR 1, LM 4)

Muñoz N, Crespi M, Grassi A, Qing WG, Qiong S, Cai LZ (1982) Precursor lesions of oesophageal cancer in high-risk populations in Iran and China. Lancet I: 876–879

Nakamura T, Matsuyama M, Kishimoto H (1974) Tumors of the esophagus and duodenum induced in mice by oral administration of N-ethyl-N'-nitro-N-nitrosoguanidine. J Natl Cancer Inst 52:519–522 (LM 4)

Napalkov NP, Pozharisski KM (1969) Morphogenesis of experimental tumours of the esophagus. J Natl Cancer Inst 42:922–940 (Macro 1, LM 8)

O'Gara RW, Horn RC (1955) Intramucosal carcinoma of the esophagus. Arch Pathol 60:95–98 (LM 5)

Olson C, Gordon DE, Robl MG, Lee KP (1969) Oncogenicity of bovine papilloma virus. Arch Environ Health 19:827–837 (Macro 11, LM 7)

Oota K, Sobin LH (1977) Histological typing of gastric and oesophageal tumours. International histological classification of tumours, no. 18. World Health Organization, Geneva (LM 26)

Paterson DR (1919) A clinical type of dysphagia. J Laryngol 34:289–291

Polk HC, Camp FA, Walker AW (1967) Dysphagia and esophageal stenosis. Manifestation of metastatic mammary cancer. Cancer 20:2002–2007 (XR 5, LM 2)

Rajindranath T, Nair KV, Devi RS, Devi NN (1984) Prolonged "in situ" stage in oesophageal carcinoma. J Assoc Physicians India 32:455–456 (LM 4)

Rector LE, Connerley ML (1941) Aberrant mucosa in the esophagus in infants and in children. Arch Pathol 31:285–294 (LM 4)

Rindi G, Bishop AE, Daily MJ, Lee FI, Isaacs P, Polak JM (1987) Presence of hormone containing cells in Barrett's oesophagus. A prospective endoscopic study of 45 cases. J Pathol 152:227A (abstract)

Robbins SL, Cotran RS, Kumar V (1984) The gastrointestinal tract. In: Robbins SL (ed) Pathologic basic of disease, 3rd edn. Saunders, Philadelphia, pp 804–806

Roberts JG (1980) Cancer of the oesophagus – how should tumour biology affect treatment? Br J Surg 67:791–797

Rosai J (1981) Gastrointestinal tract. In: Rosai J (ed) Ackerman's surgical pathology, vol 1, 6th edn. Mosby, St Louis, pp 400–569

Rywlin AM, Ortega R (1970) Glycogenic acanthosis of the esophagus. Arch Pathol 90:439–443 (Macro 3, LM 2)

Sasajima K, Kawachi T, Sano T, Sugimura T, Shimosato Y, Shirota A (1977) Esophageal and gastric cancers with metastases induced in dogs by N-ethyl-N'-nitro-N-nitrosoguanidine. J Natl Cancer Inst 58:1789–1794 (Macro 1, LM 11)

Schmidt FA (1805) De mammalium oesophago atque ventriculo. MD thesis, Halle University, Saxony

Shamma'a MH, Benedict EB (1958) Esophageal webs. A report of 58 cases and an attempt at classification. N Engl J Med 259:378–384 (XR 2, Macro 1)

Shine I, Allison PR (1966) Carcinoma of the oesophagus with tylosis (keratosis palmaris et plantaris) Lancet I:951–953 (LM 1)

Singer GM, Chuan J, Roman J, Min-Hsin L, Lijinsky W (1986) Nitrosamines and nitrosamine precursors in foods from Linxian, China, a high incidence area for esophageal cancer. Carcinogenesis 7:733–736

Smithers DW (1955) The association of cancer of the stomach and oesophagus with herniation at the oesophageal hiatus of the diaphragm. Br J Radiol 28:554–564 (Macro 1, LM 13)

Sohn D, Valensi Q, Bryk D (1965) Hepatoma metastasizing to the esophagus. JAMA 194:910–912 (XR 1, Macro 2, LM 1)

Sons HU, Borchard F (1984) Esophageal cancer. Autopsy findings in 171 cases. Arch Pathol Lab Med 108:983–988 (Macro 2)

Stanley KE (1980) Prognostic factors for survival in patients with inoperable lung cancer. J Natl Cancer Inst 65:25–32

Stout AP, Humphreys GH, Rottenberg LA (1949) A case of carcinosarcoma of the esophagus. Am J Roentgenol Rad Ther Nucl Med 61:461–469 (XR 4, Macro 3, LM 3)

Sugimachi K, Ide H, Okamura T, Matsuura H, Endo M, Inokuchi K (1984) Cytophotometric DNA analysis of mucosal and submucosal carcinoma of the esophagus. Cancer 53:2683–2687

Sugimachi K, Koga Y, Mori M, Huang GJ, Yang K, Zhang RG (1987) Comparative data on cytophotometric DNA in malignant lesions of the esophagus in the Chinese and Japanese. Cancer 59:1947–1950

Swann PF (1984) The possible role of nitrosamines in the link between alcohol consumption and esophageal cancer in man. Toxicol Pathol 12:357–360

Syrjanen KJ (1982) Histological changes identical to those of condylomatous lesions found in esophageal squamous cell carcinomas. Arch Geschwulstforsch 52:283–292 (LM 5)

Takagi I, Karasawa K (1982) Growth of squamous cell esophageal carcinoma observed by serial esophagographies. J Surg Oncol 21:57–60 (XR 11)

Takahashi K (1961) Squamous cell carcinoma of the esophagus. Stromal inflammatory cell infiltration as a prognostic factor. Cancer 14:921–933 (LM 8)

Takubo K, Tsuchiya S, Fukushi K, Shirota A, Mitomo Y (1981) Dysplasia and reserve cell hyperplasia-like change in human esophagus. Acta Pathol Jap 31:999–1013 (LM 12)

Takubo K, Nishimura H, Taniguchi Y et al. (1984) Junctions between intraepithelial carcinoma and non-neoplastic tissue of the esophagus. Light and electron microscopic studies. Acta Pathol Jap 34:785–796 (Macro 1, LM 3, EM 6)

Takubo K, Takai A, Takayama S, Sasajima K, Yamashita K, Fujita K (1987) Intraductal spread of esophageal squamous cell carcinoma. Cancer 59:1751–1757 (LM 6, EM 2)

Tateishi R, Taniguchi H, Wada A, Horai T, Taniguchi K (1974) Argyrophil cells and melanocytes in esophogeal mucosa. Arch Pathol 98:87–89 (LM 8)

Tedesco FJ, Morton WJ (1975) Lower-esophageal webs. Am J Dig Dis 20:381–383 (XR 2)

Torti FM, Dieckmann B, Beutler B, Cerami A, Ringold GM (1985) A macrophage factor inhibits adipocyte gene expression: An in vitro model of cachexia. Science 229:867–869 (Autorad 4)

Ushigome S, Spjut HJ, Noon GP (1967) Extensive dysplasia and carcinoma in situ of esophageal epithelium. Cancer 20:1023–1029 (XR 1, LM 6)

Vinson PP (1921) Hysterical dysphagia. Minn Med 5:107-108

Waldenstrom J (1938) Iron and epithelium. Some clinical observations. Part I. Regeneration of the epithelium. Acta Med Scand [Suppl] 90:380–397 (XR 8)

Waldenstrom J, Kjellberg SR (1939) The roentgenological diagnosis of sideropenic dysphagia (Plummer–Vinson's syndrome). Acta Radiol 20:618–638 (XR 22)

Weber J, Hecker E (1978) Cocarcinogens of the diterpene ester type from Croton flavens L. and esophageal cancer in Curacao. Experientia 34:679–682

Winkler B, quoted by Goldsmith MF (1984) Papillomavirus invades esophagus, incidence seems to be increasing. JAMA 251:2185–2187 (LM 2)

Wood CB, Wood RAB (1975) Metastatic malignant melanoma of the esophagus. Am J Dig Dis 20:786–789 (XR 2, LM 1)

Woodard BH, Shelburne JD, Vollmer RT, Postlethwait RW (1978) Mucoepidermoid carcinoma of the esophagus: a case report. Hum Pathol 9:352–354 (LM 2, EM 2)

Wychulis AR, Woolam GL, Andersen HA, Ellis FH (1971) Achalasia and carcinoma of the esophagus. JAMA 215:1638–1641 (XR 2, Macro 2)

Yang CS (1980) Research on esophageal cancer in China: a review. Cancer Res 40:2633–2644

Yardley JH (1987) Campylobacter pyloridis and other new infectious agents in the gastrointestinal tract. Am J Surg Pathol 11:154 (abstract)

Yates DR, Koss LG (1968) Paget's disease of the esophageal epithelium. Report of first case. Arch Pathol 86:447–452 (LM 9)

Younghusband JD, Aluwihare APR (1970) Carcinoma of the oesophagus: factors influencing survival. Br J Surg 57:422–430 (Macro 1, LM 5)

*Chapter 7*

# Surgical Resection for Postcricoid Carcinoma

D. F. N. Harrison

The hypopharynx is generally accepted as extending from the free margin of the epiglottis to the lower border of the cricoid cartilage. A horizontal line drawn at the level of the hyoid bone marks the superior border, whilst in the adult the lower border of the cricoid cartilage lies approximately at the sixth cervical vertebra. The cervical oesophagus extends from this point to the thoracic inlet and varies in length depending upon the position of the larynx. Whilst the lumen of the hypopharynx is cone-shaped superiorly, it becomes more narrow in the postcricoid region extending into the oesophagus, which from an oncological viewpoint is merely an extension of the hypopharynx.

Traditionally, and in all systems of classification, the hypopharynx is divided into pyriform fossa, posterior pharyngeal wall and postcricoid regions. Although convenient for description, there is no bar to rapid extension of squamous carcinoma from one region to another and clinically this is commonly seen at diagnosis of most hypopharyngeal tumours. No significant lymphatic or histological features distinguish these regions and pharyngeal neoplasms grow downwards as readily as cervical oesophageal lesions extend upwards.

However, in the relatively unusual early carcinomas or where clinical symptoms clearly indicate site of origin, there is a significant variation in the incidence of tumours arising within the pyriform fossa and postcricoid region. In most large series, the pyriform fossa was more frequently involved than other sites. Bryce (1967) in a series of 230 patients quoted 61% primarily in pyriform fossa, 24% postcricoid and 15% posterior pharyngeal wall. However, these figures may also reflect personal interest and expertise, particularly in relation to techniques of surgical excision and repair. Harrison and Thompson (1986) in a personal series of 101 gastric "pull up" operations reported 67% arising within the postcricoid region, 19% pyriform fossa and 9% cervical oesophagus.

# Aetiology of Postcricoid Carcinoma

A preponderance of women is found in all series although the ratio varies widely, possibly reflecting a changing pattern in aetiological factors as well as the geographical region being studied. All reports show an increased incidence in Anglo-Saxon countries over the Mediterranean area and North America (Stell 1973). This is probably unrelated to variation in radiation-induced tumours which usually follow the use of radiotherapy for thyroid disease or a previous laryngeal cancer. This figure varies between 7% and 10% (Harrison and Thompson 1986; Stell et al. 1978) and is now no longer an important factor because of time lag and abandonment of this modality.

Earlier reports of a female preponderance as high as 24:1 (Pearson 1966; Jacobs 1961) undoubtedly reflected an association between postcricoid carcinoma and the Paterson–Brown-Kelly syndrome (Plummer–Vinson syndrome). In 1919, both Paterson and Brown-Kelly reported dysphagia associated with stomatitis, glossitis and hypochromic anaemia. About the same time, in America, Plummer and Vinson studying a group of 69 patients with "hysterical dysphagia" found an associated hypochromic anaemia. Both Paterson and Brown-Kelly

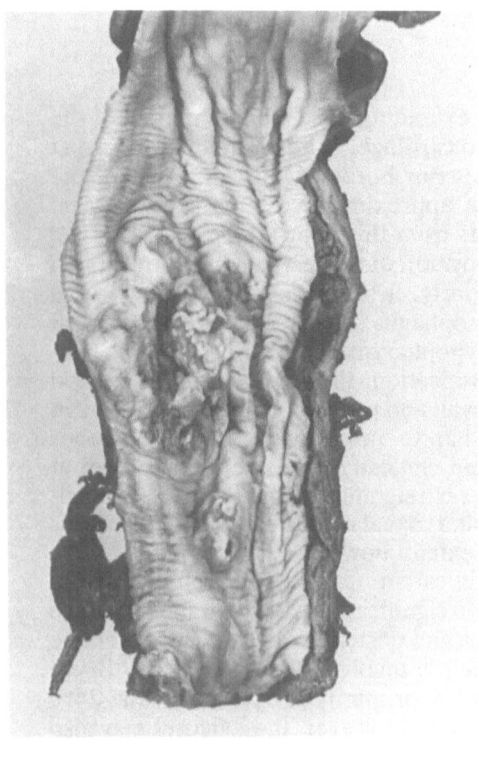

0  1  2  3  4 cm

**Fig. 7.1.** Length from excised oesophagus showing second tumour.

noticed a predominance of females and an association with postcricoid stenosis, web formation and an increased incidence of carcinoma in this region. McNab-Jones (1961) found that over one-third of patients with postcricoid carcinoma had a previous history of the syndrome. Larsson et al. (1975) reported an incidence of 40% and Pearson (1966) only 7%. There were no reports of the syndrome in the smaller number of males with postcricoid carcinoma. The duration of the dysphagia and anaemia varied between 10 and 20 years, and the patients were confined to Northern Europe despite the common incidence of hypochromic anaemia in other parts of the world.

The poor survival rates following surgery in the 1950s and 1960s were blamed on the generalised mucosal changes produced by this syndrome, although Jacobs (1961) in a careful histological study of the mucosa from 93 cases of postcricoid carcinoma found no premalignant lesions in "anaemic buccopharyngeal epithelium".

Wynder et al. (1957) investigated possible environmental factors in the production of hypopharyngeal cancer in Sweden and their associationship with anaemia. Whilst accepting a high incidence of postcricoid carcinoma in women from Northern Sweden and its relationship to iron-deficiency anaemia, they also implicated deficiencies in vitamins and animal protein.

The decreased incidence of postcricoid carcinoma in Sweden reported by Larsson et al. (1975) appears to be partly related to the disappearance of the Paterson–Brown-Kelly syndrome as well as improvements in diet. Similar reductions have been found by Stell et al. (1978) who found only 4 women with the syndrome in 114 postcricoid carcinomas and Harrison and Thompson (1986) only 7 out of 180 cases. The significance of the absence of any generalised premalignant changes in the epithelium of the upper alimentary tract is obviously of surgical importance and is substantiated by Harrison's examination of resected specimens (1970), confirming that local recurrence was primarily related to inadequate excision rather than multiple primary tumours. Examination of 125 total oesophagectomy specimens removed surgically showed only one second tumour (Harrison and Thompson 1986) (Fig. 7.1).

As with most other pharyngeal tumours the use of alcohol and tobacco probably plays a role in induction but no explanation is as yet available for the marked regional variation in incidence of postcricoid carcinoma nor the female preponderance which is still present in all large series.

# Surgical Pathology

Looser et al. (1978) have discussed the problem of "positive" margins after surgical resection concluding, not surprisingly, that positive margins lead to a higher recurrence rate at the primary site. In examining pharyngolaryngectomy specimens following resection from postcricoid and cervical oesophageal tumours Harrison (1970) found that most local recurrences were in fact regrowth of residual disease left *in situ* at the original operation. Submucosal extension measured on average 10 mm superiorly and a little less inferiorly. With the larynx lying at varying levels within the neck, superior and inferior levels of resection

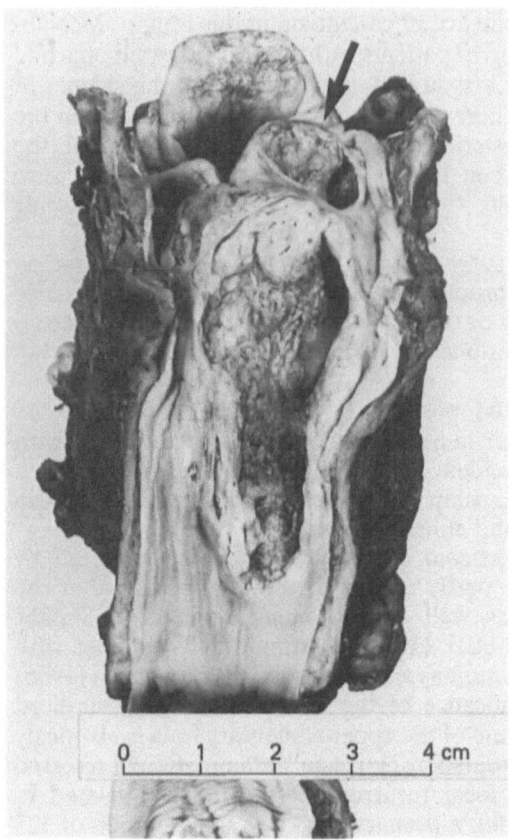

**Fig. 7.2.** Pharyngolaryngectomy specimen showing extensive hypopharyngeal tumour. Superior margin arrowed.

will be related, in part, to anatomical as well as pathological factors. Manubrial resection (Harrison 1977) gives a modest increase in accessibility inferiorly. However, extension to tongue base or posterolateral wall superiorly always limits the margins of excision (Fig. 7.2). The wall of the hypopharynx is composed of four layers: an inner mucosal lining of stratified squamous epithelium over a loose stroma, fibrous layer of the pharyngeal aponeurosis, the inferior constrictor muscle and the buccopharyngeal fascia. Loose connective tissue separates the pharynx posteriorly from the prevertebral fascia and anterior longitudinal ligament.

Extension of a postcricoid carcinoma anteriorly involves the cricoid cartilage which can easily be removed by total laryngectomy. Penetration through the muscular wall is less easily detected – adequate resection being then determined primarily by the site of extension. Whereas portions of the prevertebral fascia are removable, involvement of the carotid artery at the root of the neck results in tumour left *in situ*.

There is a rich lymphatic network draining hypopharynx and cervical oesophagus. Although the cervical lymph nodes are accessible to palpation and resection, those lying in the paratracheal region are difficult to detect and form a common site for metastases. The ultimate relationship of the upper paratracheal nodes to the lower pole of the thyroid gland and the frequency with which this gland is involved in postcricoid carcinoma (Harrison 1973) necessitates its removal in surgical excision of postcricoid carcinoma.

Much of the voluminous literature of the last two decades on the surgical management of postcricoid and cervical oesophageal cancer has been concerned with the success, or its lack, in a wide variety of operative reconstructive procedures. Although this is obviously of great importance in obtaining meaningful rehabilitation, long-term survival remains primarily related to the feasibility of adequate resection of the primary tumour and, when necessary, regional lymphatic network.

# Problems in Classification

Although several means are available for calculating "survival data", all of which produce varying arithmetic results, the input site of the "success formula" is based on the staging of the original tumour. The systems proposed by the International Union Against Cancer (UICC) and the American Joint Committee (AJC) have much in common (Table 7.1) although their accuracy and usefulness depends on the feasibility and accuracy with which the oncologist can determine three-dimensional extension while viewing the tumour two-dimensionally. Superior extension is of more significance with pyriform fossa carcinoma and inferior extension with postcricoid lesions.

**Table 7.1.**   Clinical classification for squamous carcinoma arising within the hypopharynx (UICC 1982)

| *Hypopharynx* | |
| --- | --- |
| Tis | Pre-invasive carcinoma (carcinoma *in situ*) |
| T0 | No evidence of primary tumour |
| T1 | Tumour confined to one site |
| T2 | Tumour with extension to adjacent site or region without fixation of hemilarynx |
| T3 | Tumour with extension to adjacent site or region with fixation of hemilarynx |
| T4 | Tumour with extension to bone, cartilage or soft tissues |
| TX | The minimum requirements to assess the primary tumour cannot be met |

Involvement of the adjoining larynx is of minimal significance since this organ is easily removed. Fixation of the hemilarynx (T3) invariably means involvement of cartilage (T4).

Stell et al. (1982) emphasised the importance of the vertical length of a postcricoid tumour showing that prognosis worsens when the length is more than 5 cm. However, this may be because the larger lesions are more likely to have penetrated muscular wall or metastasised to regional lymph nodes. Unfortunately, no existing classification accurately reflects the surgical pathology of postcricoid and cervical oesophageal cancer and assessment of surgical success must be correlated with adequacy of excision rather than unrealistic attempts at hypothetical classification (Willatt et al. 1987).

# Rationale for Surgical Excision

The most recent evaluation of the role of radiotherapy in the management of postcricoid carcinoma has been published by Farrington et al. (1986) based on 201 patients treated over a period of 10 years. Only half received radical treatment because of "unsuitability" and of these only 22% survived more than 5 years. Of those receiving palliative radiotherapy, 98% died within a year. Of the long-term survivors all except three had small lesions and no neck gland involvement. These poor figures are slightly worse than Pearson (1966) but better than Lord et al. (1973) who had approximately 8% 5-year survivals. Even patients whose tumour is successfully treated frequently develop post-irradiation stricture with subsequent dysphagia. No survival figures for surgery following radiation failure were available but personal experience suggests that many of these patients are unfit for surgery or prove to have unresectable neoplasms at eventual diagnosis.

Occasionally, the patient with a postcricoid carcinoma of cervical oesophagus develops rapid progressive dysphagia from an early, superficial, concentric narrowing cancer without extraluminal spread. More frequently, progressive difficulty in swallowing with consequent weight loss, coughing from overspill and excessive, sometimes bloodstained, sputum are the more common manifestations. Reduction of food intake to a more liquid form delays eventual diagnosis and early tumours are seen but rarely.

Most of the large series of this relatively uncommon neoplasm are based therefore on primary surgery for patients considered as potentially curable or suitable for "realistic" palliation. It is the improvement in reconstructive techniques which have so dramatically given new meaning to palliation, for the staged skin repairs which were the mainstay of the 1960s rarely achieved this, for the time scale greatly exceeded the duration of freedom from local recurrence.

Local surgical control necessitates obtaining clear microscopical margins above and below the macroscopical tumour and at least entails a pharyngolaryngectomy. In 1970, Harrison examined serially sectioned pharyngolaryngectomy specimens to determine the cause of failure of local control. Standard pharyngolaryngectomy is limited by anatomical structures in both its superior and inferior extent, disease being left in the residual mucosa above or oesophageal remnant below. Paratracheal nodal metastasis, thyroid gland involvement or tumour left within the tracheo-oesophageal junction will all result in "stomal recurrence" (Fig. 7.3). It was failure to control the primary tumour, even with no neck gland involvement or no extraluminal spread, that was the cause of failure in many of these patients.

Most primary postcricoid neoplasms either involve the larynx or, more seriously, grow inferiorly into the cervical oesophagus. Fortunately, the development by Ong and Lee (1960) of the pharyngolaryngoesophagectomy operation with primary pharyngo-gastric anastomosis offered unlimited inferior excision of the oesophagus, although in some patients this can be achieved within the neck.

In cases where radical excision is technically possible the ideal means of reconstructing the pharyngoesophageal defect should restore swallowing in a single stage, employ tissue outside any field of irradiation, would not require a thoracic or abdominal operation and would be accompanied by minimal mortality

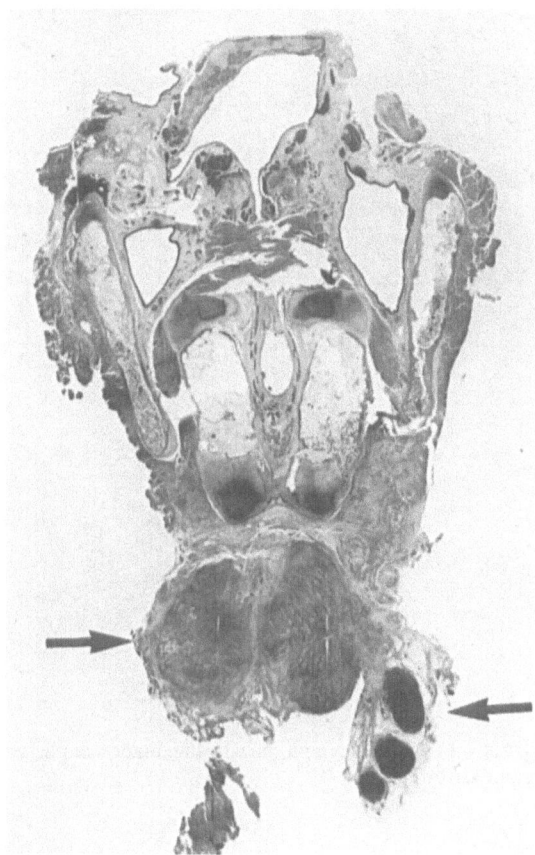

**Fig. 7.3.** Serial section at 10 μ of pharyngolaryngectomy specimen showing lower extent tumour and paratracheal lymph nodes (arrowed).

or morbidity. Such a procedure is not, as yet, available! In practice, oncology surgeons must utilise the most appropriate of the several techniques now available, choosing the one best suited to each individual patient.

Accepting that many patients present with technically incurable tumours, failure to palliate and sometimes cure has related in part to the inability of surgeons to carry out adequate resection of primary and regional metastases or effect primary reconstruction of the pharyngo-oesophageal gap (Harrison 1979).

# Excision of Primary Tumour

As with all other malignant tumours, preoperative assessment of the extent of the primary tumour and possible regional lymph node metastasis is an essential part of planning procedure.

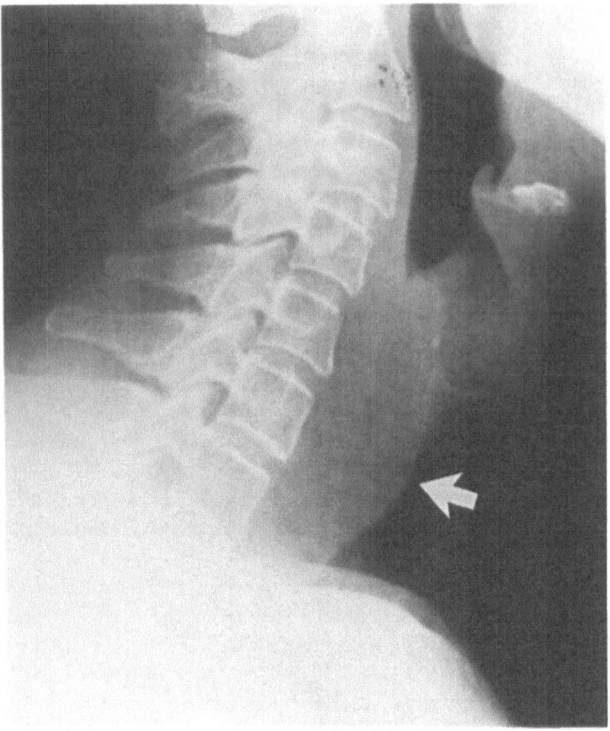

**Fig. 7.4.** Lateral radiograph showing indentation of posterior wall of trachea by crico-oesophageal tumour (arrowed).

Endoscopic examination may help to confirm the superior and inferior extent of a postcricoid tumour although the latter may be difficult because of bleeding and obstruction of the lumen. Tissue for biopsy is essential as is also the elimination of synchronous primary neoplasms within the upper alimentary system.

Lateral soft-tissue radiographs are most valuable since they can indicate possible involvement of the posterior tracheal wall from neoplasms arising within or extending into the cervical oesophagus (Fig. 7.4). If necessary, manubrial resection as described by Harrison (1977) will be necessary to allow low resection of the trachea, thus avoiding subsequent stomal recurrence (Fig. 7.5). This procedure gives access to the paratracheal lymph nodes and upper oesophagus permitting radical resection of extensive crico-oesophageal tumours.

Total thyroidectomy is considered essential in all postcricoid tumours (Harrison 1973) and invasion through the posterior pharyngeal wall on to prevertebral fascia requires local excision of this tissue, but not the anterior longitudinal ligament.

In patients with postcricoid neoplasms less than 3 cm in length, pharyngolaryngectomy with a small portion of cervical oesophagus allows adequate resection. However, most patients present with longer tumours extending superiorly to involve tongue base or upper oropharynx; or more commonly, inferiorly into

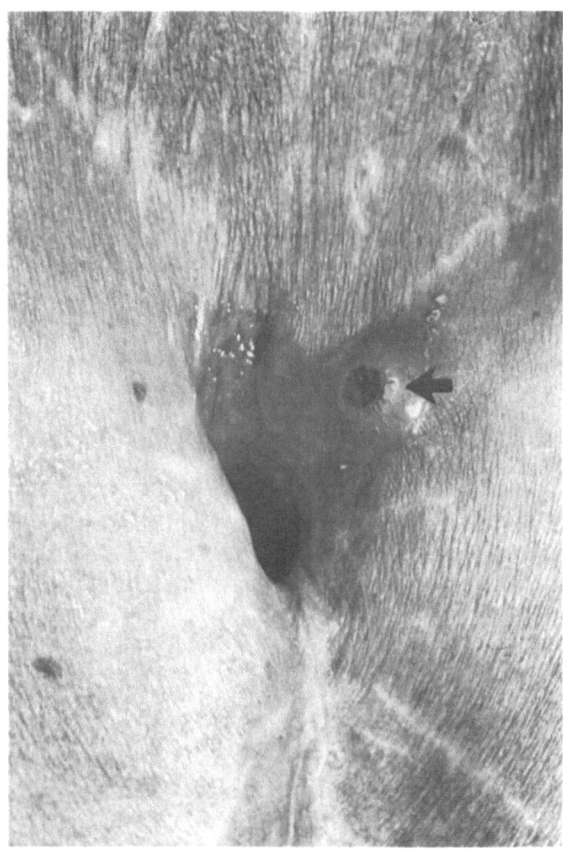

**Fig. 7.5.** Tracheostoma distorted by recurrent tumour (arrowed).

cervical oesophagus. Failure to appreciate the need for adequate local resection has led in the past to cancer left *in situ* masquerading as "local recurrence". Such inadequate resections were possibly related to the limited and inadequate means of speedily reconstructing the pharyngoesophageal defect. Much of the significant development in the past two decades has been related to a better understanding of the surgical pathology of the disease and improvement in reconstructive techniques.

## Regional Lymph Nodes

The incidence of lymph node metastasis is lower in postcricoid tumours than in other hypopharyngeal neoplasms. However, the survival curves show clearly that involved nodes, especially if bilateral or fixed, carry a very poor prognosis – no matter how the patient is treated (Stell et al. 1982). Metastases occur most commonly to the lower deep cervical and paratracheal nodes, the latter being relatively inaccessible to palpation. Palpable cervical nodes necessitate an accessory nerve-sparing radical neck dissection and if the upper paratracheal nodes are enlarged or positive on frozen section then manubrial resection with clearance of nodes down to the innominate vein is recommended (Harrison 1979). However, if positive nodes are present in the superior mediastinum, postoperative radiotherapy offers little in the way of palliation.

# Techniques for Reconstruction of Hypopharynx

Replacement of the upper food conduit after resection of a hypopharyngeal cancer is still an unsettled issue despite its being more than a century since Czerny first successfully resected an oesophageal cancer (1877) and von Mikulicz (1886) reconstructed the gullet with skin flaps. No single method is ideal for every patient as cure rates remain low whilst complication rates are high.

The two basic approaches use either a skin-lined tube or hollow abdominal viscus to close the surgically created defect.

In essence the problem is to replace a mucosal-lined cylinder sheathed in smooth muscle and cover it with skin. The new gullet will be a non-peristaltic gravity conduit and have only tongue thrust and gravity energised swallowing. An excellent, comprehensive historical review of many varied and imaginative procedures employed over the past 40 years to overcome this problem has been given by DeSanto and Carpenter (1980) and Surkin et al. (1984). Although many of these operations have long since been abandoned in favour of more sophisticated and effective procedures, radical, effective excision of the primary neoplasm still remains the most essential factor in long-term survival. Methods of reconstruction must not be allowed to influence the need for clear microscopical margins and this requires the surgeon to be able to carry out a wide range of reconstructive techniques, including microvascular anastomosis.

Table 7.2 details the various surgical techniques which have proved to be of some value although it is doubtful if any under the legend "Other" should be considered by the modern oncological surgeon.

## Cervical Skin Flaps

In 1907, Bircher tried to rebuild the entire oesophagus using anterior chest wall flaps. However, Wookey (1948) is usually credited with the successful use of cervical skin flaps following pharyngolaryngectomy. This technique was in fact a modification of methods previously used by Eggers (1925) and Trotter (1932). The Wookey modification uses a laterally based predesigned cervical skin flap usually left *in situ* with a pharyngostome and oesophagostome. After elevating the flap several times to enhance the blood supply coming from the lateral aspect, the flap is turned back on itself to form a tube and the skin defect closed with pedicled chest skin. The distance between tracheostome and oesophagostome is related to the amount of cervical oesophageal resection which may limit the lower

**Table 7.2.** Various surgical techniques used in reconstruction following pharyngolaryngectomy

| |
| --- |
| Cervical flaps |
|   Wookey-type repair |
| Tubed chest flaps |
|   Cutaneous (deltopectoral) |
|   Myocutaneous (pectoralis, trapezius) |
| Viscera |
|   Stomach |
|     Whole organ transposition |
|     Reversed gastric tube |
|     Antral autograft |
|   Colon |
|     Interposition |
|     Autograft |
|   Jejunum |
|     Autograft |
| Other |
|   Laryngotracheal autograft |
|   Tracheal autograft |
|   Skin grafts |
|   Distant skin flaps |
|   Mucosal flaps |
|   Prosthesis |

point of excision (Fig. 7.6). In post-irradiated patients delay in reconstruction was frequently greater than 6 months by which time local recurrence had appeared. Many modifications in technique were reported during the 1950s and 1960s but even when repair was completed, fistulae were common and stenosis virtually inevitable. However, the initial operative mortality and morbidity is low and in those patients where there is doubt regarding an adequate margin of excision superiorly it is wise to leave an open pharyngostome rather than bury residual disease. Later repair when the pharyngostome is considered free from disease can be carried out as a single stage using a pectoralis myocutaneous flap with a skin graft applied to the exposed muscle.

Despite the safety of using cervical skin flaps, Surkin et al. (1984) found an overall hospital mortality of 7% in 148 cases reported in the literature: complications associated with repair were 94%, including flap necrosis, fistula formation and long-term stenosis.

## Tubed Chest Flaps

It was inevitable that developments in the use of chest skin for head and neck reconstruction would be applied to the unsatisfactory use of local neck skin in repair after pharyngolaryngectomy. The use of the medially based delto-pectoral flap by Bakamjian (1965) offered a technique which was reasonably reliable, originated outside the usual radiation fields and required no surgical delay.

The basic Bakamjian flap is raised out to the shoulder, tubed with the skin-side in, placed under the cervical skin and attached end-to-end to the remaining oropharynx and to the oesophageal stump. Donor sites on chest and shoulder are covered with skin grafts (Fig. 7.7).

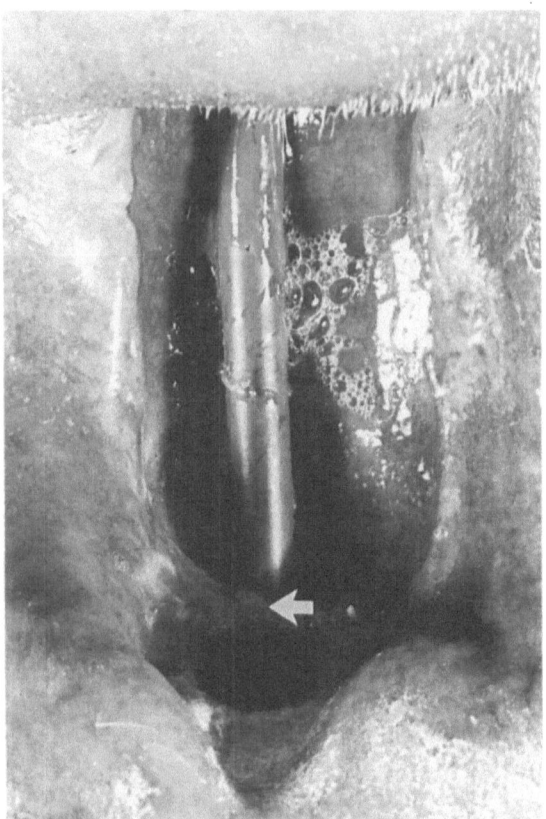

**Fig. 7.6.** Pharyngo-laryngectomy
– partition between
oesophagostome and tracheostome
(arrowed).

Whilst this was an obvious improvement over local skin flap repair, tubed delto-pectoral chest flaps also had their problems. Whilst being a safe operation, reconstructive problems were reported as 56% in 112 cases (Surkin et al. 1984), particularly related to fistula formation and stenosis. Hospitalisation was lengthy, averaging 10 weeks. Modification in technique occurred with increasing experience designed to improve the connection between skin tube and remaining oesophagus and to minimise the incidence of fistula formation. Compatibility with preoperative and postoperative irradiation depends on time interval, dosage and irradiation technique. Although De Santo and Carpenter (1980) stated that "the delto-pectoral flap should be a part of the head and neck surgeon's repertoire", it is doubtful if its use is now indicated except in exceptional circumstances.

## Myocutaneous Flap

The pectoralis myocutaneous flap has become the most widely used flap for reconstructive surgery within the head and neck. Hueston and McConchie (1968) described a compound pectoral flap in which the pectoralis major muscle was

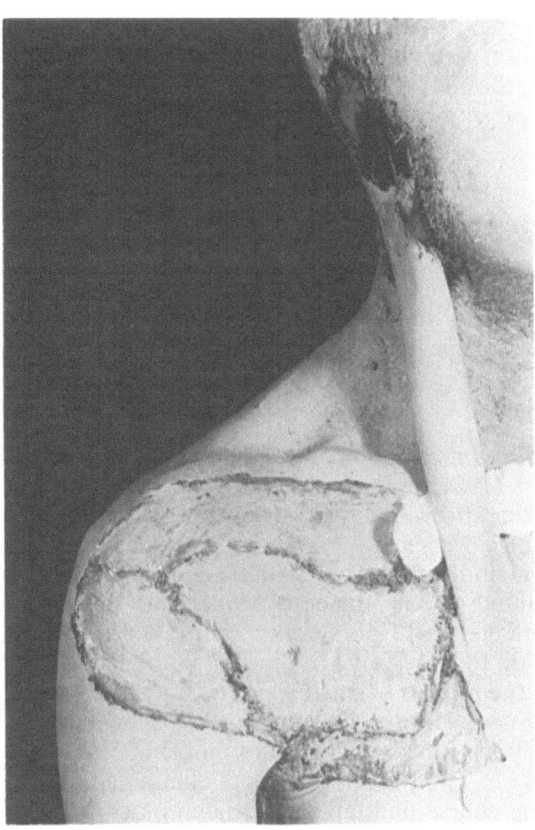

**Fig. 7.7.** Grafting of donor site following Bakamjian flap, showing cosmetic disability.

included but this technique never found favour. Ariyan (1979), using modifications of a pectoralis major myocutaneous flap, demonstrated its great versatility in repair of surgically created defects within the head and neck. This flap possesses a more reliable blood supply than the delto-pectoral flap but when used for pharyngoesophageal replacement is also associated with fistulae and subsequent stenosis. In some patients, its sheer bulk makes tubing difficult and it is difficult to see what advantage is gained by the coverage of the muscle with a quilted skin graft, as suggested by Robertson and Robinson (1984). Although a one-stage operation, unlike a similar technique described by Murakami et al. (1982), there appears to be no good reason why the flap cannot be inverted, with the skin graft then applied externally to the exposed muscle. This method has been used successfully by the author in patients undergoing a staged Wookey operation.

Fee (1984) states that "stenosis following reconstruction is a technical error in the main . . . resulting from failure to sew the mucocutaneous junction on stretch". This may be so in cases non-infected, non-irradiated and with good access. Unfortunately, if adequate excision is to be gained in cricoesophageal tumours, inferior access is often not good and although it is an extremely safe procedure, long-term results from the use of the pectoralis myocutaneous flap are far from satisfactory.

From personal experience, and reports from others, there appears to be little doubt that unless the patient is clearly unfit for abdominal surgery, visceral interposition offers the best opportunity of both cure and effective rehabilitation when surgical excision is required for postcricoid carcinoma.


## Visceral Interposition Procedures

A variety of abdominal viscera have been utilised with varying success to restore continuity following resection of postcricoid and cervical oesophageal cancer. Physiologically, only the gastric "pull up" and free revascularised bowel techniques approach the function of the hypopharynx – and neither do it as well as the original!

*Colon Interposition.* Although surgeons such as Nakayama et al. (1964), Eastcott (1964) and Grange and Quick (1978) have all attempted revascularised autografts with large bowel, colon has been most frequently used as a free pedicled segment for pharyngoesophageal interposition. Oesophageal reconstruction with an isoperistaltic or antiperistaltic loop of transverse colon brought through a subcutaneous tunnel was described in 1911 by Kelling. In 1954, Goligher and Robin described the successful transfer of the transverse and left colon to the pharynx following pharyngolaryngectomy. The interest stimulated by the reports of small series of apparently successful operations continued over the next decade. The antethoracic, subcutaneous route was abandoned since not only was it cosmetically deforming but required food to be milked down along its length. The retrosternal route eliminated the need for a thoracotomy but had a long course and left the remaining oesophagus as a blind loop. The posterior mediastinum provided the shortest pathway between pharynx and stomach whilst allowing total oesophagectomy. However, compression of the vascular pedicle by the bronchi was a danger in the posterior route and at least one sterno-clavicular joint required resection to increase the space at the exit of the anterior mediastinum.
  Colon interposition has the following advantages.

1. A long length allows easy pharyngeal anastomosis with good food transference
2. Supplying vessels are long and readily mobilised
3. Colonic-gastric anastomosis is not susceptible to peptic ulceration

However, published figures soon emphasised some of the disadvantages.

1. Considerable risk of wound infection
2. Tendency for the colon to be inert and to become distended
3. Necessity for two abdominal anastomoses

Whilst some surgeons favoured using the right colon because of the isoperistaltic nature, others felt that the better blood supply of the left colon overcame its antiperistaltic disadvantages. Of the 267 cases reported in the literature by 1984 (Surkin et al.) the operative mortality was 20%, with postoperative complications in 90% of patients. The anterior mediastinum is not designed to accommodate the bulky colon and dysphagia is common. Venous infarction is a considerable –

and invariably fatal – risk (Nicks 1967) and may relate to variations in vascularity of the colon. Selective mesenteric arteriography to select the most appropriate, well-vascularised colonic segment has been recommended by Ventemiglia et al. (1977) although this has not been commonly employed.

The isoperistaltic left colon provides the greatest length. Clamping of the left branch of the middle colic artery, leaving the colon pedicled on the left colic artery, confirms an adequate blood supply before division. Division of the transverse colon to the left of the middle colic artery and the descending colon as low as the blood supply allows should provide enough bowel to be brought behind the stomach and up through the vacant posterior mediastinum following pharyngolaryngoesophagectomy. Details of the complete procedure have been described by Griffiths and Shaw (1973), together with the various complications that may be encountered. They emphasise however the likelihood of a better swallowing mechanism following an isoperistaltic loop via the short retrosternal route and that a normal stomach is advantageous for proper nutrition and culinary enjoyment. Indeed, their comprehensive and detailed paper emphasises clearly the need for careful choice of both patient and surgical team in contemplating all types of visceral replacement surgery. With increasing experience with the gastric "pull up" operation and with small-bowel revascularisation techniques, colon has become less popular for replacement following surgical resection for postcricoid carcinoma. The information collected by Surkin et al. (1984) on 167 colonic interposition procedures included 8 of 14 publications where the number of operations was less than 10. Experience in choice of patients and technical expertise play an important part in operative mortality rates as well as long-term success.

However, in patients where the stomach is unavailable and total oesophagectomy is indicated, colonic transposition remains a valuable procedure in skilled hands.

*Gastric Transposition.* Although several surgeons had used a gastric tube in oesophoplasty by the subcutaneous route (Depage 1903) only the Heimlich (1966) reversed gastric tube, using the greater curvative antiperistaltically, had any value in pharyngoesophageal reconstruction. Even with the modifications introduced by Sugimachi et al. (1980), who divided and sutured the seromuscular and mucosal layers separately, the superior extent was limited, the blood supply distally was precarious and swallowing was poor. The first resection of a cervical oesophageal carcinoma with pharyngogastric reconstruction was reported by Shefts and Fischer in 1949. Although technically successful, the patient died of a pulmonary embolus on the sixth postoperative day. In 1960, Ong and Lee mobilised and anastomosed the stomach to the pharynx in four patients following resection of advanced laryngeal cancer which had invaded the postcricoid area by penetrating the posterior cricoid plate. There was one postoperative death but the feasibility of the procedure had been demonstrated and this operation remains the most effective means of treating advanced cricoesophageal cancers. Six years later, Le Quesne and Ranger (1966) reported 13 cases in which the fundus of the stomach was anastomosed to tongue base with two postoperative deaths but no stenosis. This technique, with minimal modifications, has now been adopted world-wide although both mortality and morbidity rates reflect the expertise and experience of the surgical teams. Stell et al. (1982) reported that 12 patients in a series of 40 patients died postoperatively (40%) whilst Harrison and

Thompson (1986) reporting 101 pharyngogastric anastomosis had 11 deaths (11%). Patient selection is obviously also of importance and even the most experienced surgeon with this technique – Lam et al. (1981) – reported an overall mortality of 31%, largely related to the poor medical condition of his patients and the advanced disease being treated.

The advantages of this operation are:

1. Total removal of the oesophagus, thus eliminating the possibility of inadequate inferior resection and multicentric lesions
2. Excision of paratracheal lymph nodes
3. No abdominal anastomosis and a one-stage operation
4. Excellent blood supply of the fundus, even in irradiated patients
5. Ready acceptance of skin graft by the cervically placed stomach, thus allowing resection of damaged or involved neck skin

Even in experienced hands, there is an unavoidable operative mortality secondary to the abdominal surgery, particularly in elderly debilitated patients or those with chronic lung or cardiovascular disease. Regurgitation of bile is common and the pharyngogastric anastomosis, although allowing trouble-free eating, is not conducive to good speech. Full feeding is usual within 7–12 days and the average period in hospital is 2–4 weeks.

*Anatomical Basis for Gastric Mobilisation.* Following the injection of the arterial tree of 22 stomachs obtained at autopsy, Thomas et al. (1979) demonstrated that the right gastroepiploic artery alone will perfuse the vessels in the fundus of the stomach, normally supplied by the left gastric artery. Perfusion is independent of the left gastric arcade and occurs through the submucosal anastomotic plexus. They conclude that, except in the presence of severe atherosclerosis, viability of the transposed fundus can be assured after preservation of only the right gastroepiploic artery.

This has been confirmed by the author's own experience of 140 gastric "pull up" operations, where gastric mobilisation by A. E. Thompson has been successful in every patient with no loss of viability of the fundus.

*Surgical Procedure (Author's Technique).* In essence the operation performed is that described by Ong and Lee in 1960 but with some important modifications based upon personal experience of 140 patients (Harrison and Thompson 1986). Thoracotomy is unnecessary since the oesophagus can be mobilised directly via the superior mediastinum and the enlarged oesophageal hiatus. It can best be described as a "synchronous combined manoeuvre", with the head and neck surgeon carrying out a pharyngolaryngectomy, as well as radical neck dissection or manubrial resection when indicated (Harrison 1977). The cervical and superior mediastinal oesophagus is mobilised from above and the abdominal surgeon then mobilises the stomach, duodenum and remaining oesophagus. The stomach can then be drawn up through the vacant posterior mediastinum allowing the fundus to be anastomosed to the open pharynx. Separation of the cut trachea from underlying oesophagus must be carried out with the balloon of the endotracheal tube deflated to minimise risk of a tear in the posterior tracheal wall. After the cardia has been divided and closed both pleural cavities are routinely drained by insertion of basal tubes. This is an essential procedure since it allows accurate assessment of postoperative blood loss from torn vessels in the posterior mediastinum. On average this amounts to 1500 ml over 36 hours and must be replaced. Particular care is taken when mobilising the duodenum and in performing a pyloromyotomy. A feeding jejunostomy tube is placed about 12 cm from the duodeno-jejunal flexure for postoperative feeding. Total thyroidectomy is carried out in all patients because of the difficulty in ensuring that the gland is not involved in cases of postcricoid carcinoma (Harrison 1973).

*Operative Mortality.* Comparisons of operative mortality rates between different centres and for varying techniques used in postcricoid ablation are hindered by numerous factors, not least of which is a lack of agreement on definition of hospital mortality (Stell et al. 1983). The most realistic definition is probably "the number of patients dying before they leave hospital, irrespective of cause".

Surkin et al. (1984), surveying the "overall mortality" for 255 gastric transpositions, quoted a figure of 15% dropping to 8% for the 146 cases reported in the last decade. Lam et al. (1981) quoted a mortality rate of 31% for 157 cases over a 14-year period, dropping to 18% during the last 2 years. The author's own experience of a mortality rate of 11% for the first 101 patients (Table 7.3) certainly confirms that poor selection was responsible for the deaths of at least 4 patients. Recent analysis of 140 patients shows an overall reduction to 9% mortality rate. It is doubtful if variations in these figures represent improved surgical experience unless a very limited number of patients are analysed. Preoperative chest infection, common in patients with obstructive lesions of the hypopharynx, is difficult to control. Poor respiratory reserve in heavy smokers or emphysema enhance the risk of any major operation whilst pulmonary emboli or myocardial infarction are hazards of all operations. Whilst haemorrhage and sepsis have not been a problem in this series, they were in the large series of Chinese patients operated upon by Lam et al. (1981).

**Table 7.3.** Hospital deaths after gastric "pull up"

| | |
|---|---|
| Operative death (aortic stenosis) | 1 |
| Pulmonary cause | |
|    Pulmonary embolism | 1 |
|    Bronchopneumonia | 1 |
|    Respiratory failure | 1 |
| Cardiovascular | |
|    Myocardial infarct | 3 |
|    Hypotension | 2 |
| Mesenteric thrombosis | 1 |
| Graft necrosis | 1 |
| Total | 11/101 (11%) |

Many patients present in poor general condition following previous unsuccessful irradiation, uncontrolled diabetes, hypertension and malnutrition. Whilst attempts must be made to improve their state prior to surgery they present as an additional operative risk. Unless a policy of rigorous selection is adopted, thereby depriving many patients of the possibility of cure or at least worthwhile palliation, it is unlikely that hospital mortality rates below 10% can be expected even in the most experienced centres.

*Postoperative Complications.* Morbidity may best be defined as non-lethal complications; such complications are present after all operations to some extent. Tables 7.4 and 7.5 show the postoperative complication rate in the experience of Harrison (1986) and of Lam et al. (1981). The marked difference between the wound infection rate may be due to a low incidence of fistula in the author's cases, possibly secondary to the routine use of metronidazole (Flagyl) as anti-anaerobic coverage (Innis et al. 1980).

**Table 7.4.**   Morbidity after gastric "pull up"

| | | |
|---|---|---|
| Pleural effusion | all | (routine drains) |
| Cardiac arrhythmia | all | (during operation) |
| Pharyngogastric fistula | 2 | (2%) |
| Sloughing of skin – stomach | 2 | (2%) |
| Wound infection | nil | |
| Abdominal wound dehiscence | 2 | (2%) |
| Colon prolapse into chest | 1 | (1%) |
| Chest infection | 15 | (15%) |
| Bile regurgitation | 22 | (22%) |
| Diarrhoea | all | |

**Table 7.5.**   Morbidity after pharyngolaryngoesophagectomy and pharyngogastric anastomosis (Lam et al. 1981)

| | | |
|---|---|---|
| Leakage | 36 | 23% |
| Sloughing of skin flaps | 19 | 12% |
| Wound infection | 43 | 27% |
| Haemorrhage | 32 | 20% |
| Partial gangrene of fundus | 4 | 3% |
| Mediastinitis | 3 | 2% |
| Bronchopneumonia | 43 | 27% |
| Pleural effusion | 24 | 15% |
| Pneumothorax | 10 | 6% |
| Chylothorax | 1 | 1% |
| Cardiac arrhythmia | 10 | 6% |

Previous radiotherapy had no influence on healing of the pharyngogastric anastomosis and any severely damaged skin was resected with a skin graft applied to the surface of the transposed stomach (Howard and Lund 1984). Chest infection remains a major problem in all series and postoperative physiotherapy is most important.

Bile regurgitation invariably ceased with oral feeding of liquids by the fifth postoperative day, but an occasional patient continued to complain of this unpleasant sensation long after full feeding. Diarrhoea occurs in all patients with jejunostomy feeding irrespective of the type of feed used and one patient had sudden intestinal obstruction from a prolapse of a colonic loop through the diaphram (Fig. 7.8).

Excellent swallowing is reported by all surgeons, although influenced in part by patient motivation since the absence of pharyngeal constriction required the sole use of the tongue to initiate deglutition. Damage to the hypoglossal nerve would seriously hamper eating – "dumping" has not been a problem possibly because many patients with postcricoid carcinomas have been "small swallowers" for many years.

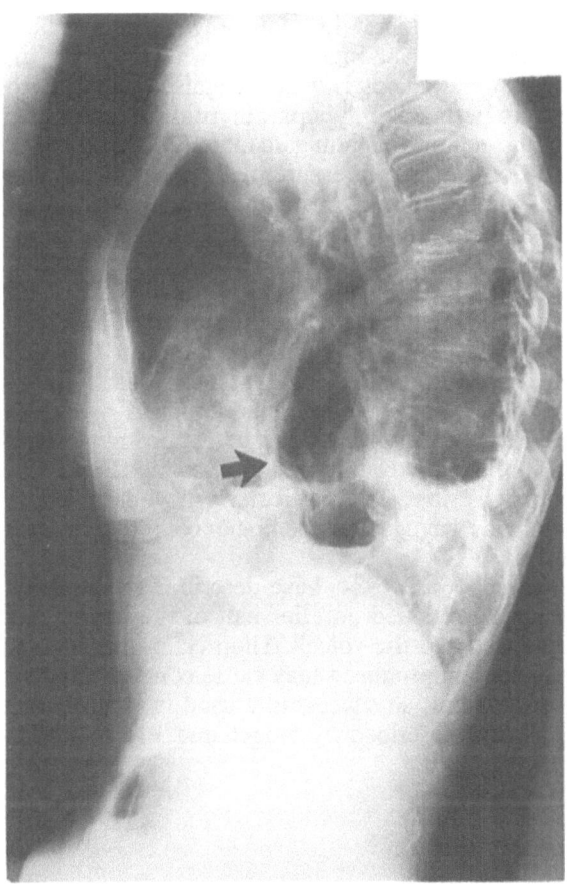

**Fig. 7.8.** Lateral chest radiograph showing colon in chest after herniating through diaphragm (arrowed).

*Long-term Problems and Survival.* In comparing the relative success of operations now used in the management of postcricoid cancer it is necessary to consider not only the intrinsic risk of the operation but the age and general condition of the patient, extent of disease and the effectiveness of the patient's rehabilitation. Patients will continue to die from further neoplasms, systemic metastases, generalised disease or other unrelated causes. Over 50% of the 109 operative survivors reported by Lam et al. (1981) died from recurrent or metastatic disease, mostly with regional lymph node metastasis. An actuarial 5-year figure of 8.9% reflected a high operative mortality rate and advanced disease. Harrison and Thompson (1986) reported an actuarial 5-year survival rate of 58% with most of the deaths occurring within the first year. With increasing experience, good follow-up and an increasing number of long-term patients, many of the earlier problems relating to calcium metabolism have disappeared (Harrison 1978; Wei et al. 1984).

Thyroid replacement is routine in our cases whilst after partial thyroidectomy, particularly following previous radiotherapy, thyroid function tests will assist in deciding whether adequate functional tissue remains. Transplantation of parathyroid tissue, as considered by Freeman et al. (1982), is ideal but has proved technically difficult in some advanced or irradiated cases and is potentially undesirable. Although the known variability in number and location of the parathyroid glands is well recognised, total thyroidectomy does not invariably lead to permanent hypoparathyroidism unless combined with superior mediastinal dissection. Calcium gluconate (20–30 ml of 10%) is added to the intravenous infusion and daily measurements of serum calcium and phosphate are continued until jejunostomy feeds commence. Often, additional amounts are needed to maintain normal levels and supplements (given as Calcium-Sandoz tablets 2.6 g/ day) may be added to oral feeds. If serum calcium remains persistently low vitamin D, usually as oral calciferol 40 000 I.U. i.v., may be required. Buchanan et al. (1975) investigated some of these refractory cases and emphasised that serum calcium levels should be monitored for at least 3 years since recovery of parathyroid function could occur, resulting in hypercalcaemia and nephrocalcinosis if supplements were continued.

The excellent cosmetic result following pharyngogastric anastomosis together with relatively trouble-free swallowing (Fig. 7.9) is, however, associated with a poor "gastric voice", particularly in women. The few good speakers either have a small pharyngogastric opening or compress the cervical stomach when regurgitating air.

Krespi et al. (1984) have described the construction of a tracheogastric shunt using the retained anterior half of the larynx and upper trachea to produce an enhanced "gastric voice". Their claim that in five patients oncological resection was not compromised may cause concern. Recent experience with the tracheogastric shunt, so successfully used in laryngectomy patients (tracheo-oesophageal) and described by Singer and Blom (1980), suggests that well-motivated

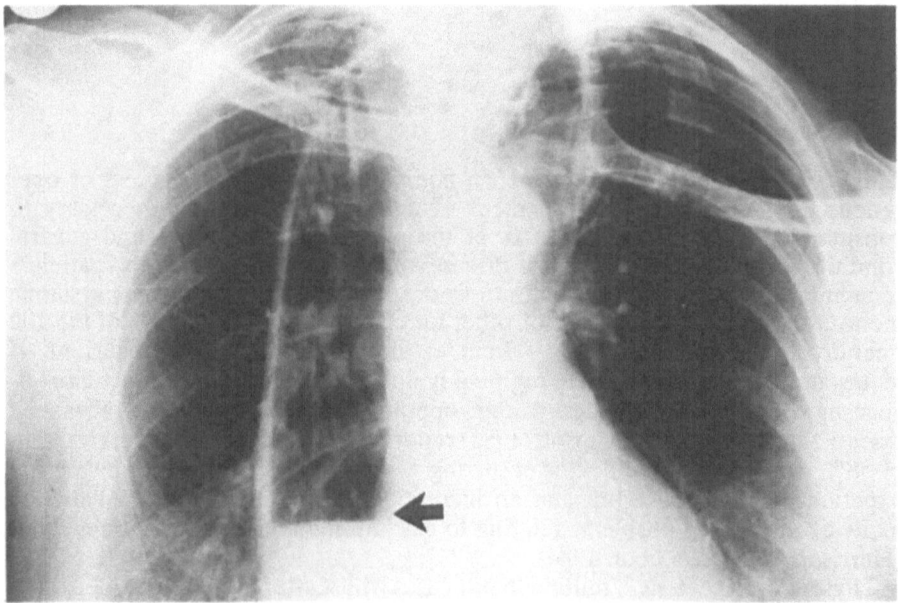

**Fig. 7.9.**   Chest radiograph showing air and fluid level in transposed stomach (arrowed).

individuals with good prognosis may benefit from this prosthesis. Surprisingly, the electrolarynx is not successful in all patients, possibly due to poor motivation, loss of tactile sensation in neck skin following previous irradiation or an inability to cope with yet another disability.

The operation of pharyngogastric anastomosis allows extensive inferior resection of cricoesophageal tumours, identical superior limitations to other procedures, and in one stage, gives good functional return of deglutition. Even in experienced hands the operation is not without risk but it does fulfil many of the criteria for the ideal reconstruction for postcricoid carcinoma.

## Revascularised Small Bowel

Pedicled viscera have long been used for oesophageal replacement but jejunum required several loops of bowel to maintain an intact pedicle when transferred into the chest. In 1959 Allison described the transposition of a Roux loop of jejunum to the pharynx following resection of a postcricoid carcinoma. This method found little favour and subsequent techniques have used revascularised autografts.

Following Seidenberg's report (Seidenberg et al. 1959) of the successful use of revascularised jejunum for oesophageal replacement in dogs and in one patient, several case reports appeared during the next decade, (Harrison 1964; Peters et al. 1971). Somewhat inexplicably the technique, although not difficult, failed to fine favour until revitalised, primarily by Gluckman et al. (1982) and Thiele et al. (1986). As with other methods of repair, reports collected from various sources of varying experience give an overall mortality rate of 8% and a 16% incidence of graft necrosis (Surkin et al. 1983). This is far greater than that reported by Gluckman et al. (1985), where there was no mortality and a graft failure of 7.6% in 52 patients.

*Surgical Technique.* This is a two-team operation with the head and neck surgeon resecting the primary tumour and preserving if possible the superior thyroid artery or, alternatively, the lingual or facial artery. The venous anastomosis is usually to the preserved external jugular or common facial vein.

For harvesting the jejunum, the second team identify Trietz's ligament and search for a suitable segment about 60 cm distal. This should have a large feeding vessel off the superior mesenteric artery which must not be damaged. The bowel segment is isolated on the feeding pedicle and is usually 6–22 cm long. After anastomosis, care being taken to arrange the segment isoperistaltically, the segment is sutured to the pharynx whilst a stapler is used for the lower anastomosis to the oesophagus (Gluckman et al. 1982). Enteral feeding via a nasogastric tube is started immediately after the ileus has recovered and oral feeding commenced 6–8 days postoperatively, after confirmation by gastrograffin swallow that healing is sound. Publications show the same variety of complications that occur after any major head and neck operation with the exception that graft necrosis can be quickly recognised and the avascular bowel removed safely. Direct inspection of the graft via the oropharynx gives adequate indication of viability and if diagnosed early enough can be replaced by a second segment. This minimises the danger of great vessel rupture which in earlier publications was associated with late diagnosis of graft necrosis.

Most patients will have some degree of graft oedema and mild dysphagia for several months. Stenosis of both upper and lower anastomosis is reported but Theile et al. (1986) found long-term swallowing for both solids and fluids to be good in 72 patients.

As with stomach and colon, tolerance to postoperative radiotherapy is good although this modality rarely succeeds in controlling neoplasm left *in situ*. In skilled hands there can be little doubt that, providing the lower oesophageal resection is amenable to anastomosis, revascularised jejunum has an important role to play in reconstruction following pharyngolaryngectomy.

The operating time depends primarily on the experience of the microvascular team. The technique is straightforward if the vessels are around 2 mm in diameter, but the time for operation may range from 5 to 17 hours. However, with increased experience, success rates will rise and this must be considered the method of choice for most postcricoid carcinomas where expert facilities are available.

## Palliation

Thirty-four patients in 114 postcricoid carcinomas seen by Stell et al. (1978) were considered as untreatable at diagnosis. This decision was reached because of the extent of the tumour, old age, poor general condition and fixed neck nodes. Only 6% survived longer than 6 months although the causes of their deaths were not recorded. Even patients considered as potentially curable will prove to have extraluminal tumour on exploration and many curative procedures are themselves palliative.

If patients' symptoms are to be improved, even if long-term cure is unlikely, then the operation must have an acceptable mortality rate and achieve restoration of swallowing quickly. Repair with a pectoralis myocutaneous flap does not always meet these requirements, particularly if disease is left within the neck. Penetration of colon or jejunum by tumour occurs quickly and only the transposed stomach has any long-term resistance to invasion – the patient usually swallowing freely for at least 6 months. However, the potential mortality and morbidity rates makes this unacceptable unless the patient is relatively young and fit. Neither radiotherapy nor chemotherapy is of any value in attaining meaningful palliation in such cases and surgery is not indicated, particularly with fixed regional lymph nodes.

## Conclusions

There is little expectation that patients with postcricoid or cricoesophageal cancer will be diagnosed at an early stage where primary radiotherapy could expect to produce long-term cure without dysphagia. Problems in obtaining local control are largely related to the extent of the tumour at diagnosis and may require pharyngolaryngectomy or pharyngolaryngoesophagectomy with manubrial resection. If the most appropriate procedure for reconstructing the resulting defect is to be offered to each patient then the surgical team should be skilled in the use of pectoralis myocutaneous flaps, gastric "pull up" operations and revascularised jejunal autografts. All have their place and only by centralisation of expertise can minimal mortality and morbidity rates be achieved.

# References

Allison PR (1959) Postcricoid carcinoma. Proc R Soc Med 52:176

Ariyan S (1979) The pectoralis major myocutaneous flap: a versatile flap for reconstruction in the head and neck. Plast Reconstr Surg 63:73–81

Bakamjian VY (1965) A two-stage method for pharyngoesophageal reconstruction with a primary pectoral skin flap. Plast Reconstr Surg 36:173–184

Bircher E (1907) Ein Beitrag zur plastischen bilding eines neuen osophagus. Zentralbl Chir 34:1479–1482

Brown-Kelly A (1919) Spasm at the entrance of the oesophagus. J Laryngol 34:285–289

Bryce DP (1967) Pharyngectomy in the treatment of carcinoma of the hypopharynx. In: Conley J (ed) Cancer of the head and neck. Butterworths, Washington DC, pp 341–346

Buchanan G, West TET, Woodhead JS (1975) Hypoparathyroidism following pharyngolaryngoesophagectomy. Clin Oncol 1:89–95

Czerney F (1877) Neue Operationen. Zentralbl Chir 4:433–434

Depage A (1903) Nouvelle methode de gastrostomie. Presse Méd 19:755–759 (abstract)

DeSanto LW, Carpenter RS (1980) Reconstruction of the pharynx and upper esophagus after resection for cancer. Head Neck Surg 2:369–379

Eastcott HNG (1964) Colonic reconstruction of the pharynx. Lancet II:1182–1187

Eggers C (1925) Removal of carcinoma of lower oesophagus: recovery. Carcinoma of the upper oesophagus and pharynx. Ann Surg 81:693–698

Farrington WT, Weighill JS, Jones PH (1986) Postcricoid carcinoma (a ten-year retrospective study). J Laryngol 100:70–84

Fee WE (1984) Hypopharyngeal reconstruction. Arch Otolaryngol 110:384–385

Freeman JL, Shaw HJ, Noyek AM, Goldberg M (1982) Parathyroid gland transplantation after total thyroidectomy with pharyngolaryngoesophagectomy. Head Neck Surg 6:610–612

Gluckman JL, McDonough S, Donegan JO (1982) The role of free jejunal graft in reconstruction of the pharynx and cervical oesophagus. Head Neck Surg 4:360–369

Gluckman J, McCafferty GJ, Black R, Coman WB (1985) Complications associated with free jejunal graft reconstruction of the pharyngoesophagus – a multi institutional experience with 52 cases. Head Neck Surg 7:200–205

Goligher JC, Robin IG (1954) Use of left colon for reconstruction of pharynx and oesophagus after pharyngolaryngectomy. Br J Surg 42:283–290

Grange TB, Quick CA (1978) Use of revascularized ileocolic autografts for primary repair after pharyngolaryngoesophagectomy. Am J Surg 136:477–485

Griffiths JD, Shaw HS (1973) Cancer of the laryngopharynx and cervical oesophagus. Arch Otolaryngol 97:340–346

Harrison DFN (1964) The use of colonic transplants and revascularized jejunal autografts for primary repair after pharyngolaryngectomy. Proc R Soc Med 57:30–34

Harrison DFN (1970) Pathology of hypopharyngeal cancer in relation to surgical management. J Laryngol 84:349–367

Harrison DFN (1973) Thyroid gland in the management of laryngopharyngeal cancer. Arch Otolaryngol 97:301–302

Harrison DFN (1977) Resection of the manubrium. Br J Surg 64:374–377

Harrison DFN (1978) Rehabilitation problems after pharyngogastric anastomosis. Arch Otolaryngol 104:244–246

Harrison DFN (1979) Surgical management of hypopharyngeal cancer. Arch Otolaryngol 105:149–152

Harrison DFN, Thompson AE (1986) Pharyngolaryngoesophagectomy with pharyngogastric anasto-
   mosis for cancer of the hypopharynx: review of 101 operations. Head Neck Surg 8:418–428
Heimlich HJ (1966) Elective replacement of the oesophagus. Br J Surg 53:913–916
Howard D, Lund VJ (1984) Skin grafting of the anterior stomach wall following pharyngogastric
   anastomosis. J Laryngol 99:273–276
Hueston JT, McConchie IH (1968) A compound pectoral flap. Aust NZ J Surg 36:61–64
Innis AS, Windle-Taylor PC, Harrison DFN (1980) The role of metronidazole in the prevention of
   fistulae following total laryngectomy. Clin Oncol 6:71–77
Jacobs A (1961) Anaemia and postcricoid carcinoma. Br J Cancer 15: 736–744
Kelling G (1911) Esophagoplastic et de ses diverses modifications. Semin Méd 31:529–531
Krespi YP, Sisson GA, Wurster CF (1984) Voice preservation in postcricoid and cervical esophageal
   cancer. Arch Otolaryngol 110:323–326
Lam KH, Wong J, Ong GB (1981) Pharyngogastric anastomosis following pharyngolaryngoesopha-
   gectomy. Analysis of 157 cases. World J Surg 5:509–516
Larsson LG, Sandstrom A, Westling P (1975) Relationship of Plummer–Vinson disease to cancer of
   the upper alimentary tract in Sweden. Cancer Res 35:3308–3314
Le Quesne LP, Ranger D (1966) Pharyngolaryngectomy with immediate pharyngogastric anastomosis. Br J Surg 53:105–109
Looser KG, Shah JP, Strong EW (1978) The significance of "positive" margins in surgically resected
   epidermoid carcinomas. Head Neck Surg 1:107–111
Lord IJ, Briant TDR, Rider WD, Bryce DP (1973) A comparison of pre-operative and primary
   radiotherapy in the treatment of carcinoma of the hypopharynx. Br J Radiol 46:175–179
McNab Jones RF (1961) The Paterson–Brown–Kelly syndrome: its relationship to iron deficiency and
   postcricoid carcinoma. J Laryngol 75:529–544
Mikulicz J (1886) Ein fall von resection des carcinomatosen oesophagus mit plastichen ersatz des
   excidirten stuckes. Prag Med Wochenschr 11:93–97
Murakami Y, Saito S, Ikari T, Haraguchi S, Okada K, Marvyama T (1982) Esophageal reconstruction
   with a skin-grafted pectoralis major muscle flap. Arch Otolaryngol 108:719–722
Nakayama K, Yamamoto Y, Tamiya T, Nakino H (1964) Experience with free autografts of the bowel
   with a new venous anastomosis apparatus. Surgery 55:796–802
Nicks R (1967) Colon replacement of the oesophagus. Br J Surg 54:124–129
Ong GB, Lee TC (1960) Pharyngogastric anastomosis after oesophagopharyngectomy for carcinoma
   of the hypopharynx and cervical oesophagus. Br J Surg 48:193–200
Paterson DR (1919) A clinical type of dysphagia. J Laryngol 34:289–291
Pearson BW (1966) Radiotherapy of the oesophagus and postcricoid region in South-East Scotland.
   Clin Radiol 17:242–257
Peters CR, McKee DM, Barry BE (1971) Pharyngoesophageal reconstruction with revascularized
   jejunal transplants. Am J Surg 121:675–678
Robertson MS, Robinson JM (1984) Immediate pharyngoesophageal reconstruction. Arch Otolaryn-
   gol 110:386–387
Seidenberg B, Rosenak S, Hurwitt ES, Som ML (1959) Immediate reconstruction of the cervical
   oesophagus by a revascularised isolated jejunal segment. Ann Surg 142:162–171
Shefts LM, Fischer A (1949) Carcinoma of the cervical esophagus with one stage total esophageal
   resection and pharyngogastrostomy. Surgery 25:849–867
Singer M, Blom E (1980) An endoscopic technique for restoration of voice following laryngectomy.
   Ann Otol Rhinol Laryngol 90:529–533
Stell PM (1973) Cancer of the hypopharynx. J R Coll Surg Edinb 18:20–30
Stell PM, Carden EA, Hibbert J, Dalby JE (1978) Postcricoid carcinoma in South-East Scotland. Clin
   Radiol 17:242–257
Stell PM, Ramadan MF, George WD (1982) Postcricoid carcinoma: the place of visceral transposi-
   tion. Clin Oncol 8:17–20
Stell PM, Missotten F, Singh SD, Ramadan F, Morton RP (1983) Mortality after surgery for
   hypopharyngeal cancer. Br J Surg 70:713–718
Sugimachi K, Yaita A, Veo H (1980) A safer and more reliable operative technique for oesophageal
   reconstruction using a gastric tube. Am J Surg 140:471–476
Surkin MI, Lawson W, Biller HF (1984) Analysis of the methods of pharyngoesophageal reconstruction. Head Neck Surg 6:953–970
Theile DE, Robinson DW, McCafferty GJ (1986) Pharyngolaryngectomy reconstruction by revascularised free jejunal graft. Aust NZ J Surg 56:849–852
Thomas DM, Langford RM, Russell RCG, Le Quesne LP (1979) The anatomical basis for gastric
   mobilisation in total oesophagectomy. Br J Surg 66:230–233

Trotter W (1932) Malignant disease of the hypopharynx and its treatment by excision. Br Med J i:510–513

Ventemiglia R, Khalil KG, Frazer OH, Mountain CF (1977) Role of preoperative mesenteric arteriography in colon interposition. J Thorac Cardiovasc Surg 74:98–110

Wei W, Lam KH, Choi S, Wong J (1984) Late problems after pharyngolaryngoesophagectomy and pharyngogastric anastomosis for cancer of the larynx and hyopharynx. Am J Surg 148:509–513

Willatt DS, Jackson SR, McCormick MS, Lubsen H, Michaels L, Stell PM (1987) Vocal cord paralysis and tumour length in staging postcricoid carcinoma. Eur J Surg Oncol 13:131–137

Wookey H (1948) The surgical treatment of carcinoma of the hypopharynx and the oesophagus. Br J Surg 35:249–266

Wynder EL, Hultberg S, Jacobsson F, Bross IJ (1957) Environmental factors in cancer of the upper alimentary tract. Cancer 10:470–487

# Chapter 8

# Surgical Resection for Intrathoracic Carcinoma

R. E. Lea

## Introduction

Once the diagnosis of carcinoma of the oesophagus has been made a decision has to be taken on the method of treatment or palliation. Available methods are:

1. Surgical removal of the tumour
2. Radiotherapy
3. Surgical bypass
4. Intubation
5. Chemotherapy
6. Laser therapy

On the information that is currently available the best treatment for an intrathoracic tumour is surgical removal. This not only offers the prospect of a cure but also gives excellent palliation. It has been suggested that radiotherapy is the treatment of choice for squamous carcinoma of the oesophagus. This is usually based on Pearson's (1969) results, which suggested a 5-year survival of 20% following radical radiotherapy. Unfortunately, no other radiotherapist has been able to produce similar results. These figures are also compared with all oesophageal resections. Evidence is emerging that the surgical results with squamous carcinoma are better than with adenocarcinoma, with a 5-year survival rate of 25% or more (Griffith and Davis 1980). Surgery, however, is a major procedure and before embarking on this course it must be ascertained that the tumour has not spread widely and that the patient has a reasonable life expectancy. If this is not the case, resection should not be considered and an alternative method of management will have to be used.

# Preoperative Assessment

Factors that should be considered are:

1. Age
2. Size and extent of the tumour
3. General fitness of the patient

## Age

Carcinoma of the oesophagus is more common in the elderly. Age alone is not important and surgery can be successful in patients in their ninth decade. What is of more importance is their activity and general interest in life. An active 80-year-old with a will to recover has a much better prospect of recovery than a sedentary 60-year-old with little interest in life. It is helpful to try and assess a patient's likely life expectancy if he did not have carcinoma and, if this appears to be good, surgical treatment should be considered. Therefore, although no specific age should be considered as a bar to an operation, it should be remembered that any surgical complication is more serious in the older patient.

## Size and Extent of Tumour

The size of the tumour is important as the larger the tumour the more likelihood there is of full thickness penetration of the wall and local invasion. The length of the tumour can be fairly accurately assessed by a barium swallow, but lateral extent is more difficult. Occasionally, this can be seen on a barium swallow (Fig. 8.1). Computerised tomography is of more help but is not infallible in assessing local invasion (Thompson et al. 1983). It will also give some indication of nodal involvement both in the chest and abdomen. Bronchoscopy will give some indication of lateral spread in tumours of the proximal two-thirds of the oesophagus and should always be done. The important area to examine is the medial wall of both main bronchi but particularly the left. Metastases in the liver should be excluded by CT scanning or ultrasound; the latter is slightly more sensitive.

## General Fitness of the Patient

Apart from the extent of the tumour, the general fitness of the patient is important. Major points to consider are:

   1. *Cardiovascular.* As many of the patients are elderly and also have a history of smoking, cardiovascular problems are common. A previous myocardial

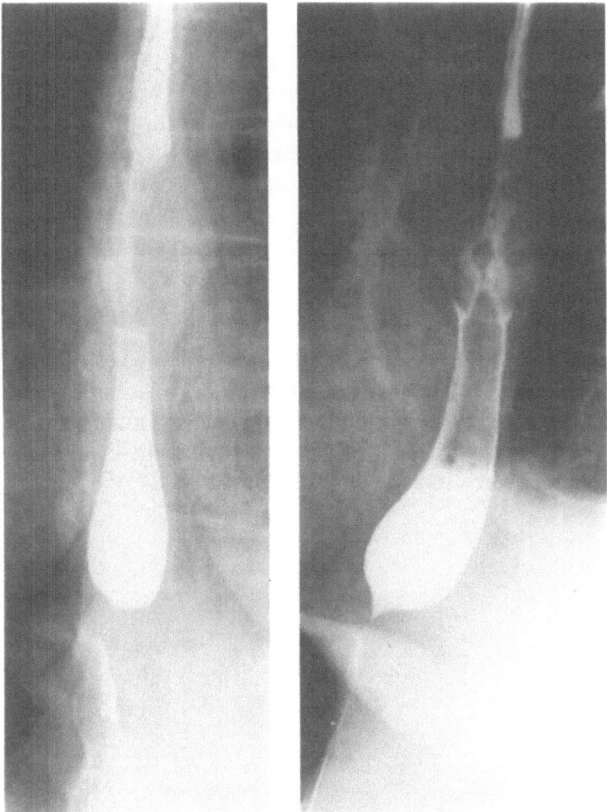

**Fig. 8.1.** Barium swallow showing lateral extent of the carcinoma.

infarction is not a contraindication provided the patient has made a good recovery. A cerebrovascular accident is more serious and does appear to increase the risk of an operation, with a high chance of further cerebral problems.

2. *Pulmonary Function.* As the majority of patients with carcinoma of the oesophagus have smoked, all have a degree of lung damage. It is helpful to do simple spirometry tests which give an indication of lung function. Although there are no absolute figures which would contraindicate an operation, a patient with a FEV$_1$ below 1.0 l should be very carefully assessed.

Aspiration pneumonia may occur as the result of dysphagia, but it is usually only a complication of total dysphagia. It is serious as it will delay or even prohibit an operation.

3. *Renal Function.* Although the patient may not have any renal disease, urinary output may be reduced due to a restricted fluid intake. Any degree of dehydration must be corrected, either by increased oral fluids or, if this is not possible, intravenously.

4. *Nutrition.* Almost all patients at the time of presentation have lost weight but most are still in a reasonable physical state. Many articles have been written

on nutrition but there is no convincing evidence that intensive preoperative feeding improves postoperative mortality or morbidity apart from wound infections (Heatley et al. 1979). In most cases, all that is required is to correct dehydration. Occasionally, in a patient who is extremely wasted, a short course (a week is probably adequate) of intravenous feeding and vitamin supplements is indicated. In a small trial on nutritional status carried out by the author the postsurgical morbidity and mortality were no different in patients with impaired nutrition (Lea et al. 1986).

## Selection of Patients for Operation

Clearly, many patients are not fit for an operation. Although the operability rate varies, in the United Kingdom probably only 25% of all patients are submitted to an operation. Some excellent statistics are provided by the West Midlands Cancer Registry (Matthews et al. 1987). Over a twenty-five-year period 4680 patients with carcinoma of the oesophagus were included. Of these 1143 (24.4%) had a resection.

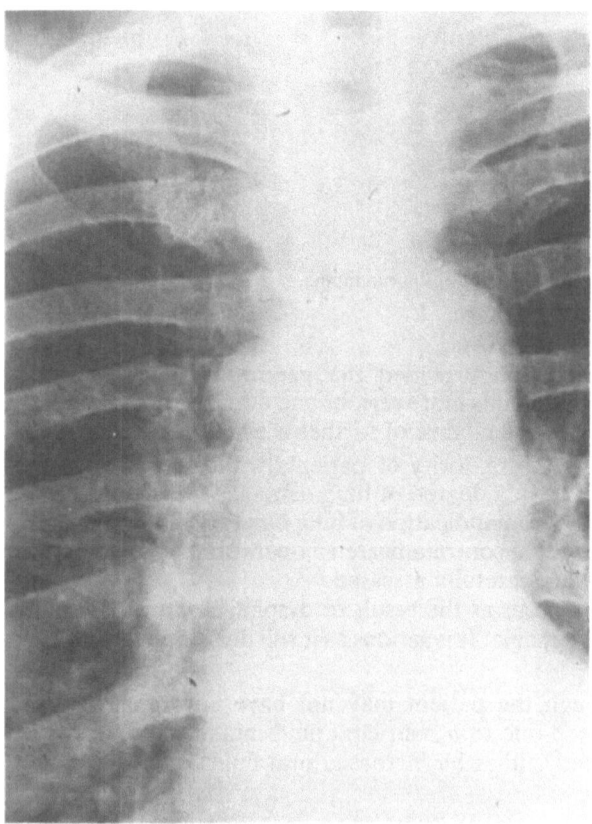

**Fig. 8.2.**   Chest radiograph showing tumour in the azygos vein.

Patients are either inoperable due to the extent of the disease or because of their poor general health. The general health of the patient is part of his or her initial assessment. Some patients are borderline and only experience of similar cases will provide an answer. Provided there is no evidence of metastases or local invasion of vital structures the patient should be treated by an operation (Fig. 8.2).

# Preoperative Treatment

The patient should be admitted 2–3 days prior to the operation. When previously seen he should have been told to stop smoking. A chest radiograph should be done to exclude any lung complications or possible tumour spread. Physiotherapy is important before operation and is vital after operation.

Fluid input and output should be measured and if inadequate intravenous fluids are given. Plasma urea, creatinine and electrolytes are measured and liver function tests carried out.

Although the stomach is generally used in reconstruction it is occasionally necessary to use the jejunum or colon. It is therefore helpful to have the colon empty as a final decision may not be made till operation. This also avoids the discomfort of constipation after the operation. A low-residue diet is given together with a stimulant laxative. Sodium picosulphate with magnesium sulphate (Picolax) is most effective.

The operation is covered by antibiotics which are either given with the premedication or when the intravenous line is established in theatre. Cefuroxime 750 mg 8-hourly for 48-hours is effective in most cases.

# Types of Operation (with Use of Stomach)

### Anaesthesia

It is extremely helpful to have a double lumen endobronchial tube, allowing one-lung anaesthesia. Exposure is enhanced and retraction of the lung by the assistant is not necessary.

Full postoperative monitoring should be done and therefore radial artery and central venous pressure lines and a urinary catheter are inserted. In many cases, intensive monitoring may appear excessive as the patient makes an uneventful recovery. However, by strict observation any complication can be promptly detected and early corrective measures applied.

Deep vein thrombosis and pulmonary embolism are potential complications and preventive measures should be taken. Compressed stockings and Flowtron boots on the operating table are simple to use and appear to be of value. Subcutaneous heparin has been recommended but in the author's experience is associated with increased bleeding.

## Surgical Approach

There is no ideal approach for all cases and the method used depends on the site of the tumour. The main procedures available are:

Left oesophago-gastrectomy
Ivor Lewis/Tanner operation
McKeown operation
Left oesophago-gastrectomy with left cervical anastomosis
Transhiatal oesophagectomy without thoracotomy
Bilateral thoracotomy

All these procedures usually use the stomach for reconstruction but it is possible to use the jejunum or colon.

A major factor in deciding which approach to use is the site of the tumour. Because the arch of the aorta is on the left side, tumours involving the proximal three-quarters of the oesophagus have usually been treated from the right side. On this side, the only structure covering the oesophagus is the mediastinal pleura and the arch of the azygos vein. Apart from the site of the tumour, the philosophy of the surgeon is a factor. An example of this is the recent vogue for an oesophagectomy without a thoracotomy. Although good results are claimed, many surgeons consider this a poor cancer operation. Such a surgeon is unlikely to use this technique.

A straightforward approach is to treat tumours at or just above the oesophago-gastric junction from the left and more proximal tumours from the right.

### *Left Oesophago-gastrectomy*

This procedure is indicated for tumours around the oesophago-gastric junction and is ideal for a total gastrectomy. It is usually confined to tumours at 35 cm from the incisor teeth or beyond. The patient must be accurately placed on the operating table, lying on the right side. The shoulders should be at right angles to the table but the pelvis is rotated backwards to 45 degrees. The simplest method to maintain this position is a vacuum bean bag. Pressure points should be carefully padded, in particular to protect the right common peroneal nerve. Undue pressure at this point can result in a postoperative foot-drop.

A thoraco-abdominal incision is made through the seventh intercostal space. To give the best exposure the incision should be mainly a thoracotomy with a short extension onto the abdomen (Fig. 8.3). The abdominal portion should be made first so that operability can be assessed. Spread to the left gastric lymph nodes is common and fixity at this point or distant spread suggests it is unwise to proceed. If resection is feasible the incision is extended onto the chest fully dividing the latissimus dorsi muscle. The costal margin is divided, with excision of a 2-cm segment. This is to prevent overriding of the cut ends when the wound is closed. The diaphragm is partially divided around the circumference for 8–10 cm leaving 1 cm attached to the chest wall, to allow closure. This incision, instead of a radial incision in the diaphragm, avoids cutting the phrenic nerve. A rib spreader is inserted and the full extent of the tumour assessed. In the majority of cases a

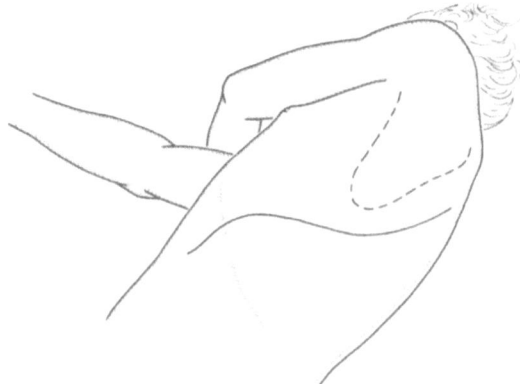

**Fig. 8.3.** Line drawing of left thoraco-abdominal incision.

partial oesophago-gastrectomy will give adequate clearance but extensive gastric involvement will require a total gastrectomy.

When part of the stomach is to be retained it is mobilised by dividing the left gastric artery and preserving the right gastric vessels with the gastro-epiploic arcade. This requires division of the left gastro-epiploic artery and the omental branches (Fig. 8.4). If the omentum is very fatty, it is better to remove it otherwise fat necrosis may occur due to ischaemia. The short gastric vessels are also divided although sometimes the spleen should be removed to give adequate clearance. After the greater curve has been freed, the stomach can be retracted upwards and the left gastric vessels divided. If there are involved nodes around the artery it may be necessary to divide the pancreas. A Payr's clamp is placed across the body of the pancreas, which is then divided on the distal side of the clamp. Interlocking non-absorbable mattress sutures are placed proximal to the clamp and ligated after removal of the clamp. After dividing the lesser omentum

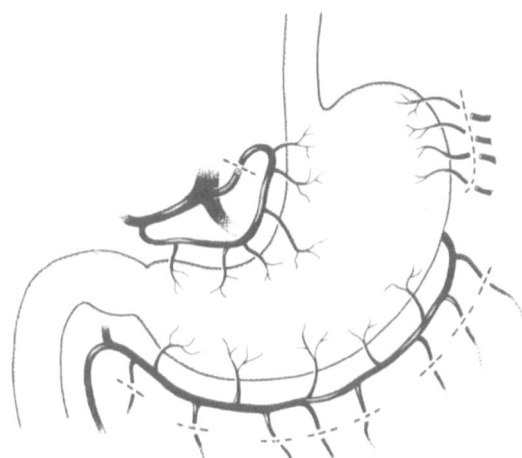

**Fig. 8.4.** Line drawing of gastric vessels.

the stomach is quite mobile and easily brought into the chest. The stomach can then be divided to create a gastric tube. The simplest way to achieve this is to place a 90-cm stapling gun from lesser to greater curve ensuring adequate clearance from the tumour. After dividing the stomach the suture line is covered with a Lembert suture of continuous 2/0 catgut or polyglycolic acid (Dexon). The oesophagus is divided a minimum of 5 cm above the upper limit of the tumour (Table 8.1) and the tumour removed.

**Table 8.1.**   Proximal resection margin and anastomotic recurrence (Wong 1987)

| Length of margin (cm) | Patients | | |
|---|---|---|---|
| | No. affected | Total | % |
| 0–2 | 1 | 4 | 25 |
| 2–4 | 2 | 11 | 18 |
| 4–6 | 2 | 13 | 15 |
| 6–8 | 2 | 26 | 8 |
| 8–10 | 1 | 15 | 7 |
| >10 | 0 | 26 | 0 |

As a result of dividing the oesophagus a vagotomy will have been done. A decision therefore has to be made about the pylorus and whether to do a drainage procedure. Many surgeons do not do anything and in most cases there is no problem. In a small number of cases gastric stasis occurs and a pyloroplasty is then required. This clinical observation has been confirmed in a prospective randomised trial (Cheung et al. 1987). The disadvantage of a pyloroplasty is the biliary reflux which can follow. To overcome both these problems a pyloromyotomy is preferable and will avoid delayed gastric emptying. It does not appear to be associated with excessive biliary reflux.

The gastric remnant is brought into the chest through the hiatus and a small opening made in the anterior wall just below the new fundus. An end-to-side oesophago-gastric anastomosis is made. The technique will depend upon the surgeon's preference but it is essential to obtain complete mucosal apposition. A satisfactory method is a single layer of interrupted non-absorbable braided polyester sutures (3/0 Mersilene). All the posterior sutures are inserted before tying. When the posterior portion is completed, the sutures are tied with the knots on the inside. The anterior sutures are tied as they are inserted with the knots on the outside. To avoid devascularising the oesophagus at the suture line only a short segment of the oesophagus should be mobilised above the suture line – 1–1.5 cm is recommended as the maximum.

After completion of the anastomosis the diaphragm is repaired with a continuous polyglycolic acid suture (Dexon). Provided the lung has not been damaged only a basal chest drain is required. The remainder of the wound is closed in layers with continuous absorbable sutures.

## Lewis/Tanner Operation

This operation was described by Lewis (1946) and Tanner (1947). As originally described by Lewis it was a two-stage operation with an interval of two weeks between stages. Although still frequently called a two-stage operation, both stages are now done at the same operation. The first stage is mobilisation of the stomach and the second stage a right thoracotomy. A disadvantage of this approach is that the tumour is not seen until half the operation has been done. In practice, this is rarely a problem as the tumour is usually removable. In a personal series of 149 Lewis operations it was not possible to remove the tumour in only 3 patients. Should it be impossible to remove the tumour, the stomach can still be used to bypass the obstruction.

The patient is placed supine on the operating table and an epigastric incision made. This would normally be a midline incision but a left or right paramedian or a transverse incision is quite satisfactory. After a full abdominal exploration the stomach is mobilised as previously described and a pyloromyotomy performed. Division of the left triangular ligament allows the left lobe of the liver to be retracted to expose the oesophagus and hiatus. The peritoneal reflection around the hiatus should be divided. The abdomen is then closed and the patient placed in a full lateral position lying on the left side. The chest is opened through a fifth intercostal space posterolateral thoracotomy. With a double lumen endobronchial tube in place the anaesthetist is able to collapse the right lung and this will provide excellent exposure to the whole of the intrathoracic oesophagus. The only structures crossing it are the mediastinal pleura and the arch of the azygos vein. The arch of the vein is ligated and divided. The oesophagus is then mobilised from well above the tumour to the hiatus. Below the arch of the aorta the blood supply to the oesophagus is direct from the descending aorta. These vessels are often short and should be sutured. Care should also be taken in separating the oesophagus from the trachea. The posterior wall of trachea is membranous and very thin. The other structure to be aware of is the thoracic duct. Because the patient has had nothing to eat the duct is difficult to identify. Damage to the duct will be recognised by the continuous pooling of serous fluid in the mediastinum. All that is required is ligation of the two cut ends.

Traction on the oesophagus will bring the stomach into the chest and care should be taken not to rotate it. The oesophago-gastric junction can then be divided using a stapling gun and sutures as previously described. Proximally the division should be well above palpable tumour (Table 8.1). A small opening is then made on the posterior wall of the stomach just below the fundus and the anastomosis is performed using a single layer of interrupted sutures. By inserting all the posterior layer without tying the sutures, the anastomosis can easily be made at the apex of the chest, with only 3 cm of intrathoracic oesophagus. Therefore, in the majority of cases there is little to be gained by extending the exposure into the neck. There must be no tension on the suture line. After inflation of the lung, the wound is closed and one basal drain is inserted.

The intrathoracic stomach makes an excellent tube and frequently is barely visible on a radiograph (Fig. 8.5a,b).

## McKeown Operation

This procedure is also known as the three-stage operation. First carried out by McKeown in 1961, a third cervical stage was added to the Lewis/Tanner operation. Initially, this was on the left side of the neck but was subsequently changed to the right side to avoid damage to the left recurrent laryngeal nerve.

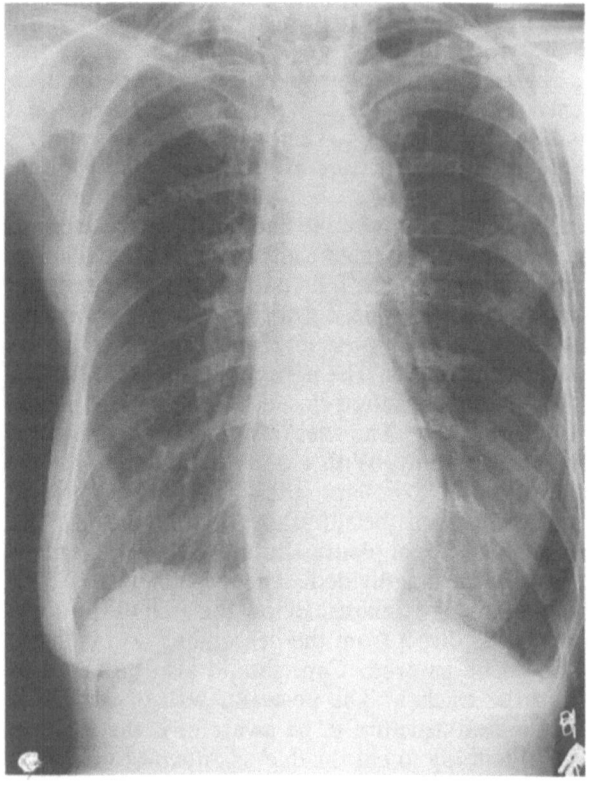

**Fig. 8.5a,b.** Chest radiographs showing intrathoracic stomach. **a** Plain radiograph. **b** Barium swallow.

According to McKeown (1979) the advantages of his operation are:

1. The wide excision which diminishes the risk of local recurrence. This is true but it is not always necessary to extend into the neck to achieve an adequate excision. If the anastomosis is high in the right chest only an extra 2–3 cm will be obtained by the third stage.

2. Ease of anastomosis and therefore a diminished incidence of anastomotic leak. Unfortunately, it is not proven that the anastomotic leak rate in his series is reduced as no statistics are available. It is also stated that a leak in the neck is less serious than an intrathoracic leak. Although this is true if there has been no operation, for example after endoscopy, it is not true after oesophagectomy. The tissue planes are wide open and any cervical leak will inevitably gravitate into the chest. In spite of these reservations it is sometimes necessary to extend into the neck.

If the McKeown procedure is to be used there is some advantage in changing the order of the three stages as originally described. The second thoracotomy stage should be done first. The advantage of this is that the tumour can be immediately assessed and resectability confirmed, unlike the Lewis operation.

**Fig 8.5** (*continued*)

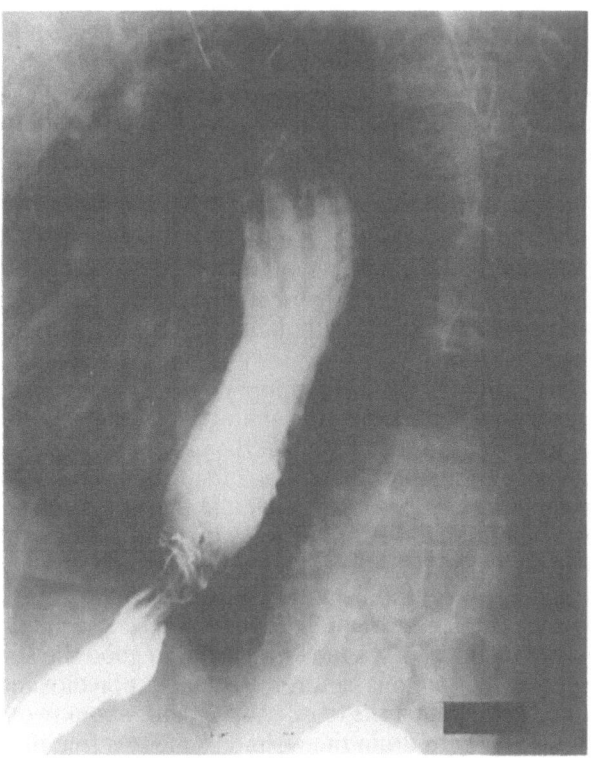

b

After the thoracotomy and mobilisation of the oesophagus the chest is closed. The patient is turned onto his back and the laparotomy and cervical incisions made simultaneously. This sequence also shortens the operating time.

## Left Oesophago-gastrectomy with Left Cervical Anastomosis

If there is an indication to transect the oesophagus in the neck then a preferable approach to the McKeown operation is a left-sided thoraco-abdominal incision with a left cervical incision. This was described by Belsey (1965) and has recently been favoured by Matthews (1986b). The initial part of the operation is exactly as described for a left oesophago-gastrectomy with a thoraco-abdominal incision through the seventh intercostal space. The oesophagus is mobilised to the arch of the aorta. It is then freed from behind the arch which is easily done with the finger, together with traction on the oesophagus. The mediastinal pleura is incised above the arch and the oesophagus encircled with a tape. It may be necessary to divide the superior intercostal vein. Traction on the oesophagus above the arch will allow the stomach to be pulled through the mediastinum until the fundus lies above the arch. Occasionally, at this stage it is apparent that the stomach will not reach the neck. If this is the case it is feasible to divide the right gastric vessels without causing ischaemia. Although this leaves the right gastro-epiploic arcade as the sole blood supply to the stomach this, surprisingly, is adequate. Before placing the stomach in the mediastinum it should be divided and closed at the oesophago-gastric junction. This is easier to do at this stage than through the cervical incision. The oesophagus is then attached to the stomach with two or three linen sutures so it can be drawn into the neck. Once the stomach has been placed in the superior mediastinum the incision can be closed. It is advisable to insert both an apical and a basal intercostal drain before closing the chest. When the neck is opened, the lung will tend to drop away creating an apical pneumothorax which without an apical drain may persist when the cervical wound is closed.

The patient is placed in supine position and the oesophagus exposed through a left cervical incision. Unfortunately, a synchronous incision cannot be made as the left arm is in the way when the patient is in the lateral position. The incision runs along the anterior border of sterno-mastoid, from the suprasternal notch upwards for 5–7 cm. After dividing the platysma muscle, the sterno-mastoid is retracted laterally. Both the omo-hyoid muscle and the middle thyroid vein are divided. With the internal jugular vein retracted, the oesophagus is clearly seen. Provided the oesophagus has been fully mobilised, traction will deliver the stomach into the wound. The oesophagus is divided and an oesophago-gastric anastomosis made. As the exposure is so good the simplest method is to use two layers of continuous suture. Recently, polydioxanone (PDS) an absorbable suture which retains its tensile strength for about two months, has been used. It is not necessary to drain the wound as there is free drainage into the chest.

## Bilateral Thoracotomy

This method has been used by Dark et al. (1981). In a series of 499 resections a bilateral thoracotomy was used in 30 cases with high tumours. The stomach was mobilised through a left thoracotomy with incision of the diaphragm, followed by a right thoracotomy for the anastomosis. It is not apparent what advantages this method confers over other techniques.

## Oesophagectomy without Thoracotomy

Although this is a standard technique for postcricoid tumours, some surgeons have used it for intrathoracic growths. First described by Denk (1913) it has recently been used by Orringer and Sloan (1978) and appears to be gaining popularity in the USA.

The technique is to expose the oesophagus simultaneously from above and below, using blunt dissection to free the oesophagus from the mediastinum. Surprisingly haemorrhage, as reported by Orringer (1986), is not a major problem. Although freedom from respiratory complications is claimed as a major justification for this approach, major respiratory problems are not a feature of a thoracotomy in units experienced in a transthoracic approach. The principle of good exposure and ability to see what is being dissected is paramount, unless it can be shown that by blind dissection both early and late results are better. It is too early to make a decision about this technique but the present position is excellently reviewed by Wong (1986). Until further results are known the only definite indication would appear to be a patient who has had a previous pneumonectomy or disease confined to the cervical oesophagus (see also Chapter 9).

# Use of Other Organ Substitutes

In all the operations so far described the stomach is the best organ substitute for the oesophagus. It has an excellent blood supply, mobilisation is straightforward and only one anastomosis is required. The only significant problems associated with its use are the loss of its reservoir function and the occurrence of reflux. Most patients adapt fairly quickly to eating smaller meals. Reflux can be a nuisance but not as commonly as one would expect. The higher the anastomosis the less is the problem of reflux. The stomach is not always suitable – in particular if there has been a previous partial gastrectomy. In these circumstances jejunum or colon can be used.

1. *Jejunum* This is an ideal replacement if a total gastrectomy has been required to remove the tumour. A Roux-en-Y loop should be created. If an interposition graft is to be inserted between oesophagus and stomach, jejunum is not ideal. The blood supply is variable and most surgeons find it difficult to obtain sufficient length. Furthermore, a troublesome alkaline oesophagitis may occur (Belsey 1965).

2. *Free Jejunal Graft.* This requires the mobilisation of a segment of jejunum with its blood supply. The vessels are re-anastomosed in the chest or neck. Suture of the vessels requires a microvascular technique. At present, the only indication for this procedure would appear to be when it is not possible to obtain an adequate length of stomach, jejunum or colon to reach from the abdomen to above the tumour.

3. *Colon.* The colon has many of the advantages of stomach. It is easily mobilised and the blood supply is usually reliable. A disadvantage is that preoperative preparation is required to ensure an empty clean colon. This is one reason why a stimulant laxative should be part of the preoperative preparation for any patient undergoing oesophageal resection. The best part of the colon to use is the left half of the transverse colon with the splenic flexure. The blood supply is based on the ascending branch of the left colic artery (Fig. 8.6). The use of this portion results in an isoperistaltic graft which can be long enough to reach the neck. The only disadvantage is that three anastomoses are required. The approach is a left thoraco-abdominal incision through the seventh intercostal space.

The oesophagus is mobilised and the length of colon required is measured. The stomach is transected at the oesophago-gastric junction and closed. To give adequate exposure it is usually necessary to divide the short gastric vessels. The

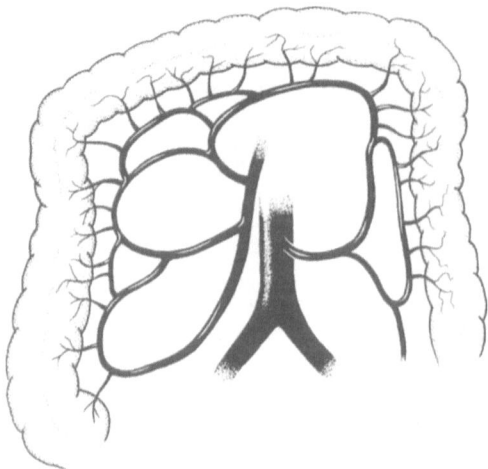

**Fig. 8.6.** Line drawing of colonic blood supply.

colon graft is prepared by dividing the attachment of the omentum over the relevant portion of the colon. The left colic, midcolic and marginal arteries are identified. The best method to identify the vessels is to lift the colon out of the wound and transilluminate the mesocolon. The mesocolon is incised and the vessels divided as indicated. If a long length is required, the midcolic artery will require ligation. The colon is divided and the proximal end taken through the lesser sac and hiatus into the chest. An end-to-end oesophago-colic anastomosis is made using a single layer of interrupted sutures. The distal portion of the graft is anastomosed to the posterior wall of the stomach about 7 cm from the fundus. There is then a good length of intra-abdominal colon which prevents reflux. Usually two layers of continuous catgut are used. Finally an end-to-end colo-colic anastomosis is made, again using two layers of continuous catgut. The wound is closed with a single basal chest drain. The postoperative management is the same as after the other procedures already described.

4. *Skin Tubes*. These are mainly of historical interest and only have application to tumours in the cervical oesophagus.

## Postoperative Management

In many centres it has not been the general practice to nurse all patients following oesophagectomy in an intensive care unit. The reasons are various; often there is a lack of facilities but not infrequently it has been considered not necessary. That this is a misconception has been partly borne out by past results. Many of these patients have impaired lung function and are elderly. The critical period is the first twelve hours when the patient is vasoconstricted, cold and not fully recovered from the effects of the anaesthetic. Hypoxia, due to inadequate ventilation and sputum retention can easily occur and this will have a harmful effect on the anastomosis. By monitoring blood gases this complication can be avoided. The patient must also be encouraged to cough at this early stage to prevent subsequent chest complications. If the patient is unable to cooperate in this early period, there should be no hesitancy in using ventilatory support. Usually all that is required is overnight ventilation with extubation early the following morning. By then the patient should be alert and able to cooperate.

At the end of the operation, provided there is no history of chest disease, the patient is extubated and transferred to the intensive care unit. Oxygen is administered via a face mask. The pulse rate, blood pressure and blood loss from the intercostal drain are recorded initially every 15 minutes, but provided these are stable the frequency of observation can be reduced. Urinary output should be measured hourly and should be 30–40 ml/hour. Urinary output is a good parameter to assess progress. A reduction in output may be an early warning that tissue perfusion is not adequate and corrective measures may need to be taken. Venous pressure should also be recorded but this is less useful unless fluid replacement has been inadequate, when it can be invaluable. Arterial blood gases are measured and, if abnormal, are repeated. A chest radiograph at this stage is helpful to confirm that both lungs are fully expanded and that there is no pneumothorax or fluid collection in the opposite chest (Fig. 8.7). During the operation it is common for the mediastinal pleura on the opposite side to be

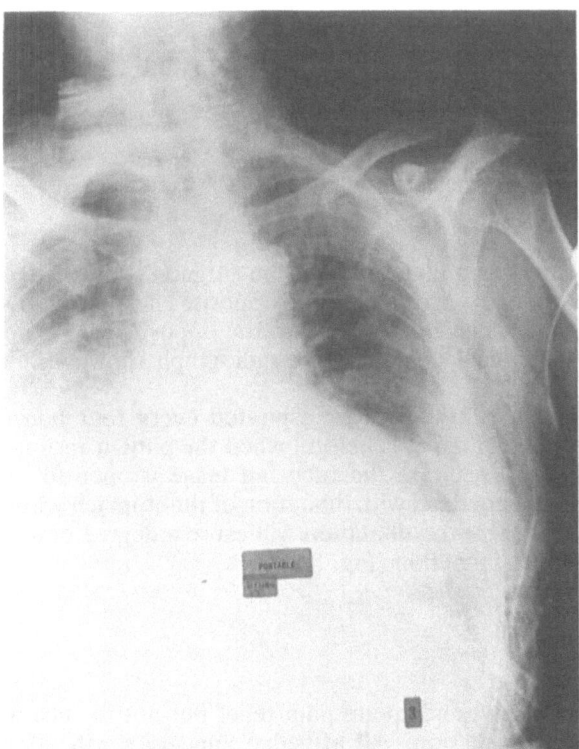

**Fig. 8.7.**   Chest radiograph showing postoperative haemothorax on opposite side.

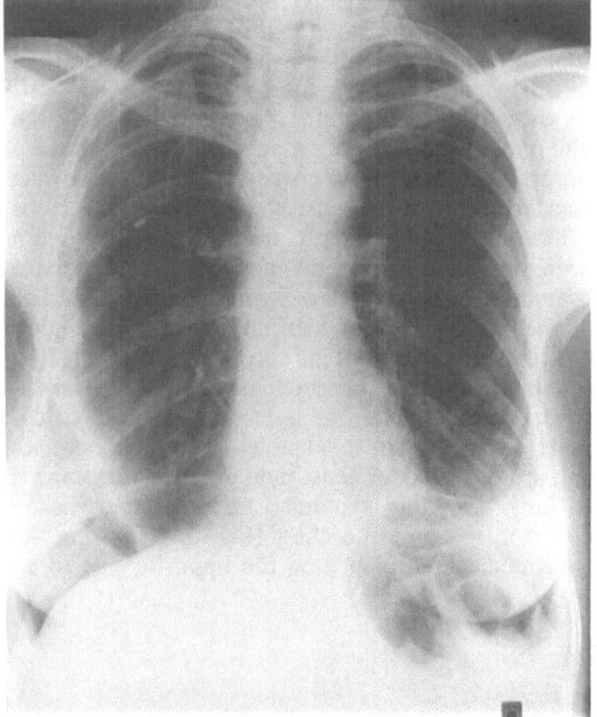

**Fig. 8.8.**   Chest radiograph showing gastric dilatation.

opened. Blood and air can then accumulate without the surgeon's knowledge. Should the pleura have been opened a sucker into the opposite chest to remove any accumulated fluid is all that is needed. A drain to the opposite side is not necessary. However, if the immediate postoperative radiograph shows a fluid collection, a drain must be inserted.

A nasogastric tube is advisable and should be aspirated every four hours. Although initially of little convincing use it is helpful when the patient resumes oral fluids. Some surgeons do not aspirate the tube but leave it open to the atmosphere. This occasionally is associated with dilatation of the stomach within the chest and should be avoided as gastric dilatation will cause a degree of lung compression and loss of pulmonary function (Fig. 8.8).

## Pain Relief

It is essential that the patient receives adequate pain relief but not to such an extent as to cause respiratory depression. All effective analgesics will affect respiration. Papaveretum (Omnopon), although not ideal, is the best available. It is preferable to give small frequent doses rather than large doses. Initially, because of vasoconstriction, absorption is poor and the first dose should be given intravenously, followed later by intramuscular injections. Although reasonably satisfactory, pain control does fluctuate as blood level falls. It has been shown that by combining opiates with a non-steroidal anti-inflammatory drug (NSAID), much better pain control is obtained with less fluctuation (Keenan et al. 1983). The two drugs that have been used are indomethacin and diclofenac. The latter is perhaps not quite so effective but probably has fewer side effects. The drug is given rectally in a suppository for the first three days. As NSAIDs affect renal blood flow they should not be used in patients with renal or cardiovascular disease, particularly hypertension or low output states. The advantage of this method is that it is simple to use and avoids excessive respiratory depression. For the patient it is extremely effective.

## Fluid Replacement

The patient should have nothing by mouth for the first two postoperative days. Fluids are given intravenously in the form of a crystalloid solution. To make postoperative care as simple as possible a solution of 0.18% sodium chloride and 4% glucose is used with 1 g potassium chloride added to alternate 500 ml units. The rate of infusion is approximately 35 ml/kg/24 hr. In practical terms this means 2–3 l a day depending upon the weight (lean muscle mass) of the patient. It has not been found advantageous to start intravenous feeding at this stage. Continuing blood loss from the chest drain must be measured and replaced with blood.

## First Postoperative Day

Provided all parameters are normal the patient may be returned to the ward. The chest drain is removed if the chest radiograph is satisfactory, though if drainage persists (which is unusual) the drain should remain in place. The arterial line and peripheral intravenous line are also removed, just leaving the central venous line. The urinary catheter is left for 48 h both for monitoring and for the convenience of the patient, particularly if female. It is difficult to cope with a bed pan on the first day!

Physiotherapy is most important and should be reinforced with hot inhalations of a volatile substance. Menthol and eucalyptus, 15 ml in 500 ml of hot water, is soothing and encourages deep breathing. This should be given 2–3 times a day for the first three days or whilst there is respiratory embarrassment.

Early mobility is encouraged to prevent deep vein thrombosis and therefore the patient is allowed out of bed for a short period.

## Second Postoperative Day

Provided urinary output is adequate the urinary catheter is removed but the input and output of all fluids must still be measured. A further chest radiograph is taken to confirm clear lung fields. Chest physiotherapy and inhalations are continued.

## Third and Subsequent Days

By now the patient should be well on the way to recovery and fairly mobile. Oral fluids are started, initially 30 ml of water hourly. Provided this is being absorbed it can be increased to 60 ml and by the end of the day to free fluids. An advantage of a nasogastric tube is that it is easily confirmed that fluids are being absorbed although gastric stasis at this stage is unusual. The choice of three days is arbitrary and the patient does swallow saliva from the time of the operation. However, the stomach takes a little time to regain motility and in practice three days has been satisfactory. Some surgeons insist on a radiographic contrast study before allowing oral fluids. This is a rather negative approach and of little value. If the patient has an anastomotic leak it will be apparent without the help of radiographs.

As oral fluids start, intravenous fluid must be appropriately reduced. Particularly in the elderly it is possible to cause cardiac failure due to excessive intravenous fluid. Once oral intake is adequate the intravenous line can be removed.

Over the following days the diet is increased from fluids to a soft diet. There will be some oedema around the anastomosis and swallowing may be a little uncomfortable but this soon subsides.

Sutures are removed on the 8–10th postoperative day and the patient discharged on the 10–12th day.

# Postoperative Complications

The majority of patients make a straightforward recovery and 80% are discharged by the 13th postoperative day. Nevertheless, with this type of extensive surgery and the advanced age of many of the patients there is an associated morbidity and mortality.

On return to the intensive care unit the patient is cold with associated vasoconstriction. Over the next few hours vasodilatation and a good peripheral circulation should occur. The pulse and blood pressure should be stable, with an hourly urinary output of 30–40 ml. If this does not occur there is a problem which requires correction.

### Blood Loss

Blood lost during the operation should have been replaced immediately. It is essential that blood loss should be accurately measured during operation by weighing swabs and measuring the amount in the sucker. Subsequent loss is measured in the chest drain bottle but as the abdomen is not drained it is possible for there to be undisclosed bleeding in this area. If hypovolaemia is thought to be the problem the response to a bolus of fluid should be observed. Should bleeding continue there should be no delay in returning the patient for re-operation.

## Cardiac Tamponade

Cardiac tamponade may occur and may be missed if not considered. The presentation is of a low output state but with a raised central venous pressure. It can result from blood clot in the mediastinum pressing on the back of the heart or, if the pericardium has been opened, bleeding into the pericardial space. If there is any doubt the patient should be returned to theatre.

## Low Output State

A low output state is likely to be due to hypovolaemia but it may be secondary to poor cardiac function. Provided fluid replacement has been adequate, cardiac support will be required. Dopamine, a cardiac stimulant, acts on sympathetic receptors in cardiac muscle, increasing contractability with little effect on rate. A low dose, the so-called renal dose, produces vasodilatation and increased renal perfusion but a higher dose (more than 5 µg/kg body weight/min) can produce vasoconstriction. It is given as an intravenous solution at the initial rate of 2 µg/kg body weight/min. Any dysrhythmia must be corrected. Improvement should occur but, if it does not, ventilatory support will be necessary. An endotracheal tube is inserted and intermittent positive pressure ventilation (IPPV) commenced and continued until improvement ensues.

## Pulmonary Complications

The pulmonary complications that may follow operation are:

Sputum retention and infection
Aspiration pneumonia
Pulmonary embolism

### Sputum Retention and Infection

With adequate prophylactic measures these problems should be avoidable. Any patient with chronic sputum production should be given intensive preoperative physiotherapy. A week in hospital with vigorous chest physiotherapy can make an enormous difference. Occasionally this is reinforced with a broad spectrum antibiotic but usually this is held back to cover the operation. Following operation this type of patient should be ventilated for the first postoperative night to overcome the period when the patient has difficulty in coughing. Patients with poor respiratory reserve require an elective tracheostomy. A minitracheostomy appears to be as satisfactory though the patient cannot be ventilated through this unless a jet ventilator is available. Should sputum retention occur which cannot be relieved by suction there should be no delay in performing a bronchoscopy under local anaesthesia. Prompt treatment of sputum retention will prevent lobar collapse and pneumonia.

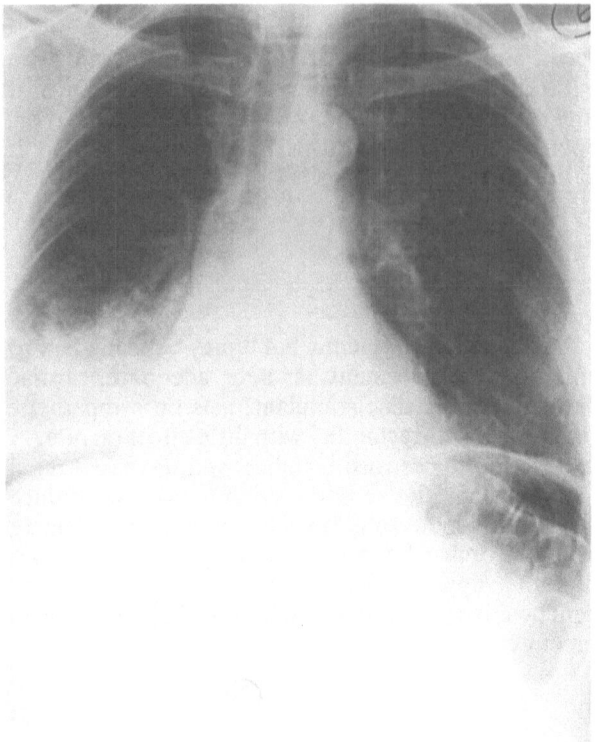

**Fig. 8.9.** Chest radiograph showing aspiration pneumonia.

## Aspiration Pneumonia

Aspiration pneumonia (Fig. 8.9) is due to loss of the lower oesophageal sphincter as a result of the operation and the intrathoracic stomach. Reflux is more of a problem with a lower oesophagectomy. Reflux is a positional problem and therefore the patient should be sat up as soon as possible. Even at night the patient should sleep propped up, as sedation may result in a lack of awareness of reflux. Should an aspiration pneumonia occur it will take 2–3 weeks to resolve. In the long term, reflux and aspiration become less of a problem and eventually the patient can try sleeping flat.

## Pulmonary Embolism

Pulmonary embolism is secondary to venous thrombosis. The latter is a complication of any major surgery and particularly malignancy. Measures to prevent thrombosis must be taken. The simplest and most important are to ensure adequate hydration and early mobilisation. Thrombosis probably starts on the operating table. To promote venous return intermittent calf compression should be used during the operation (Roberts and Cotton 1974) by the use of compression boots placed on the legs when the patient is positioned on the operating table. They can also be used afterwards but they are not very comfortable and not necessary if the patient is fairly mobile. Compression stockings are probably of some value.

Heparin, particularly subcutaneous heparin, has been extensively used in major surgery (Kakkar et al. 1972). This was used extensively in a personal series with no occurrence of pulmonary emboli. Unfortunately, there was excessive postoperative blood loss, particularly when indomethacin was used for pain relief, possibly due to a synergistic effect. Since discontinuing subcutaneous heparin, and using the above measures, no patient has had a clinically obvious pulmonary embolism.

Should a deep vein thrombosis develop, immediate treatment is given with intravenous heparin and oral anticoagulation which is continued for three months.

## Renal Complications

Oliguria during the immediate postoperative period is most likely to be due to a low output state. Provided this is corrected, urine should soon start to flow. This is assuming that any water depletion was adequately corrected before operation. If, after eliminating these causes, urinary output is still inadequate a small dose of frusemide is given, followed if necessary by a larger dose. If there is still no response it must be assumed that some renal damage has occurred. This is treated in the routine manner with fluid restriction and, if necessary, peritoneal dialysis, though this is not commonly needed.

## Anastomotic Leaks

In many series an anastomotic leak is a major cause of morbidity and mortality. This complication is very serious as there is an associated high mortality. With care the incidence of a leak should be low especially when stomach is used for reconstruction. To avoid a leak certain principles should be adhered to.

1. Both the remaining oesophagus and stomach should have a good blood supply. Ischaemia at the suture line will cause failure. In the lower two-thirds of the oesophagus only a short length should be mobilised above the anastomosis to avoid ischaemia. In the upper third blood supply is from above from the inferior thyroid arteries.

2. Hypoxia must be avoided at all times.

3. Mucosa must be accurately apposed without undue tension nor must the sutures be tied too tight.

4. Local infection should be prevented. When the oesophagus is divided care should be taken to avoid soiling the mediastinum with oesophageal contents.

There is no evidence that the use of ring stapling guns is advantageous and they are expensive.

Should a leak occur it usually becomes apparent on the fifth to eighth day. In most cases it is clinically obvious in that the patient's general condition deteriorates. Initially this may not be so and the only abnormality may be a pleural effusion or a hydro-pneumothorax. If there is any doubt about the diagnosis it can be confirmed by a radiographic contrast swallow. It has been known for this to be normal but to show a leak on subsequent re-examination (Fig. 8.10). Treatment must be immediate if the patient is to survive and not succumb to infection. Fluid must be drained by an intercostal drain of at least 24FG size. Oral feeding should be stopped and a high-calorie intake started either enterally via a fine bore tube or intravenously by a central catheter tunnelled

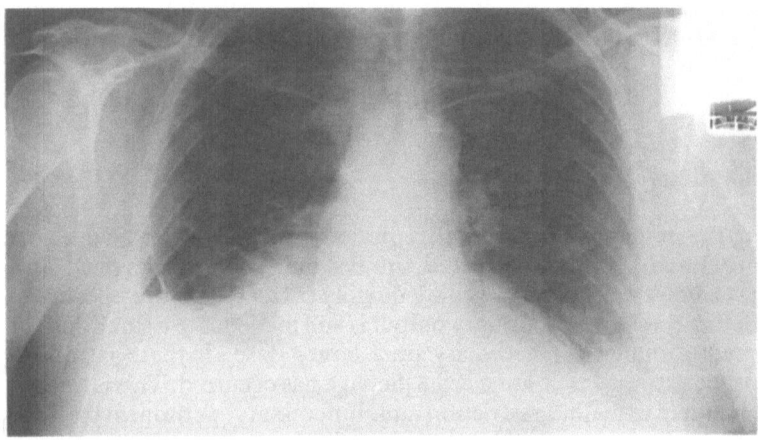

a

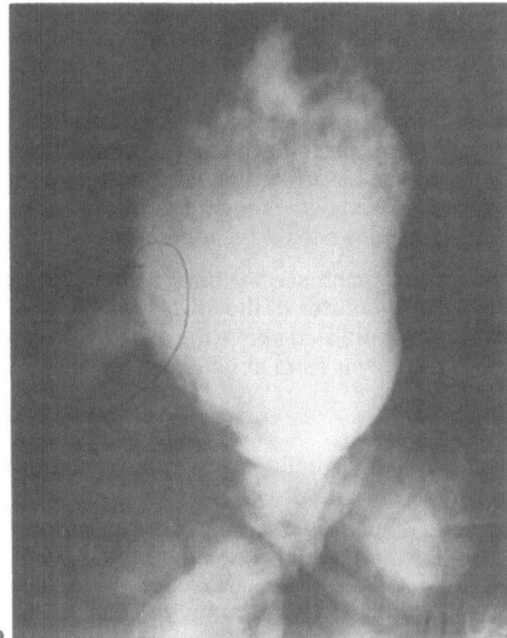

b

**Fig. 8.10a,b.** Radiographs with contrast, showing leak. **a** Plain radiograph showing fluid level. **b** Contrast showing oesophageal leak.

subcutaneously to reduce the risk of infection. If enteral feeding is used it is essential that the tube is passed beyond the stomach into the small bowel to prevent the problem of reflux. Broad spectrum antibiotics should be given, but if possible discontinued after a few days to avoid the problems of pseudomonas or fungal infections. Provided the pleural cavity is well drained and the lung fully expanded infection is not a major problem. With time the anastomosis should heal.

## Chylothorax

Considering the proximity of the thoracic duct, it is surprising that a chylothorax is not more common after oesophagectomy. Although it can occur following any operative approach, in the author's own series it has only occurred after a right thoracotomy. The incidence has been low at 1% and it has not been seen for some considerable time. This is due to an awareness of the thoracic duct and ensuring that after mobilisation of the oesophagus, serous fluid is not accumulating in the mediastinum. If it is, the duct must be identified and the two ends ligated. Should a divided duct be missed, it may not become apparent for a few days as the patient is not eating. If it is not immediately diagnosed the chest drain will have been removed and a pleural effusion will be the first sign. This will not necessarily have the appearance of chyle if the patient is not eating. Although the fistula may heal, only 50% do so and this is unpredictable (Ross 1986). The patient can lose a considerable amount of fluid from the fistula and soon develop an electrolytic imbalance. Although this complication can be treated conservatively it is preferable to operate and ligate the duct, a procedure which is well tolerated and does not significantly delay recovery.

# Late Complications

## Dysphagia

Recurrent dysphagia is due to an anastomotic stricture or recurrent tumour. A stricture usually occurs 4–6 weeks after operation. It is related to healing and is usually trivial. There is some difficulty in eating meat and bread. This usually settles but occasionally the dysphagia becomes worse and dilatation is necessary. In a minority of patients further dilatation is required. In this group it appears that reflux is a contributory cause as there is usually an associated oesophagitis. Further treatment is with antacids and $H_2$ antagonists.

Dysphagia due to recurrent tumour is unlikely before six months and is associated with failure to thrive after the operation. It is due to tumour within the oesophagus which indicates an inadequate operation or mediastinal tumour causing compression. In a study by Wong (1987) the incidence of anastomotic recurrence in relation to the length of clearance obtained at operation was examined. If the margin was more than 10 cm, there was no anastomotic recurrence (Table 8.1).

Clearly, it is not always possible to obtain 10 cm clearance but the principle must be to resect the oesophagus as far above the upper limit of the tumour as is possible.

A hoarse voice is often an early sign of recurrence due to involvement of the left recurrent laryngeal nerve by tumour. A chest radiograph may not help but oesophagoscopy should provide an answer. Treatment is by radiotherapy regardless of the histological type. The only exception would be a small cell carcinoma (which is rare in the oesophagus) when chemotherapy would be the first choice. If there is no response to radiotherapy a tube can be inserted.

Occasionally a recurrence of the tumour may be small and occur some considerable time after the original treatment. In the author's own series there have been two patients who developed a second tumour or recurrence 5 and 12 years later. In one this was tumour at the site of anastomosis which was again resected and he remains well ten years later. The second was a woman with a postcricoid carcinoma, treated by radiotherapy and twelve years later developed

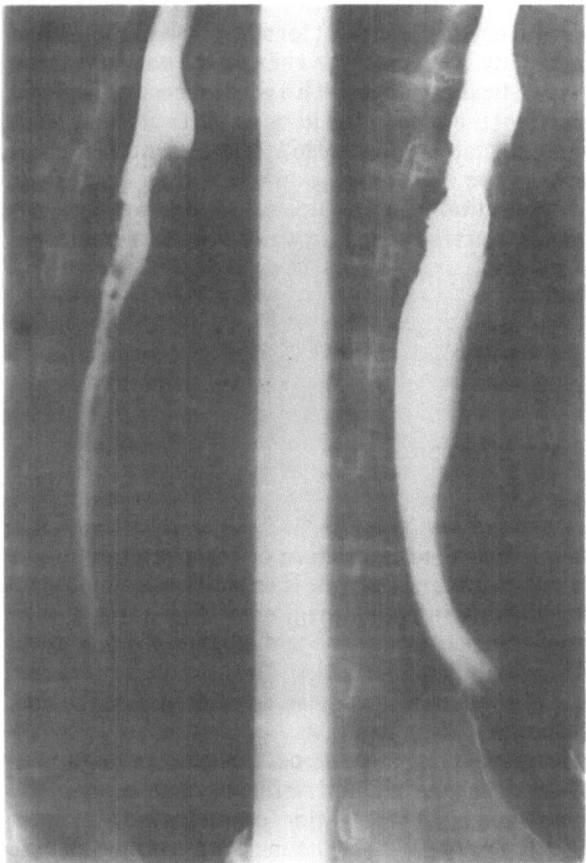

**Fig. 8.11.** Barium swallow – second primary after radiotherapy for a postcricoid carcinoma 12 years previously.

a carcinoma at the level of the aortic arch (Fig. 8.11). After an Ivor Lewis operation she remains well five years later.

### Diarrhoea

Loose bowel motions are common in the immediate postoperative period but fortunately usually resolve after a few days. In some patients the diarrhoea is persistent and is related to the rapid transfer of food from the stomach to the small bowel and also to the vagotomy which is the result of the oesophagectomy. Treatment with codeine phosphate or diphenoxylate hydrochloride (Lomotil) is usually effective. If there is little improvement further investigation is required to exclude a malabsorption syndrome. Latent coeliac disease may become apparent after operation.

### Failure to Thrive

Prior to and during the operative period weight loss occurs. After hospital discharge there is frequently further slight weight loss; weight should stabilise after two weeks and then slowly rise. Weight gain is slow and it is unusual to reach the former weight. It is helpful to weigh the patient at each follow-up appointment to confirm that the weight is increasing or stabilised. A decrease is ominous and is usually the first indication of recurrent tumour, even when there is no dysphagia.

### Cough

A persistent cough suggests bronchial involvement with tumour which can be confirmed by bronchoscopy. Just occasionally the intrathoracic stomach appears to act as an irritant focus particularly if dilated. Coughing is aggravated by the ingestion of food (Fig. 8.12).

# Results

The incidence of carcinoma of the oesophagus has an enormous variation in different parts of the world. In England and Wales there is little geographic difference with an incidence of 9.1/100 000 in males and 7.5/100 000 in females (1983). There is thus little sex difference although this is not true in other countries where there is often a male predominance. What is difficult to ascertain is the operation and resection rates. From an extensive review by Earlam and Cunha-Melo (1980) of 83 783 patients the operation rate was 58% with 39% resections. For the United Kingdom these figures are probably too high. Unfortunately, there are no figures available for the total number of operations each year.

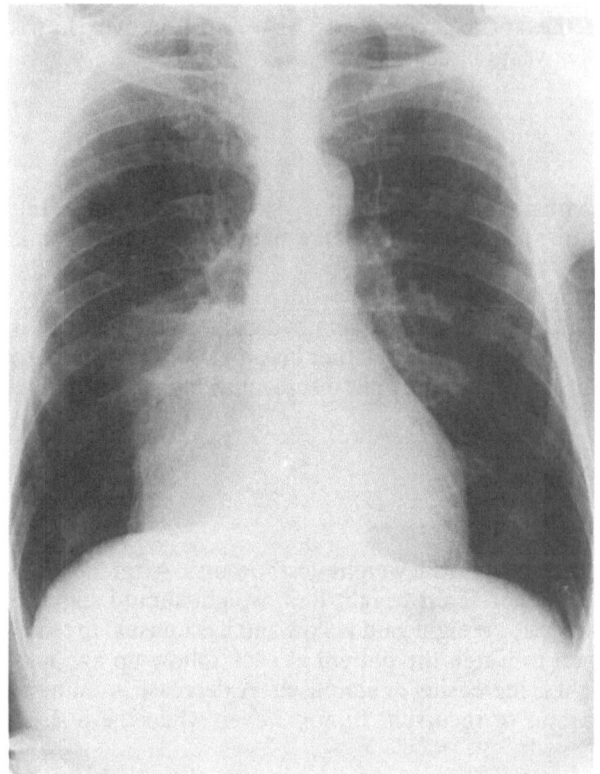

**Fig. 8.12.** Chest radiograph showing persistently dilated stomach causing chronic cough 5 years after operation.


Although each region has a cancer registry, most are unable to provide accurate statistics. An exception is the West Midlands Cancer Registry which has recently published a monograph on cancer of the oesophagus (Matthews et al. 1987). In a twenty-year-period, 1957–76, 4680 patients were registered with a diagnosis of carcinoma of the oesophagus, of whom only 1143 (24.4%) had a resection. Certainly, there are a large number of patients who, for various reasons, are not treated surgically.


## Hospital Mortality

Death following operation may be classified as any death occurring in hospital or any patient dying within 30 days. It is important to know the number of patients who die as a result of the operation and therefore death within hospital is usually the more realistic figure. This and other problems are discussed by Earlam in his paper. The mean figure for early death in this collected series was 29%. It would be wrong to assume that this is the current position. The series consists of 122 papers with a range of mortality from 1% to 69%, from all parts of the world; it includes papers published as long as 30 years ago in which the operations must have been carried out up to 40 years ago. It is also not realistic to include figures from Asia where the disease is of a different pattern and where early lesions which are just confined to the mucosa and submucosa, are common. In the western world these early tumours are rare.

Since 1980 the Society of Cardiothoracic Surgeons of Great Britain and Northern Ireland have made an annual return to the Society and the results collated. The response rate has been 96%. These figures (Table 8.2) give an accurate indication of the present situation.

**Table 8.2.**  Resections and mortality data taken from the UK Thoracic Surgical Register

|                | 1979 | 1980 | 1981 | 1982 | 1983 | 1984 | 1985 |
|----------------|------|------|------|------|------|------|------|
| Resections     | 1122 | 724  | 786  | 773  | 824  | 891  | 693  |
| Mortality (%)  | 17.4 | 15.5 | 19.1 | 11.6 | 10.8 | 8.9  | 7.8  |

There are, however, a considerable number of patients treated by general surgeons for which no detailed statistics are available. From the above figures it is interesting to note how hospital mortality has fallen since the results have been collected. This is presumably due to improved selection of patients (as the numbers have decreased) together with better postoperative management.

Surgical experience has to be recognised as a major factor in treating this disease when the patient is so often in such a poor clinical state. This was demonstrated in a personal series of 400 resections by Collis (1971). His results (Table 8.3) show that with greater experience hospital mortality can be reduced.

**Table 8.3.**  Collis (1971) – personal series

| Cases    | Hospital mortality (%) |
|----------|------------------------|
| 1–50     | 52                     |
| 51–300   | 15                     |
| 301–400  | 12                     |

This improvement with experience has also been seen in the author's own series of 395 resections (Table 8.4).

**Table 8.4.**  Lea – personal series, 1974–1988

| Cases     | Hospital mortality (%) |
|-----------|------------------------|
| 1–99      | 10                     |
| 100–199   | 16                     |
| 200–299   | 6                      |
| 300–395   | 5                      |

In an interesting study from the West Midlands Cancer Registry, Matthews (1986b) reported on the effect of surgical experience. From 1957 to 1976 resections were performed on 1119 patients. These were divided into two groups of 581 and 538 patients. In the first or occasional group the operations were performed by 127 surgeons who averaged three or fewer resections a year. In the second or frequent group there were only four surgeons who averaged six or more resections a year. Operative mortality for the occasional group was 39.4% and 21.6% for the frequent group. This adds strong support to the argument that carcinoma of the oesophagus should only be treated in centres where there is sufficient experience in treating the disease.

## Late Results

Although a cure may be obtained following resection the majority of operations must be considered as palliation. Swallowing following resection is superior to any other method of palliation and may provide a considerable period of symptom-free life. There is, in addition, the bonus of a cure in some patients. The reason for the poor long-term results is not that carcinoma of the oesophagus has a different behaviour pattern but that by the time of operation the tumour is already advanced. What is disappointing in so many patients is the long interval between the first symptom and treatment. In England, Le Roux (1962) found that the mean interval was 7.5 months, and there is little to indicate that this has improved over the last 25 years. The cause of the delay is usually the patient failing to seek medical advice. Unfortunately, when the patient does see the doctor it is not uncommon for treatment with an antacid or $H_2$ antagonist to be given without investigation. Dysphagia must always be regarded as a serious symptom and promptly investigated. In spite of this delay there is no correlation between duration of symptoms and long-term survival.

## Five-Year Survival

In considering five-year survival it is essential to compare comparable figures. This can be difficult as an author may only consider those patients who survived the operation and not consider hospital mortality. Earlam in his series found that 12% of those resected survived five years. This is a similar to the figure from the West Midlands Registry where the crude survival rate was 11% in 1143 resections. Crude five-year survival from other large series is given in Table 8.5.

**Table 8.5.** Late results of surgical resection

|                | No. of cases | Five-year survival (%) | Hospital mortality (%) |
|----------------|--------------|------------------------|------------------------|
| Dark (1981)    | 449          | 18                     | 7.6                    |
| Griffith (1980)| 211          | 15                     | 11.4                   |
| Jackson (1979) | 216          | 14                     | 18                     |
| Lea (1987)     | 205          | 15                     | 10                     |

It is unfortunate that McKeown (1985) was unable to complete a long-term follow-up on his patients. He claimed that an advantage of the three-stage operation was the wide excision possible and by inference the improved long-term results but this still requires confirmation.

All these figures are for overall survival and do not take account of histology. Griffith discusses this factor and gives a 25% survival for squamous carcinoma but only 8% for adenocarcinoma. The important factors in long-term survival are, however, the degree of wall penetration and lymph node spread (Skinner et al. 1986). Regrettably it is unusual to see cases where the tumour has not involved the full thickness of the wall. Until methods of early detection become available it is unlikely that the surgical results can be improved in any major way. What the present day surgeon must ensure is an adequate resection margin, meticulous anastomotic technique and a high standard of postoperative care to ensure that patients submitted to an operation have the best possible surgical results.

# References

Belsey R (1965) Reconstruction of the oesophagus with left colon. J Thorac Cardiovasc Surg 49:33–55

Cheung HC, Siu KF, Wong J (1987) Is pyloroplasty necessary in oesophageal replacement by stomach? A prospective randomised controlled trial. Surgery 102:19–24

Collis L (1971) Surgical treatment of carcinoma of the oesophagus. Br J Surg 58:801–804

Dark SF, Mousalli H, Vaughan R (1981) Surgical treatment of carcinoma of the oesophagus. Thorax 36:891–985

Denk W (1913) Zur radikaloperation des osophaguskarzinoms. Zentralbl Chir 40:1065

Earlam R, Cunha-Melo JR (1980) Oesophageal squamous cell carcinoma: 1. A critical review of surgery. Br J Surg 67:381–390

Griffith JL, Davis JT (1980) A twenty-year experience with the surgical management of carcinoma of the oesophagus and gastric cardia. J Thorac Cardiovasc Surg 79:447–452

Heatley RV, Williams RHP, Lewis MH (1979) Pre-operative intravenous feeding – a controlled trial. Postgrad Med J 55:541–545

Jackson JW, Cooper DKC, Guvendik I, Reece-Smith H (1979) Surgical management of malignant tumours of oesophagus and cardia. Br J Surg 66:98–104

Kakkar VV, Corrigan T, Spindler J et al. (1972) Efficacy of low doses of heparin in prevention of deep-vein thrombosis after major surgery: a double blind, randomised trial. Lancet II:1133

Keenan DJ, Cave K, Langdon L, Lea RE (1983) Comparative trial of rectal indomethacin and cryoanalgesia for control of early post-operative pain. Br Med J (Clin Res) 287(6402):1335–1337

Lea RE, Archer T, Royce C (1986) Abstract International Oesophageal Week, Munich

Le Roux BT (1962) The influence of resection on the natural history of carcinoma of the hypopharynx, oesophagus and proximal stomach. Surg Gynecol Obstet 115:162–170

Lewis I (1946) Surgical treatment of carcinoma of oesophagus with special reference to new operation for growths of middle third. Br J Surg 34:18–31

Matthews HR (1986a) Effects of surgical experience on the results of resection in oesophageal carcinoma. Br J Surg 73:621

Matthews HR (1986b) Left-sided subtotal oesophagectomy for carcinoma. Abstract International, Oesophageal Week, Munich

Matthews HR, Waterhouse JAH, Powell J, McConkey CC, Robertson JE (1987) Cancer of the oesophagus. Macmillan, London (Clinical cancer monographs, vol 1)

McKeown KC (1972) Trends in oesophageal resection for carcinoma. Ann R Coll Surg Engl 51:213–238

McKeown KC (1979) Carcinoma of the oesophagus. J R Coll Surg Edinb 24:253–274

McKeown KC (1985) The surgical treatment of carcinoma of the oesophagus. J R Coll Surg Edinb 30:1–14

Orringer MB (1986) Transhiatal oesophagectomy without thoracotomy for carcinoma of the oesophagus. Adv Surg 19:1–49

Orringer MB, Sloan H (1978) Oesophagectomy without thoracotomy. J Thorac Cardiovasc Surg 76:643–654

Pearson JG (1969) The value of radiotherapy in the management of oesophageal cancer. AJR 105:500–513

Roberts VC, Cotton LT (1974) Prevention of postoperative deep vein thrombosis in patients with malignant disease. Br Med J i:358–362

Ross K (1986) Thoracic surgery. Butterworths, London, pp 59–62 (Rob and Smith's Operative surgery, 4th edn)

Skinner DB, Ferguson MK, Soriano A, Little AG, Staszak VM (1986) Selection of operation for oesophageal cancer based on staging. Ann Surg 204:391–401

Tanner NC (1947) The present position of carcinoma of the oesophagus. Postgrad Med J 23:109–139

Thompson WM, Halvorsen RA, Foster WL, Williford ME, Postlethwait RW, Korobkin M (1983) Computed tomography for staging oesophageal and gastro-oesophageal carcinoma – reevaluation. AJR 141:951–952

Wong J (1986) Transhiatal oesophagectomy for carcinoma of the thoracic oesophagus. Br J Surg 73:89–90 (editorial)

Wong J (1987) Oesophageal resection for cancer: the rationale of current practice. Am J Surg 153:18–24

*Chapter 9*

# Transhiatal Oesophagectomy without Formal Thoracotomy

R. M. Kirk

## Historical

Surgery within the chest was difficult until techniques were developed to inflate the lungs with the pleural cavity opened. Denk (1913) first suggested the possibility of coring out the oesophagus from within the mediastinum by a cervico-abdominal approach. Alton Ochsner (1978) reports seeing Clairmont performing this procedure in 1923 in Zurich, which was published in 1924.

Grey Turner (1933) reported a patient on whom he carried out the operation, subsequently creating a skin tube oesophageal substitute. Eventually the technique was replaced by transpleural and thoracoabdominal approaches. Blunt oesophagectomy was later used following pharyngolaryngectomy, providing a route for the stomach to be brought into the neck for pharyngogastrostomy (Le Quesne and Ranger 1966).

The technique was revived for the palliative excision of incurable intrathoracic carcinoma (Kirk 1974) and has become increasingly popular in sick and elderly patients with advanced disease as an alternative to other procedures. When cure is considered possible, most surgeons employ formal right thoracotomy as described by Ivor Lewis, or as modified by McKeown.

## Indications

Many surgeons, including Belsey (1978), reasonably claim that there are no indications for tearing out the oesophagus from among the many vital and delicate structures within the mediastinum. The technique offends against the tenets of good surgery, risking damage to the fragile posterior wall of the trachea, the thoracic duct, and risking uncontrollable haemorrhage from the major pulmonary vessels or vena azygos. If it is misapplied to potentially curable patients it denies them the radical surgery they need. Suggestions that the operation may diminish the pulmonary complications associated with formal thoracotomy have not been confirmed (Lancet 1986). Whatever the theoretical arguments, blunt oesophagectomy can be safely performed without calamitous operative disasters even in elderly patients (Williamson 1985).

The prognosis following resection for oesophageal carcinoma is said to be depressingly poor (Earlam and Cunha-Melo 1980)* except when the disease is identified before it has produced symptoms, using cytological screening as reported from China (Collaborating Group 1976). The high incidence of supraclavicular node involvement (Sannohe et al. 1981) often vitiates hopeful attempts at intrathoracic radical surgery (Kirk 1983). Blunt oesophagectomy was initially reserved for palliation of oesophageal squamous carcinoma but more recently has been used for adenocarcinoma affecting the lower oesophagus.

Clinical assessment, radiology and oesophagoscopy with biopsy and cytology are carried out. Tumour length and the presence of "skip" lesions are noted (Kirk and McLaughlin 1985). At the minimum, ultrasound scanning of the liver is performed to exclude obvious liver secondaries. Those in whom radical resection is not possible but who are expected to survive months rather than weeks are considered for blunt oesophagectomy. Patients who appear to have early growths are scanned by computed tomography from the midcervical region to the midabdomen to exclude tumour extension, obvious enlarged nodes and intra-abdominal deposits. If there is no evidence of spread these patients are normally submitted to right thoracotomy with a view to radical resection.

Blunt oesophagectomy can be applied to resecting the oesophagus for benign disease such as recurring or resistant stricture and extensive neuromuscular dysfunction (Orringer 1985).

# Preoperative Preparation

Cardiorespiratory function is assessed since many of these patients are borderline and must be discussed with the anaesthetist. Undernourished patients are given high protein, high calorie diet, liquidised if necessary, while awaiting operation. For those with severe dysphagia the stricture is dilated at the time of diagnostic oesophagoscopy. If necessary, a normal sized or small bore nasogastric tube is inserted to allow liquid feeds to be given. Expensive parenteral nutrition is less effective and is rarely indicated.

A single injection of antibiotic is given intravenously by the anaesthetist at the start of the operation. The choice varies but at present a cephalosporin and metronidazole are considered the most effective.

---

*But see p. 16 – Editor.

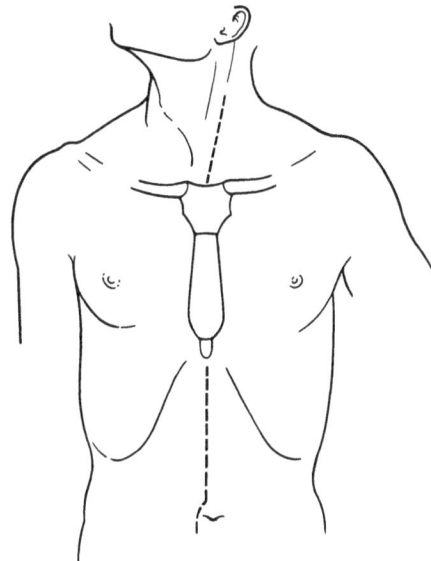

**Fig. 9.1.**   The sites of the abdominal and
cervical incisions are indicated by broken lines.

# Operative Approach

The intubated, anaesthetised and catheterised patient lies supine, head on a
rubber ring. The anaesthetist inserts a central venous cervical line on the side
opposite to that on which the anastomosis will be made. Electrocardiography
leads are applied well away from the midline. The skin is prepared from the angle
of the jaw down to the pubis. Head towels are applied, the neck is extended and
the head is turned away from the side of the intended anastomosis. Towels are
applied to leave the neck, sternum and midline abdomen exposed (Fig. 9.1).

The abdomen is opened through an upper midline incision skirting the
umbilicus. Complete abdominal exploration is carried out to exclude concomitant disease and spread of tumour, starting in the pelvis and working upwards to
avoid disseminating tumour cells. If there is no obvious spread that precludes
palliative resection, the oesophageal hiatus is now opened anterior to the
oesophagus and a finger is inserted into the posterior mediastinum to separate the
pericardium from the upper surface of the diaphragm, which is then incised
anteriorly from the crus after securing, ligating and dividing the inferior phrenic
vessels. This procedure is unnecessary if the hiatus is patulous. The phreno-
oesophageal ligament is widely incised so that a hand may be introduced into the
posterior mediastinum (Fig. 9.2).

Tumours of the lower thoracic and intra-abdominal oesophagus can be
assessed and the lower end of higher tumours can be identified, to decide if they
are likely to be resectable. A broad-bladed retractor is inserted behind the heart
to lift it gently anteriorly, often allowing a view up to the level of the tracheal
carina.

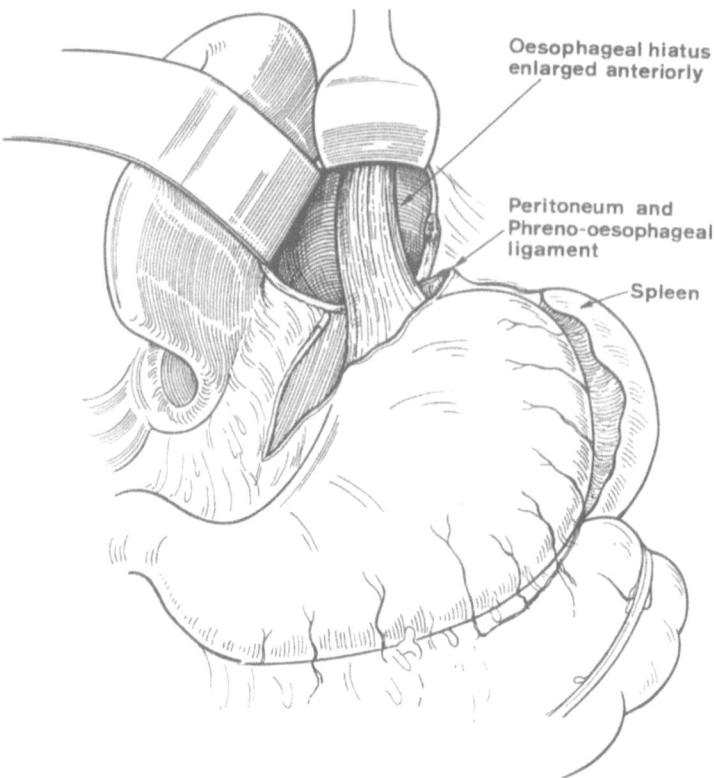

Oesophageal hiatus
enlarged anteriorly

Peritoneum and
Phreno-oesophageal
ligament

Spleen

**Fig. 9.2.** The diaphragmatic hiatus viewed from below after incising the crus.

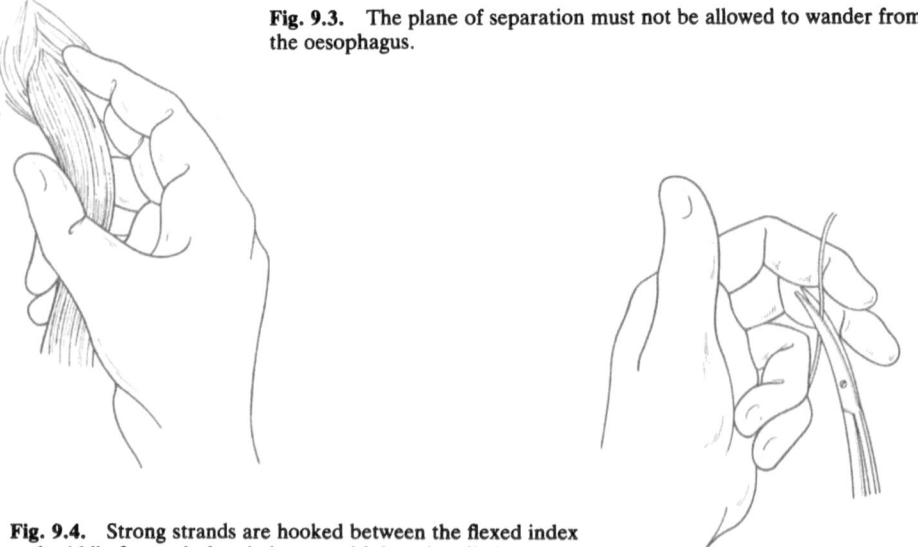

**Fig. 9.3.** The plane of separation must not be allowed to wander from the oesophagus.

**Fig. 9.4.** Strong strands are hooked between the flexed index and middle fingers before being cut with long-handled scissors.

## Mobilisation from Below

Dissection starts from the area of the cardia. In patients with associated sliding hiatal hernia the cardia lies in the posterior mediastinum enclosed by stretched phreno-oesophageal ligaments.

There is but one vital rule in carrying out blunt oesophageal resection and that is to keep in intimate contact with the oesophagus at all times, not allowing the plane of separation to wander away from this. While the thumb and medial fingers encircle the oesophagus, the index and middle fingers extend upwards to separate structures from it (Fig. 9.3). At the level of the tracheal bifurcation strong strands of vagal nerve pass from the root of the lung to the oesophagus. These should be hooked by the flexed index and middle fingers which are then slightly separated so that the tips of long-handled scissors can be passed within the protection of the fingers to cut the nerves (Fig. 9.4). Sharp dissection is best avoided unless the structures have been identified as safe to divide and surrounding viscera have been protected from damage.

Dissection is first posterior, then anterior, then lateral. A small artery passes from the aorta directly to the lower oesophagus: it is usually ruptured without being recognised and seals spontaneously but when it is identified it should be ligated on the aorta before being divided.

Great care is necessary when starting the separation of the trachea from the oesophagus since it is possible to damage the flimsy membranous posterior wall of the trachea. If the line of cleavage is difficult to find it is usually best to begin the separation from above through the neck.

## Gastric Mobilisation

It is wise to defer gastric mobilisation until it is certain that the tumour is resectable or can be bypassed. The spleen is preserved unless it is inadvertently damaged.

A hole is made through an avascular part of the gastrocolic omentum and the posterior wall of the stomach is separated from the pancreas and posterior abdominal wall. The gastrocolic ligament is now divided, while taking great care to preserve intact the right gastroepiploic vessels along the gastric greater curve. In particular, the right gastroepiploic vein can easily be damaged near the pylorus since it lies more to the left than is often expected. The left gastroepiploic and short gastric vessels are carefully divided between ligatures. The gastrophrenic ligament is divided.

The stomach is lifted forwards. Posteriorly, a vein arches between the upper border of the pancreas and the gastric cardia from the diaphragmatic crus.

The lesser omentum is incised through an avascular part and this is extended upwards towards the diaphragm, after ensuring that any accessory hepatic vessels accompanying the hepatic branches of the vagus are first ligated. The lesser omentum is incised distally taking care to stop short of the vital structures at its distal end.

As the gastric lesser curve is now drawn forwards the arching peritoneal fold is seen that contains the left gastric vessels, lymphatics and the coeliac branch of the posterior vagus. The lymph nodes around the coeliac axis are mobilised into the left gastric pedicle which is then doubly ligated and divided flush on the posterior wall.

The duodenal loop is fully mobilised by Kocher's manoeuvre so that the pylorus can be drawn up to the hiatus, being restrained only by the tension in the right gastroepiploic vein and the structures in the free edge of the lesser omentum. The pylorus is examined for scarring and a finger invaginates the anterior gastric antral wall through the ring to exclude stenosis or a mucosal diaphragm. If this can be accomplished, pyloroplasty is unnecessary.

## Approach from Above

The patient's chin is turned away from the side of the incision, the neck is extended and an incision is made along the lower half of the anterior border of sternomastoid muscle. Originally, the approach was from the patient's left side, subsequently the right side was used for fear of damaging the thoracic duct, but as this did not appear to present a problem, a left-sided approach is now advised. The upper oesophagus veers to the left and during bimanual dissection a right-handed person can conveniently insert the right hand into the posterior mediastinum while mobilising the oesophagus from above with the left hand inserted through the cervical incision. The incision is deepened into the groove between the carotid sheath laterally, identified by the arterial pulsations, and the central mass of trachea, oesophagus and thyroid gland (Fig. 9.5). Three structures are encountered – the omohyoid muscle which is divided, the middle thyroid vein which is divided between ligatures, and the inferior thyroid artery which is preserved if possible. As the plane is deepened the prevertebral muscles are reached.

The central mass of thyroid gland, trachea and oesophagus is gently rotated to the opposite side, exposing the groove between the trachea and oesophagus. The recurrent laryngeal nerve is identified and preserved as the oesophagus is carefully separated from the trachea by using Moynihan or Lahey forceps. Since the opposite recurrent laryngeal nerve cannot be seen it is particularly important to be gentle in separating the oesophagus. The oesophagus is encircled with a tape.

The oesophagus is first pushed forward from behind and then separated from the back of the trachea with an index finger, down into the posterior mediastinum. In some patients it is possible to reach to the tracheal bifurcation.

When carrying out a combined operation of pharyngolaryngectomy for postcricoid carcinoma the otolaryngologist usually deals exclusively with the cervical approach but cooperates with the general surgeon working from below to free the upper thoracic oesophagus.

## Combined Mobilisation from Above and Below

At this stage synchronous bimanual separation of the remaining attachments of the oesophagus around the root of the lungs may be valuable. A right-handed surgeon should stand on the patient's right side. The right hand is inserted through the abdominal wound up into the posterior mediastinum from below,

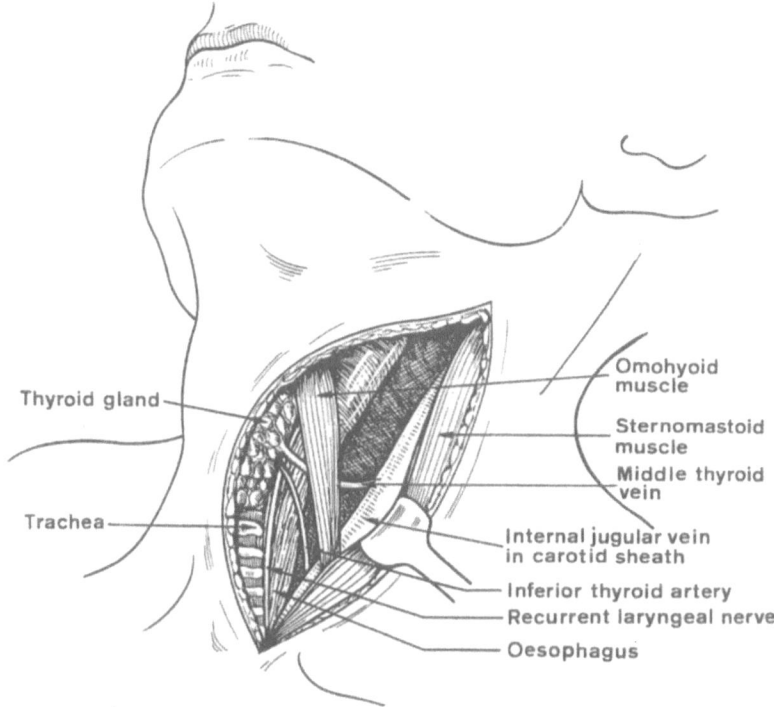

**Fig. 9.5.**   The carotid sheath is separated laterally from the central mass of trachea, thyroid gland and oesophagus.

while the fingers of the left hand reach down from the neck. The fingers meet and identify intervening structures, gently separating them from the oesophagus. This is often the most delicate and difficult part of the dissection, especially if the tumour is midoesophageal. When all the attachments have been divided, traction on the cervical oesophagus freely draws the gastric cardia upwards and traction on the stomach draws down the cervical oesophagus.

## Resection

If the tumour is in the upper third of the oesophagus the upper palpable margin of the tumour is identified so that transection can be carried out at least 6–7 cm higher up. If the tumour is in the mid or lower oesophagus, the lower cervical oesophagus is gently drawn up so that the transection can safely be made through the upper thoracic oesophagus. Natural retraction places the anastomosis in the lower neck.

A non-crushing bowel clamp is placed across the oesophagus above the selected resection line. A strong ligature is firmly tied around the oesophagus 2–3 cm below the line of resection. The oesophagus is transected. Alternatively, a line of staples may be applied across the oesophagus below the resection line. A long tape is attached to the lower cut end of the oesophagus.

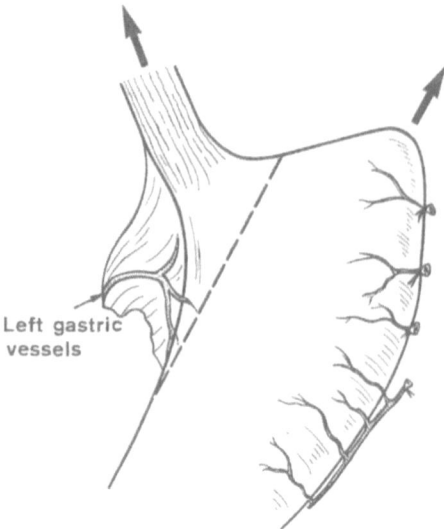

**Fig. 9.6.** Traction is applied on the gastric fundus and the lower greater curve so that a straight 90-mm stapler can be placed to reach from the lower lesser curve to the right side of the gastric fundus. The line of the stapler is indicated by the broken line.

Left gastric vessels

The free end of the tape is secured in the neck while the oesophagus is drawn down from below. The tape is freed below and now lies in the track of the oesophagus.

The transection line through the stomach at the lower end of the oesophagus depends upon the site of tumour. For upper-third growths it is usual to cut straight across the cardia. For mid and lower-third growths the cardia, gastric lesser curve, left gastric vessels and attached lymph nodes should be removed. The technique of Akiyama (1980) can almost always be performed and is advisable even in the presence of high tumours which, nevertheless, may produce neoplastic glands at the cardia. The fundus of the stomach, grasped at its highest point, is drawn upwards and to the left, outside the costal margin, placing it slightly on stretch. The oesophagus is drawn to the right, slightly tenting the lesser curvature of the stomach. A 90-mm straight stapling device is placed to cross the mid lesser curvature below and the angle of His above (Fig. 9.6).

The stapler is actuated and before removing it the specimen is excised by cutting along its right edge. Initially the staple line was invaginated with a running suture but this is no longer considered to be necessary.

## Oesophagogastrostomy

The gastric fundus should reach to the neck without tension when laid on the anterior chest wall. The lower end of the tape is now sutured to the highest point of the fundus. It acts as a guide as it is drawn upwards from the neck. Meanwhile, the stomach is gently fed through the enlarged hiatus from below while making sure that there is no twisting. As the gastric fundus emerges, it is gently grasped with swab-holding forceps to draw it into the neck.

The origin of the right gastroepiploic artery is checked to be pulsating, with no traction on the right gastroepiploic vein. The abdomen is examined to exclude continuing bleeding or inadvertent damage. The colour of the gastric fundus is assessed. It may be slightly congested but the veins should not be excessively dilated. If they are, it is possible that a twist has been allowed to occur as the stomach was pulled up. In case of doubt the stomach should be withdrawn and carefully repassed.

If all is well, the cut upper end of oesophagus and gastric fundus are laid together. The tape is freed. An incision is made into the gastric fundus to match the oesophageal lumen. The non-crushing clamp is removed from the upper cut oesophagus. For many years 2/0 chromic catgut was used for the anastomosis but now absorbable 4/0 polyglycolic acid, polyglactin and polydioxanone or non-absorbable silk and polyamide sutures are used. The all-coats stitch picks up each end of the oesophageal and gastric openings (Fig. 9.7). The stitches are drawn apart to stretch the openings.

The most usual method of anastomosis is by a single layer of interrupted stitches, though a continuous over and over absorbable suture has also been used. All-coats sutures are inserted along the posterior wall, apposing the mucosal edges, with knots tied within the lumen, 2 mm apart, taking 2-mm bites on each side.

Before the anterior sutures are inserted, a closed, long, curved forceps is passed up through the oesophagus into the pharynx and the tips are pushed laterally against the skin of the neck. A small incision is made over the tips of the forceps which are then pushed through to grasp the end of a nasogastric tube. The tube is drawn down and the tip is guided well down into the stomach. The outer end of the pharyngostomy tube is fixed by a stitch to the skin. The anterior wall of the oesophagogastric anastomosis is completed with the knots of interrupted stitches tied on the outside.

The exact method of stitching does not matter so much as the perfection with which it is accomplished. Sutures must be tied just tightly enough to appose but not strangle the enclosed tissue. The oesophagus is capable of enormous distension and stitches placed close together when it is slack may be widely separated when the patient swallows a bolus of fluid or food. Some surgeons, including the author, often insert a second layer of sutures, picking up the oesophageal muscularis and submucosa, and also the gastric seromuscularis, so as to invaginate the all-coats stitch.

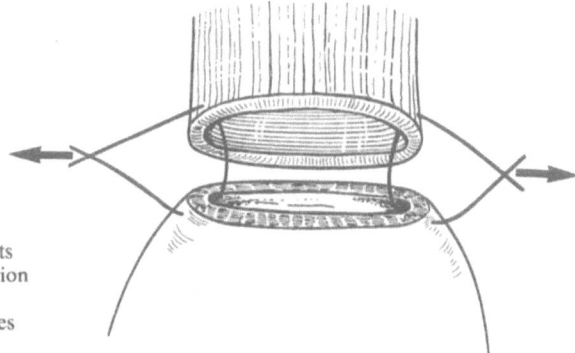

Fig. 9.7. Preparation for the oesophagogastrostomy. An all-coats stitch is placed at each end as traction stitches in order to stretch the anastomosis gently while the sutures are inserted.

Although circular stapling instruments may be used to accomplish the anastomosis, it is difficult to draw up sufficient stomach to insert the head and safely close the hole subsequently. In the neck, suturing is so easy to perform that mechanical aids are unnecessary.


## Technical Considerations

The attachments of the lesser omentum to the lesser curve may restrict it so the larger lesser curve assumes the shape of a reversed "C". The stomach can be straightened and lengthened by ligating and dividing the lesser omental attachments along the lesser curve.

Access can be difficult in the upper abdomen, to mobilise the stomach, to assess the growth through the hiatus, and to carry out the dissection in a controlled manner. If there is any difficulty an immediate subcutaneous midline lower sternotomy (Foley and Kirk 1976; Kirk 1987a,b) will improve the exposure. At the upper end of the abdominal incision the skin and subcutaneous tissues are separated from the anterior aspect of the sternum, the diaphragmatic slips to the xiphoid process are divided, and a finger is inserted behind the sternum in the midline to separate the pericardium and pleura. A large straight bone-cutting forceps is used to cut the xiphoid and sternum in the midline as far as is necessary to improve the access, if necessary up to the manubriosternal junction. An index finger protects the tip of the deep blade from contact with the anterior mediastinal contents. A large pack is wedged into the gap to separate the two halves and also to stop bleeding from the bone edges. This exposes the upper abdomen, allows safe mobilisation of the gastric fundus without inadvertent damage to the spleen, facilitates safe dissection around the coeliac glands and offers a good view through the enlarged hiatus into the posterior mediastinum (Fig. 9.8). It is unnecessary to re-appose the sternal halves. The upper stitch of the abdominal wound closure picks up the diaphragmatic slips that were separated from the xiphoid process.

A problem that is sometimes encountered is when the tumour proves at operation much more extensive and fixed than is anticipated from X-rays, endoscopy or scanning techniques. It is well known that oesophageal carcinoma may spread longitudinally within the oesophageal wall or in peri-oesophageal lymphatics (Kirk and McLaughlin 1985). Fixation may be discovered in the mid or upper thorax when the lower oesophagus is already mobilised. It is then often difficult to reach down from the neck to tackle the dissection from above. Another problem is that although the gastric fundus usually reaches comfortably to the neck, occasionally there is unacceptable tension on the right gastroepiploic vein which partially obliterates it and threatens to congest the stomach. It is also sometimes necessary to resect the gastric fundus so that the conduit is shorter than planned. The shortened conduit threatens safe anastomosis.

The neck incision can be carried over the middle of the suprasternal notch and down the midline of the sternum to 5–7 cm below the manubriosternal joint. A finger is inserted between the sternothyroid and sternohyoid muscles, down behind the sternum to separate the deep structures. The sternum is split in the midline using a sternal saw or Lebsche's knife, to 5 cm below the manubriosternal joint (Orringer 1984; Fig. 9.9). The halves are separated with a ratchet sternal

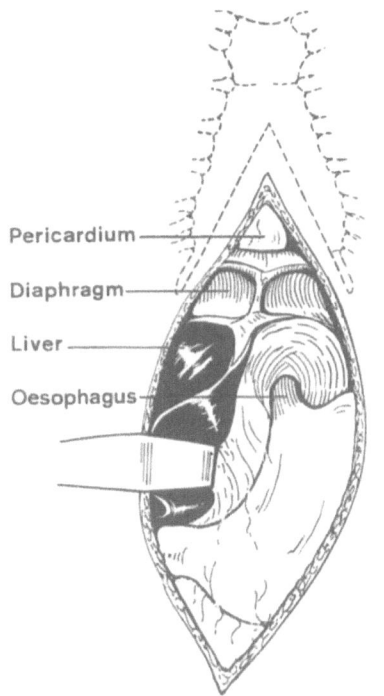

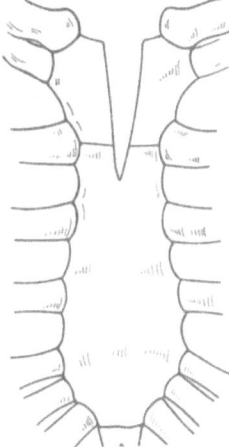

◀ **Fig. 9.8.** Subcutaneous midline sternotomy improves the view of the upper abdomen and hiatal region.

Pericardium

Diaphragm

Liver

Oesophagus

**Fig. 9.9.** Upper midline partial sternotomy.

retractor. If necessary, the left innominate vein can be divided between ligatures. The oesophagus is seen projecting to the left of the trachea and dissection is easily carried out. Care is taken not to injure the left recurrent laryngeal nerve. Safe dissection is possible and, provided the upper oesophagus has not been extensively mobilised, the anastomosis can be made using a shorter than expected conduit in the superior mediastinum instead of the neck.

A lower subcutaneous midline sternotomy is frequently performed and it is often preferable to convert this into a complete midline sternotomy (Ong et al. 1978; Kirk 1987). It is important to make the decision early so that the full benefit of the excellent exposure is gained throughout the operation and especially if the intrathoracic dissection is likely to be difficult. The lower end of the cervical and the upper end of the abdominal incisions are joined along the midline over the sternum (Fig. 9.10). The structures deep to the sternum are separated with a finger passed from above and below. The sternum is split in the midline using a sternal or Gigli saw and the halves are separated with a ratchet sternal retractor (Fig. 9.11). The exposure is excellent, both to facilitate dissection and for the anastomosis. When the gastric conduit is short, it can be brought anteriorly or posteriorly and anastomosed to the upper third of the intrathoracic oesophagus. The exposure can be further increased by making a longitudinal incision in the right pleura and dividing the azygos vein between ligatures to gain access to the oesophagus from the thorax. Subsequently the pleura is repaired and an extra drain inserted if necessary.

On occasion the stomach cannot be employed for the anastomosis because it proves to be extensively involved with tumour, or the lymph nodes along the

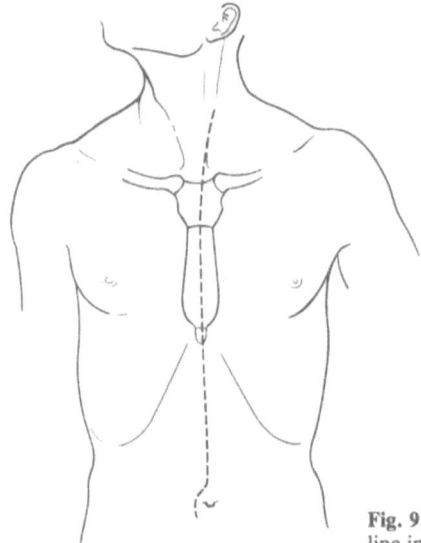

**Fig. 9.10.** Complete midline sternotomy. The broken line indicates the incision.

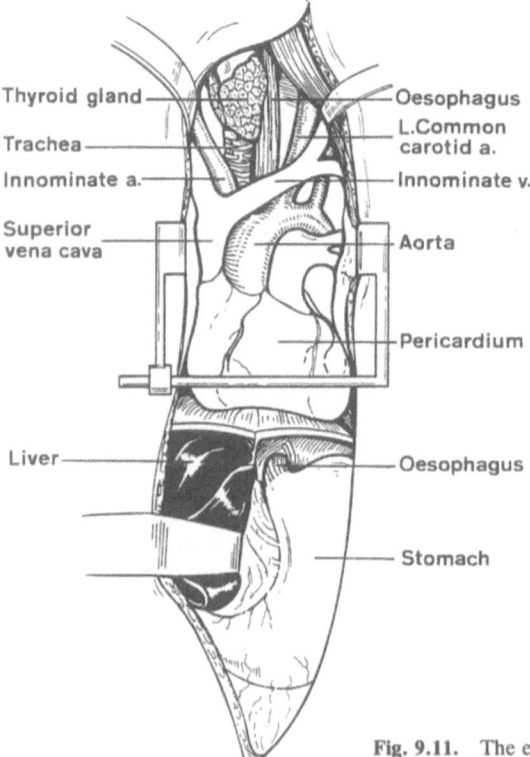

**Fig. 9.11.** The exposure provided by complete midline sternotomy.

lesser curve extend down towards the pylorus too far to allow the stomach to remain. In this case a Roux-en-Y loop of jejunum or colonic conduit can be brought up anteriorly or posteriorly.

The sternotomy is closed using nylon threads mounted on stout trocar pointed needles that pass through the marrow cavity and out through the outer cortex of the sternum.

Two additional methods of blunt oesophageal resection have been described in the literature, but have not been used by the author. The oesophagus may be stripped out with a vein stripper, but in practice most tumours produce a swelling that would not pass through the largest stripper available. Another technique is to invaginate the oesophagus from above into itself by traction from within, but again the tumours are usually too large to allow inversion of the oesophagus through the restricted lumen. Both of these methods could be used when removing a normal oesophagus during the performance of blunt oesophagectomy for a benign condition or when excising it during pharyngolaryngectomy – but in these conditions blunt oesophagectomy is easy.

## Closure

The colour of the gastric fundus is checked and if it is congested the right gastroepiploic vein should be examined to see if it is obstructed. Residual bleeding is controlled. The pleura is checked as thoroughly as possible to detect tears which are repaired when possible. It is wise to insert bilateral chest drains for 24 hours, either through the intercostal spaces or through the hiatus. The abdominal wound is closed using looped O nylon by mass closure. The neck is closed after inserting a drain which is attached to a vacuum suction bottle before being removed after 24–48 hours.

# Postoperative Care

Most patients are kept in the intensive care unit overnight until they are extubated and are breathing satisfactorily. Daily chest X-rays are taken and the chest drains are removed after 24–48 hours. Fluid, electrolyte and nutritional requirements are infused intravenously. The stomach is aspirated until the patient can be sat upright, for fear of overspill. On the 4th or 5th postoperative day the anastomosis is usually checked radiologically using a water-soluble contrast medium. If this is satisfactory oral feeding is started and the pharyngostomy tube is removed.

# Results

Blunt oesophagectomy has been carried out in 83 patients, aged 35–88 years (mean 62.7). There were 26 females, 57 males. In 46 the tumour was adenocarcinoma or undifferentiated, one affecting the whole oesophagus. In 37 the tumour was squamous with 31 intrathoracic, four cervical involving pharyngolaryngectomy in association with otolaryngologists, and two proving to involve the whole oesophagus. Resection had to be abandoned in 15 patients because of extension of the tumour discovered at operation. Of these two were suitable for Kirschner's operation of subcutaneous presternal gastric bypass, two had substernal gastric bypass, one had subcutaneous Roux loop bypass and in one patient who had a tumour extending into the stomach, a left thoraco-abdominal anastomosis was performed. In five patients intubation was attempted but successful in only three and in four patients no procedure was carried out.

There were surprisingly few complications attributable to the method of oesophageal resection. No patient bled into the thorax – and one patient required to be returned to theatre for ligation of the inferior thyroid artery from which the initial ligature had slipped following pharyngolaryngectomy. Five patients had laryngeal nerve palsy which improved sufficiently in four to require no intervention but in one patient Teflon was injected into the cord to restore normal phonation. The feared complication of tracheal laceration has not occurred and there were no patients with evidence of thoracic duct damage.

There were 22 in-hospital deaths (24%), 11 of which were cardiorespiratory. Leaks accounted for four deaths (three of which occurred early in the series) and in four cases there was a minor leak that healed spontaneously. One patient developed a late leak following complete sternotomy, requiring reopening and the insertion of a per-antral feeding tube and reclosure of the sternotomy. An additional patient required a mucocutaneous pectoralis major flap repair of a persistent neck fistula.

Two of the patients in whom resection had to be abandoned died rapidly from septicaemia and one developed an early broncho-oesophageal fistula and died. One other patient died from septicaemia without demonstrable leak. The three final deaths were accounted for by one patient who died following the relief of simple postoperative intestinal obstruction, one with rapid recrudescence of tumour and a final patient in whom the cause of death was not established.

Because the operations were all performed as palliative procedures in patients considered to be incurable, routine long-term follow-up was not carried out.


# Conclusions

The results in this series are not a source of pride but should not be compared with operations carried out in the hope of curing apparently limited disease. Surgeons dealing with oesophageal carcinoma can obtain good results only by rejecting for treatment those patients who are likely to fare badly because of the extent of the disease or because of infirmity. This makes up the majority of the patients seen by the author. The terminal stages of untreated oesophageal carcinoma are extremely distressing and intubation, radiotherapy and chemotherapy are unreliable in relieving the symptoms while successful resection and anastomosis offers good short-term palliation.

*Acknowledgment.* Figures 9.8 to 9.11, inclusive, are reproduced, with permission, from the British Journal of Surgery (1987).

# References

Akiyama H (1980) Surgery for carcinoma of the oesophagus. Curr Probl Surg 17:52–150
Belsey R (1978) Discussion of Orringer MB, Sloan H: Esophagectomy without thoracotomy. J
    Thorac Cardiovasc Surg 76:643–654
Clairmont P (1924) Zur Radikaloperation des Oesophaguskarcinoms. Zentralbl Chir 51:42–46
Collaborating Group for Research on Esophageal Cancer, Linhsien County, Honan (1976) Early
    diagnosis and surgical treatment of esophageal cancer under rural conditions. Chin Med J [Engl]
    2:113–116
Denk W (1913) Zur Radikaloperation des Oesophaguskarcinoms (Vorlaufige Mitteilung). Zentralbl
    Chir 40:1065–1068
Earlam R, Cunha-Melo JR (1980) Oesophageal squamous cell carcinoma. I. A critical review of
    surgery. Br J Surg 67:381–390
Foley RJE, Kirk RM (1976) Subcutaneous midline sternotomy for upper abdominal access. Proc R
    Soc Med 69:851–852
Kirk RM (1974) Palliative resection of oesophageal carcinoma without formal thoracotomy. Br J Surg
    61:689–690
Kirk RM (1983) Double indemnity in oesophageal carcinoma? Br Med J i:582–583
Kirk RM (1987a) Gastroduodenal surgery. In: Kirk RM, Williamson RCN (eds) General surgical
    operations, 2nd edn. Churchill Livingstone, Edinburgh, pp 63–64
Kirk RM (1987b) Partial and complete sternotomy for blunt oesophagectomy. Br J Surg 74:685–687
Kirk RM, McLaughlin JE (1985) Oesophagus. In: Hadfield GJ, Hobsley M, Morson B (eds)
    Pathology in surgical practice. Edward Arnold, London, pp 48–64
Lancet (1986) Transhiatal oesophagectomy without thoracotomy. Lancet II:376 (editorial)
Le Quesne LP, Ranger D (1966) Pharyngolaryngectomy with immediate pharyngogastric anastomo-
    sis. Br J Surg 53:105–109
Ochsner A Jr (1978) Discussion of Orringer MB, Sloan H: Esophagectomy without thoracotomy. J
    Thorac Cardiovasc Surg 76:643–654
Ong GB, Lam KH, Lam PHM, Wong J (1978) Resection for carcinoma of the superior mediastinal
    segment of the oesophagus. World J Surg 2:479–504
Orringer MB (1984) Partial median sternotomy: anterior approach to the upper thoracic esophagus. J
    Thorac Cardiovasc Surg 87:124–129
Orringer MB (1985) Transhiatal esophagectomy for benign disease. J Thorac Cardiovasc Surg
    90:649–655
Sannohe Y, Hiratsuka R, Doki K (1981) Lymph node metastases in cancer of the thoracic esophagus.
    Am J Surg 141:216–218
Turner GG (1933) Excision of the thoracic oesophagus for carcinoma with construction of an
    extrathoracic gullet. Lancet II:1315–1316
Williamson RCN (1985) Abdominocervical oesophagectomy in the elderly. Ann R Coll Surg Engl
    67:344–348

# Resection using Stapling Instruments

R. J. Donnelly

## Introduction

Oesophagogastrectomy is the procedure of choice in many patients with carcinoma of the lower and middle thirds of the oesophagus, offering the best chance
of cure and an effective means of palliation. It has, however, been associated
historically with a high incidence of morbidity and mortality. The length of the
procedure, often in elderly debilitated patients, and a significant incidence of
anastomotic leakage have been largely responsible for disappointing results in
many reported series.

Clinical results have improved in recent years due to improvements in
anaesthetic management and perioperative care. Surgical techniques have also
advanced with better suture materials and, in recent years, with the development
of stapling instruments. The use of stapling instruments in oesophageal surgery
has been the subject of lively debate and will remain so for some time to come.
There is little argument that, for many surgeons, they speed up the process of
resection and anastomosis and reduce the overall operating time, and this still
remains an important consideration in the surgical care of the old and infirm. It is
also claimed by the proponents of stapling that the anastomotic leakage rate is
reduced, that tissue handling and soiling is reduced and that patients recover
more quickly and can therefore be discharged home sooner. These latter
advantages are more difficult to substantiate because so much depends on the
skills and experience of the individual surgeon.

To date there has been no controlled prospective randomised clinical trial to
assess the relative merits of stapling versus hand suturing for oesophageal
anastomosis with respect to complications, blood loss, cost, operating time and

hospital stay. Until such a trial has been done, it will remain a matter of individual preference as to which method is used. Many will continue to prefer and take pride in traditional suturing techniques. Others will be attracted by the clean, quick and effective nature of stapling instruments.

In the author's view, staplers not only have an advantage in terms of time but also specifically in making the anastomosis high in the thorax. The hand-sewn cervical anastomosis is recommended by some so that, if a leak should occur, it will be extrathoracic and therefore less serious. The authors experience is that, using the EEA stapling gun, a high intrathoracic anastomosis can be safely achieved with a very low leak rate, eliminating the time and the scar associated with a separate cervical incision. It is also the author's preference to mobilise the stomach through an incision in the diaphragm rather than the traditional thoracoabdominal incision and staplers have certainly facilitated this and further contributed to a reduced operating time.

Staplers do not in any way reduce the care and attention required to achieve good results with oesophageal resection. They do, however, reduce surgeon fatigue and thereby help concentration, particularly if the dissection is long and difficult. Because the procedure is quicker, the surgeon is also freed for other work and can use his time more effectively, particularly if his caseload is high.

# Historical Aspects

A comprehensive account of the history of the use of mechanical stapling instruments in surgical practice is given in the book Stapling in Surgery (1984) by Felicien Steichen and Mark Ravitch. Various mechanical devices have been in use since the earliest days of abdominal surgery but stapling instruments, as we know them today, were pioneered in the Soviet Union by Dr N. M. Amosov (Amosov et al. 1958). During a visit to Russia in 1958 Dr Ravitch observed this work and, with some difficulty, obtained an instrument and took it back with him to the USA. There, he and his colleagues began to experiment and, in association with the United States Surgical Corporation, redesigned and further developed the full range of stapling instruments having introduced them into clinical practice at an early stage (Ravitch et al. 1959, 1964; Ravitch and Steichen 1972a,b).

A circular stapling instrument for end-to-end anastomosis, similar in concept to the modern instruments, was developed by the Russians in the early 1960s (Katinina et al. 1962) and a similar instrument was later described by the Chinese (Wu Ying-K'ai and Huang Kuo-chun 1979). The EEA instrument, with a double row of staples, was subsequently developed in association with the United States Surgical Corporation. This instrument was introduced into the United Kingdom in 1979 by a subsidiary of this company now known as Autosuture Company UK.

Stapling techniques for restoring continuity of the gastrointestinal tract after oesophagectomy were pioneered in the West by Ravitch, Steichen, and Chassin before the advent of the circular end-to-end anastomotic device (Steichen 1971; Ravitch and Steichen 1972; Steichen and Ravitch 1979; Chassin, 1978). However, it was not until the advent of the EEA instrument in 1979 that mechanical suture of the oesophagus became widely accepted. Early experiences using this device appeared in a flurry of reports extolling the merits of the new technique (Hugh 1980; Molina et al. 1980; Graham et al. 1981; Sugimachi et al. 1981; Hirashima et al. 1982; Fabri and Donnelly 1982). Stapling using the EEA proved to be simple, time-saving and reliable (Hopkins et al. 1984; Steichen and Ravitch 1984; Donnelly et al. 1985) and now has an established role in modern surgical practice.

# Technique

Several instrument companies are now producing stapling instruments but the author's experience in oesophageal surgery has been with the EEA, LDS, TA, Surgiclip and Pursestring instruments (Autosuture Company UK) and these will be described here.

A variety of surgical approaches to the oesophagus are in current use. The author's preference is for a left thoracotomy through the bed of the seventh rib. Access to the abdomen is obtained through an incision in the diaphragm. The costal margin is not divided unless exposure is limited as a result of previous abdominal surgery or by the bulk of the tumour. The anastomosis is carried out above and lateral to the aortic arch except in cases where resection is clearly only palliative.

If the tumour is considered resectable, the stomach is fully mobilised along the greater and lesser curvatures. This is rapidly accomplished using the LDS instrument which simultaneously applies two staples and cuts between them. It is preferable to take the short gastric vessels with individual applications of the Surgiclip instrument and division with scissors. The left gastric artery is tied with a a stout ligature and divided with the LDS.

Pyloroplasty is only carried out if the pylorus is narrowed, contracted or scarred. This can often be achieved through the incision in the diaphragm but, if there is difficulty, the skin incision should be extended on to the abdomen and the costal margin divided.

After mobilising the oesophagus up to and above the aortic arch, the stomach is delivered into the chest. The site for gastric transection is chosen and the stomach stapled at this point, in a transverse direction, with the TA90 instrument. A clamp is applied to the proximal stomach to prevent spillage and the stomach divided with scissors along the face of the TA90 before the instrument is removed. The cut edge may then be oversewn for added security.

The Pursestring instrument is applied to the oesophagus at the point chosen for transection. The oesophagus is cut with scissors distal to the clamp leaving a small 4-mm cuff of tissue. This is essential to prevent subsequent pulling out of the pursestring suture. The resected specimen is then removed. A 1/0 Prolene suture is passed through the eyes of the pursestring clamp and left lying without tension on a small artery clip. A non-crushing clamp is placed on the oesophagus proximal to the pursestring clamp which is then removed. Three stay sutures are inserted into the free end of the oesophagus at 12, 5 and 7 o'clock, making sure that all layers of the oesophageal wall are incorporated.

A longitudinal incision is made in the anterior wall of the stomach away from the transverse staple line. The EEA instrument (Fig. 10.1), which will fit

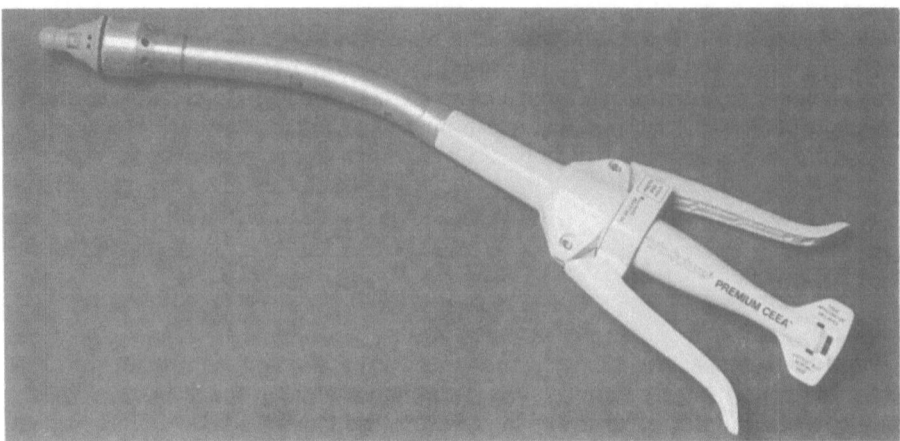

**Fig. 10.1.**   The Autosuture stapling instrument.

comfortably in the lumen of the oesophagus, is chosen for the anastomosis. It is important not to be too ambitious in the size of instrument selected. Sizers can be used but these can cause trauma to the oesophageal wall and it is better to make a visual judgement based on experience. The EEA, without the anvil, is inserted through the gastrotomy and the central rod brought through the posterior wall of the stomach, away from the previous staple line and free from any of the staples used to mobilise the stomach. The rod is extended and the anvil attached and lubricated. With assistance from the stay sutures, the anvil is manipulated with great care into the lumen of the oesophagus. This is often more easily achieved if the posterior wall is first brought over the edge of the anvil followed by the anterior wall.

The stay sutures must be relaxed when the pursestring suture is firmly tied down around the central column. The EEA instrument is then closed, allowing the stomach to come upwards to the oesophagus and thereby avoiding unnecessary tension on the oesophagus. Correct compression is achieved by observation of the control on the handle of the instrument. This is then fired and two rows of staggered interrupted staples are applied in a circular fashion between the oesophagus and the stomach. Simultaneously, a circular knife cuts out the core of tissue contained within the rows of staples. The instrument is opened again and removed with a gentle rotatory movement. The staple line is inspected through the gastrotomy for haemostasis and to ensure that the mucosa has been incorporated all round. A nasogastric tube is placed through the anastomosis from above and the gastrotomy closed with a TA instrument. This staple line may also be oversewn.

The doughnuts of tissue removed by the EEA are examined and a satisfactory anastomosis is indicated if all layers of both stomach and oesophagus are incorporated.

The patient is given nil by mouth until the fourth postoperative day and thereafter advanced to a soft diet over a period of a few days. A postoperative gastrografin swallow is only carried out if an anastomotic leak is suspected or if there has been undue difficulty in performing the anastomosis.

Following discharge from hospital, patients are followed-up in clinic at regular intervals and assessed for evidence of recurrent tumour or of anastomotic narrowing. Any patient with dysphagia is readmitted for oesophagoscopy.

# Results

The author first used the EEA instrument for oesophagogastric anastomosis in January 1980 and has used it in every case since that time except for two patients who required a cervical anastomosis performed by hand suture. Over the next 7½ years 176 patients underwent resection using the EEA stapler; 166 of these were for malignant disease (91%). The mean age was 63 years (range 33–84 years). The male to female ratio was 2:1. Operative mortality, defined as death within 30 days or during initial hospital stay, was 8.5%.

## Anastomotic Leaks

There were no anastomotic leaks in the first 100 patients (Donnelly et al. 1985) but three subsequent leaks brought the overall leakage rate to 1.7%. Two of the leaks occurred after attempting to insert too large a stapler into a non-compliant oesophagus. One of these patients died but the other patient, who was also managed conservatively, survived after a long and complicated postoperative course. The third patient was re-explored and found to have a leak where a portion of the gastric wall had not been included in the stapled anastomosis. The gastric doughnut must have been incomplete at the original operation but this had gone unnoticed. A simple stitch was all that was required and the patient made a good recovery.

Leakage from sutured oesophago-gastric anastomoses has an average reported incidence in the literature of 10% (range 0%–41%) (Chassin 1978). The average reported anastomotic leak rate using modern stapling techniques is 1.4% (range 0%–3.3%) (Donnelly et al. 1985). A technical fault is usually identifiable and careful attention to detail should keep this complication to a minimum.

## Strictures

Patients were closely questioned about dysphagia during follow-up and the overall postoperative incidence was 17.4%. All patients complaining of any degree of dysphagia were oesophagoscoped and dilated as necessary. Only patients who had some degree of anastomotic narrowing and who benefited symptomatically from dilatation were categorised as having an anastomotic stricture.

Anastomotic stricture due to recurrent tumour caused dysphagia in 6.2% of patients undergoing resection for malignant disease. The rate of benign anastomotic narrowing in all discharged patients, excluding those with recurrent anastomotic disease, was 12.5%. The majority of these (84%) had a lumen diameter greater than 10 mm as assessed by the Olympus Q10 endoscope. The highest rate of narrowing occurred in patients who underwent resection for benign stricture. The incidence in these patients was 37.5% compared to 9.6% for resections in patients with malignant disease ($P<0.05$).

There was a trend towards a higher incidence of stricture formation with a smaller head size; 17% for the 25-mm head, 13.5% for the 28-mm head and 5.4% for the 31-mm head. However, these differences did not reach statistical significance.

The vast majority of strictures occurred within the first six months and 79% of patients obtained permanent relief from two or fewer dilatations. The narrowing, when it occurs, appears to be of a much softer, more localised and less severe variety than that seen after hand-sewn anastomoses and to respond much more readily to dilatation.

The rate of benign stricture formation in our patients (12.5%) is lower than the 20% reported by Wong and colleagues (Wong et al. 1987) using the EEA stapler, but is more in line with those reported by West and colleagues (12.9%) (West et al. 1981) and Hopkins and colleagues (13.3%) (Hopkins et al. 1984) who, like ourselves, made corrections for hospital deaths and recurrent anastomotic disease.

## Age

There is a reluctance by many physicians to refer patients over 70 years of age for oesophageal surgery. In our series 46 patients were over the age of 70 years and 16 of these were over 75 years. Operative mortality in these 46 patients was 13.0% but in patients over 75 years the operative mortality was 6.3%. There was no statistically significant difference in mortality between these two groups or compared with the mortality of 8.5% in the 166 patients of all ages described earlier. There were no anastomotic leaks and average hospital stay was 13.4 days. These figures compare favourably with those reported in the literature in this age group (Wong 1981; Behl et al. 1983; Keeling et al. 1988; Mitchel 1987) and may be attributable in part to a simpler surgical approach (left thoracotomy alone) and speedier and less complicated surgery resulting from the use of stapling instruments. Oesophageal surgery can be carried out in this age group with acceptable results.

# Conclusions

Stapling instruments now have an established part to play in modern oesophageal surgery. They have been shown to be safe, speedy and simple to use, to the benefit of both patient and surgeon. They remain expensive, however, and their true cost benefit has yet to be established.

# References

Amosov NM, Berezovsky KK, Zabroda GS (1958) Experience of 100 resections of the lungs with UKL-60. Eksp Khirurg 6:3

Behl PR, Holden MP, Brown AH (1983) Three years experience with the esophageal stapling device. Ann Surg 198:134–136

Chassin JL (1978) Oesophagogastrectomy: data favouring end-to-side anastomoses. Am Surg 188:22–27

Donnelly RJ, Sastry MR, Wright CD (1985) Oesophagogastrectomy using the end-to-end anastomotic stapler: results of the first 100 patients. Thorax 40:958–959

Fabri B, Donnelly RJ (1982) Oesophagogastrectomy using the end-to-end anastomosing stapler. Thorax 37:296–299

Graham HK, Johnston HW, McKelvey TD, Kennedy TL (1981) Five years experience in stapling the oesophagus and rectum. Br J Surg 68:697–700

Hirashima T, Hara T, Benetani A et al. (1982) A new stapling device in oesophageal mucosal transection. J J Surg 12:160–162

Hopkins RA, Alexander JC, Postlethwait RW (1984) Stapled oesophagogastric anastomosis. Am J Surg 147:283–287

Hugh TB (1980) Simplified EEA stapled anastomosis by the end insertion technique. Am J Surg 139:449–450

Katinina TV, Babkin SI, Kasulin VS, Astafiev GV (1962) Mechanical sutures for oesophago-intestinal (gastric) anastomoses. Clin Surg [Moscow] 8:81

Keeling P, Gillen P, Hennessy TP (1988) Oesophageal resection in the elderly. Ann R Coll Surg Engl 70:34–37

Mitchel RL (1987) Abdominal and right thoracotomy approach as standard procedure for esophago-gastrectomy with low morbidity. J Thorac Cardiovasc Surg 93:205–211

Molina JE, Lawton BR, Avance D (1980) Use of circumferential stapler in reconstruction following resection for carcinoma of the cardia. Ann Thorac Surg 31:325–328

Ravitch MM, Steichen FM (1972a) Techniques of staple suturing in the gastrointestinal tract. Ann Surg 175:815–824

Ravitch MM, Steichen FM (1972b) Experience with a second generation of stapling instruments in general and thoracic surgery. Bull Soc Int Chir 31:502

Ravitch MM, Brown IW, Daviglus GF (1959) Experimental and clinical use of the Soviet bronchus stapling instrument. Surgery 46:97–108

Ravitch MM, Steichen FM, Fishbein RH, Knowles PW, Weil P (1964) Clinical experience with the Soviet mechanical bronchus stapler (UKB-25). J Thorac Cardiovasc Surg 47:446–454

Steichen FM (1971) Clinical experience with autosuture instruments. Surgery 69:609–615

Steichen FM, Ravitch MM (1979) Mechanical sutures in esophageal surgery. Ann Surg 191:373–381

Steichen FM, Ravitch MM (1984) Stapling in surgery. Year Book Medical Publishers, Chicago, pp 3–77, 220–257

Sugimachi K, Ikeda M, Ueo H et al. (1981) Clinical efficacy of the stapled anastomosis in esophageal reconstruction. Ann Thorac Surg 33:374–378

West PN, Marbargar JP, Martz MN, Roper CL (1981) Esophagogastrectomy with the EEA stapler. Ann Surg 193:76–81

Wong J (1981) Management of carcinoma of the oesophagus: art or science? Ann R Coll Surg Edin 26:138–149

Wong J, Cheung H, Lui R, Fan YW, Smith A, Sui FK (1987) Esophagogastric anastomosis performed with a stapler: the occurrence of leakage and stricture. Surgery 101:408–415

Wu Ying-K'ai, Huang Kuo-chun (1979) Chinese experience in the surgical treatment of carcinoma of the oesophagus. Ann Surg 190:361–365

# Chapter 11

# Palliative Therapy

A. Watson

## Introduction

Palliative treatment, in one of its various forms, is appropriate in three types of clinical situation. Firstly, a patient with a potentially operable tumour may be considered too old, infirm or to have such serious intercurrent disease as to render the risks of resection unacceptably high. Secondly, the tumour may be considered unresectable, or incurable by virtue of the presence of metastatic disease or of gross involvement of contiguous structures, such as the presence of tracheo-oesophageal fistula, recurrent laryngeal nerve paresis or extensive mediastinal spread demonstrated by CT scanning. Thirdly, there is a small but finite group of patients who are considered to be fit for resection, to have a localised, resectable tumour, but who at operation are found to have either undetected metastases or an unexpected degree of tumour extension into contiguous structures which makes resection hazardous or technically impossible.

The extent to which the various palliative modalities are deployed depends, in many centres, on the degree of preselection before referral to surgeons and on the aggressiveness of the surgeon to whom patients are referred. Reported resection rates vary between 16% and 90% (Earlam 1984; Keeling et al. 1988), which is likely to reflect referral pattern, selection criteria and the operative mortality which the surgeon is prepared to accept, as it is well recognised that mortality increases with increasing resectability rate (Ong et al. 1978; Belsey and Hiebert 1974).

In Lancaster, our unit initially or ultimately sees all referred cases of oesophageal carcinoma from a well-defined catchment population of approximately 200 000 people, which has one of the highest incidences of the disease in the United Kingdom. All patients are assessed with regard to fitness for surgery and staged to exclude, as far as possible, obvious metastatic or incurable disease such as recurrent laryngeal nerve paresis, tracheo-oesophageal fistula or extensive mediastinal spread, and we find, using these criteria, that only 40% of all referred cases meet the criteria for an attempt at curative resection. This selection process has resulted in a resectability rate of 97% with an operative mortality of around 10% (Watson 1987). Attempts to increase the rate of operation frequently result in a reduction in resectability rate or an increase in operative mortality. The large retrospective review of Earlam and Cunha-Melo (1980) reported a mean operation rate of 58% but a resectability rate of 39% – thus one-third of patients were operated on unnecessarily. Similar results were published in a large series from the Mayo Clinic, where 67% of patients were submitted to surgery, but only 45% underwent resection (Gunnalaugsson et al. 1970). Ong et al. (1978) showed that as resection rate increased from 45% to 58%, operative mortality increased from 18% to 44%.

It appears, therefore, that if operative mortality is to be kept at a respectable level, and resectability rate constitutes a high proportion of operability rate, then palliative treatment will be appropriate in 50%–60% of all referred patients. The various palliative modalities which may be employed are discussed below.


# Palliative Resection


The distinction between palliative surgery and "curative" surgery is less easy in oesophageal cancer than in some other tumours. In Britain, over 70% of tumours have metastasised to lymph nodes at the time of surgery, and fewer than 20% are confined to the oesophageal wall (Watson 1984), and as a consequence, overall 5-year-survival rate is disappointing (see Chap. 8). In these circumstances, many take the view that any surgical treatment is essentially palliative (Belsey 1980; Wong 1981). The principal reasons for offering resection to the group of patients who do not have obviously incurable disease and are considered fit to withstand the operation are firstly that it is difficult to predict the small proportion of patients who will survive 5 years, and secondly, to restore ability to swallow. Progressive dysphagia, with impairment of nutrition and ultimately an inability to swallow even saliva leads to a particularly distressing demise, and resection offers superior palliation to all other modalities, with restoration of normal swallowing in over 90% of patients (Watson 1982).

At operation, it is usually possible to make a reasoned judgement as to whether the operation is likely to be purely palliative, or an attempt at cure. In extreme cases, where the tumour is locally advanced, and cannot be completely removed, and where lymph nodes are obviously grossly involved, most surgeons would consider their efforts to be purely palliative, and would limit these to local tumour excision. In less extreme cases, some surgeons, notably Skinner (1983), perform an ultra-radical operation with excision not only of the majority of the oesophagus and gland fields but adjacent pleura and pericardium. Our practice is in accord with that of Wong (1987) in that subtotal oesophagectomy with lymphatic clearance is attempted in all cases, and the operation is deemed palliative or "curative" depending on whether these objectives are considered to have been fulfilled.

The results of palliative resection are, as one might expect, less favourable than where the procedure has been deemed potentially curative. In Wong's study (1987), mean survival of 232 resected patients at 3.5 years was 24.4%. However, of those patients considered to have had a curative resection, survival was 41.3%, compared to 7.3% in those whose operation was felt to be palliative. Skinner et al. (1986) reported a similar trend, with more favourable survival data for those undergoing radical en-bloc oesophagectomy, compared with those undergoing a more localised resection. It is possible that this difference does not reflect the radical nature of the operative procedure, but reflects the selection of relatively favourable tumours which are likely to have a better prognosis. In our practice, where a similar operative procedure is conducted in all but very advanced tumours, an overall 5-year-survival rate of 13% comprised 50% in node-negative cases and 6% in node-positive cases, indicating that it is the biology and staging of the tumour rather than the nature of operation which influences survival.

# Surgical Bypass Procedures

Surgical bypass has declined in popularity in Britain as a palliative modality since the development of intubation and laser techniques. However, it is more commonly employed in the United States and in the Far East, where these latter modalities are used less frequently. When it is possible to determine by preoperative staging that the tumour is likely to be unresectable, or has metastasised, most workers in this country would now favour a non-operative approach. However, despite increased emphasis on preoperative staging there is still a small proportion of patients initially deemed operable, whose tumour proves to be unresectable at operation. In these circumstances, a palliative bypass procedure may be considered a reasonable alternative to intubation, in that the surgery is not of greater magnitude once the chest is opened, and the quality of palliation is comparable to that following resection. Bypass procedures may also provide useful palliation in the presence of tracheo-oesophageal fistula, although there is no evidence that this is superior to that provided by endoscopic intubation.

## *Oesophago-gastrostomy*

The simplest form of bypass procedure is to anastomose the mobilised gastric fundus end-to-side to the oesophagus proximal to the tumour. However, superior results are claimed by dividing the oesophagus proximal to the tumour, closing the distal end and performing an end-to-end anastomosis between the proximal oesophagus and the gastric fundus (Johnson and Clagett 1970).

## *Reversed Gastric Tube*

Heimlich and Winfield (1955) described the construction of a tube from the greater curvature of the stomach, based on the left gastro-epiploic vessels, of sufficient length to bypass the entire oesophagus and perform an oesophago-gastric anastomosis in the neck. Postlethwait (1979) reported the use of this technique in 20 patients, in whom the gastric tube was placed substernally, with good functional results.

## Kirschner Operation

This is another variant of cervical oesophago-gastrostomy in which the mobilised stomach is brought subcutaneously or retrosternally into the neck for end-to-end anastomosis, the distal oesophagus being anastomosed to a Roux-en-Y loop of jejunum.

## Colonic and Jejunal Interposition

A vascularised colonic or jejunal conduit may be brought retrosternally or subcutaneously to bypass the oesophagus, the proximal end being anastomosed to the cervical oesophagus and the distal end to the stomach. Colon is preferred to jejunum, as preservation of its blood supply is more predictable, but the principal disadvantage of these procedures is the magnitude of the operation, with multiple anastomoses, in a debilitated patient.

### Disadvantages of Surgical Bypass

The main disadvantage of surgical bypass procedures is the application of major surgery to patients, who by definition have advanced tumours and are usually debilitated, and who have a limited life span. This is reflected in reported results of these procedures, with operative mortality ranging between 21% and 41%, with mean survival of approximately five months (Postlethwait 1979; Wong et al. 1981). It is debatable whether such high mortality is justified when subsequent survival is poor, particularly when other less invasive means of palliation are available.

# Intubation

Intubation has taken various forms over the last century, the main objective being to avoid an unpleasant demise from starvation in those patients who, by virtue of age, general condition or tumour extent, are considered inappropriate for resection. The various intubation procedures are less invasive than surgical bypass, and therefore, have some attraction in those frail, elderly patients with advanced disease who clearly would not tolerate major surgery, but in whom restoration of the ability to swallow at least a soft diet would make the remaining weeks more comfortable. The principal disadvantage of intubation procedures is that the degree of palliation obtained rarely equals that of resection or surgical

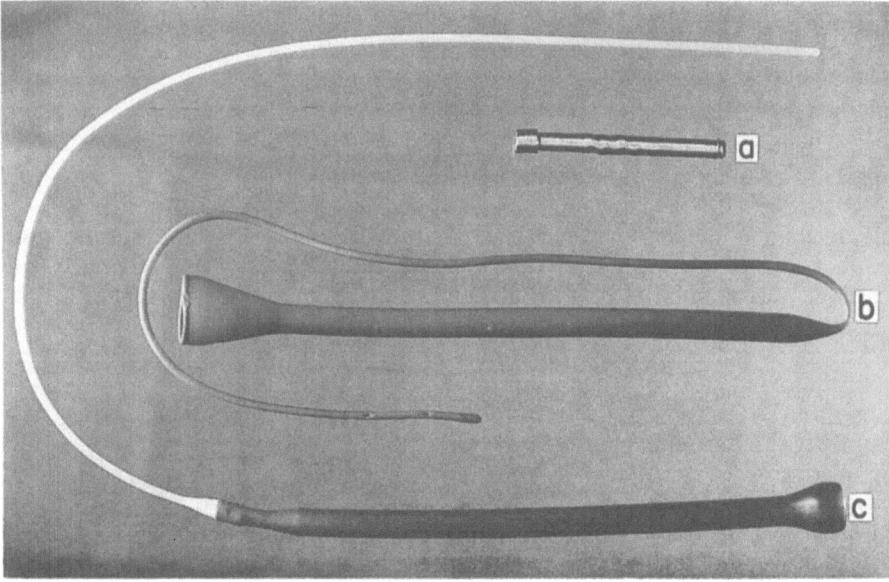

**Fig. 11.1.** Three different types of tube for internal bypass palliation of an oesophageal carcinoma. Souttar tube (**a**); Mousseau–Barbin tube (**b**); Celestin tube (**c**). Reproduced, with permission, from Hurt R, Bates M (1986) *Essentials of Thoracic Surgery*. Butterworths, London.

bypass, and mechanical complications associated with the prosthetic tubes themselves may occur.

There have been various designs of prosthetic tube over the years and various means devised of inserting them. The common features of the tubes employed are strength, in order to withstand tumour compression, flexibility in order to allow passage, an expanded upper end to prevent distal tube displacement and an internal diameter of 10–12 mm to allow the passage of an adequately masticated or soft diet (Fig. 11.1). More recent tubes have been made with a distal flange in order to prevent proximal displacement. Both pulsion and traction methods of introduction of the tubes have been employed, the former using either a rigid oesophagoscope or fibreoptic endoscope, and the latter by traction on a pilot extension which is passed through the tumour from above and then through a small gastrotomy.

## Intubation Using the Rigid Oesophagoscope

This technique, by definition, requires general anaesthesia and the use of a tube sufficiently narrow to allow placement via the rigid oesophagoscope through the tumour. The most widely used tube in this context is the Souttar tube (Fig. 11.1), which is manufactured as a non-compressible coil of silver wire. The tumour is first dilated and the tube then introduced over a bougie. The internal diameter of Souttar tubes is between 6 and 10 mm and thus the quality of palliation is not as great as with other tubes of greater diameter. The other major problem associated with this rigid tube is pressure necrosis, with resulting haemorrhage, perforation and fistula formation and, occasionally, migration of the tube into the mediastinum (Proctor 1980).

## Surgical (Traction) Intubation

This technique evolved as a result of dissatisfaction with the results and complications of the use of rigid tubes passed via the rigid oesophagoscope. The technique was popularised by Mousseau et al. (1956) and Celestin (1959), the principle being the passage of a more flexible, wider tube, by initially passing a narrow pilot guide through the tumour, on which traction was applied at laparotomy and gastrotomy to position the tube. The Mousseau–Barbin tube is made of Neoplex and the Celestin tube of polyethylene, both being strong, yet flexible, with internal diameter of 10 mm (see Fig. 11.1).

The advantages of surgical intubation are that it allows the passage of a wider calibre tube than is feasible via the rigid endoscope and avoids many of the complications associated with such tubes. Furthermore, it is a much less invasive procedure for the palliation of inoperable tumours than is surgical bypass. However, although the surgical procedure is relatively simple, surgical intubation is associated with an operative mortality between 25% and 40% (Diamantes and Mannell 1983; Lishman et al. 1980). This probably reflects the immuno-depressive effect of surgery on an already debilitated patient, but it is likely also that perforation, due to splitting of the tumour, occurs more frequently than is realised. The quality of palliation following surgical intubation is inferior to that following resection or surgical bypass, with only 15% being restored to normal swallowing, although over 60% are able to take a soft or puréed diet (Watson 1982). Mean survival following surgical intubation in our series was 8 months.

### Insertion of Celestin or Mousseau–Barbin Tube at Laparotomy

When inoperability is confirmed at laparotomy, the objective is to pass the tail of the tube *per oram* through the neoplastic stricture into the stomach. When obstruction is incomplete, and particularly if a naso-gastric tube has passed into the stomach, the tail of the Celestin or Mousseau–Barbin tube can be passed by the anaesthetist and its passage observed into the stomach by the surgeon. Where the lumen is small, dilatation of the neoplastic stricture may be necessary first. In some cases where the tumour is both tight and tortuous, particularly at the cardia, it is sometimes easier for the surgeon to pass a bougie from below after performing a gastrotomy and then to fix the tail of the prosthetic tube to the bougie and railroad this into the stomach. Once the tail has been passed into the stomach, by whichever mechanism, having performed a small gastrotomy, gentle traction is applied to the tail and the passage of the prosthetic tube through the oesophagus felt. Once resistance is encountered as the distal end of the tube proper is felt at the upper margin of the tumour, further traction should be slow and gentle in order to enable the gradual widening of the prosthetic tube progressively to dilate the neoplastic stricture, in order to reduce the risk of perforation when the full diameter of the tube traverses the tumour. Resistance is felt for a second time as the proximal funnel of the tube reaches the upper limit of the tumour, and once this stage is reached, no further traction is applied. The distal end of the prosthetic tube is cut off at an appropriate level in the stomach, so that it does not abut against the gastric wall. The tube should be secured to the gastric wall to prevent proximal displacement, distal displacement being prevented by the funnel shape of the proximal portion of the tube. The gastrotomy is then closed.

## Fibreoptic Endoscopic Intubation

The advent in the last two decades of fibreoptic endoscopy has enabled not only visualisation of the upper gastrointestinal tract without the need for general anaesthesia, but it has enabled therapeutic procedures, including dilatation of benign and malignant strictures, and intubation to be performed relatively non-invasively. The principle underlying fibreoptic endoscopic intubation is the passage, under sedation with diazepam with an analgesic such as pentazocine, of a steel guide-wire through the tumour under direct vision, utilising the biopsy channel of the endoscope. The neoplastic stricture is then dilated using Eder–Puestow or Celestin bougies, following which a tube on an introducer is passed over the guide wire and through the tumour under fluoroscopic control. Special tubes have been devised for this purpose, manufactured from silicone (see Fig. 4.13) (Atkinson and Ferguson 1977) and latex reinforced with concentric stainless-steel wire (Celestin, 1978) (see Fig. 4.14). Each of these tubes has an internal diameter of 12 mm, which is larger than previously described tubes, and each has a distal flange to prevent proximal migration.

The avoidance of surgery and general anaesthesia means that fibreoptic endoscopic intubation is less invasive than other palliative procedures, which is an important consideration in the management of debilitated patients whose life expectancy is short. However, the procedure is not without its risks, and procedure-related mortality between 6% and 11% is reported (Watson 1984; Ogilvie et al. 1982). In our series comparing the technique with surgical intubation, mean hospital stay was 7.6 days compared to 13.0 days for surgical intubation in a similar group of patients, and mean survival following the procedure was 11 months. The quality of palliation was better than with surgical intubation, 33% being restored to normal swallowing with over 60% of the remainder being able to tolerate a soft or puréed diet. However, once more, the degree of palliation falls short of that achieved by resection or surgical bypass.

The principal complications of fibreoptic endoscopic intubation are perforation, tube migration and blockage of the tube. Early perforation occurred in 11% of patients in the series of Ogilvie et al. (1982) and was frequently, but not invariably, fatal. Late perforation occasionally occurs in patients who have subsequently received radiotherapy. Tube migration is less common since the design of tubes was modified to include a distal flange. Tube blockage may be caused by bolus obstruction or by tumour overgrowth above or below the tube.

Fibreoptic endoscopic intubation, because of avoidance of surgery and general anaesthesia, is currently the most attractive of the intubation techniques in those patients for whom resection is inappropriate. It is associated with less procedure-related mortality, fewer complications and a better quality of palliation. It also provides useful palliation in those patients with tracheo-oesophageal fistula, with persistent dysphagia after radiotherapy and where local recurrence is a late complication of surgical resection. In these circumstances, surgical intubation would appear only to have a place in the small number of patients in whom fibreoptic endoscopic intubation is not feasible because of extreme tortuosity or gross narrowing of the neoplastic stricture, or where the tumour is discovered to be unresectable at operation (Watson, 1985). The results of surgical and endoscopic intubation are shown in Table 11.1.

**Table 11.1.** Relative mortality, hospital stay and restoration of normal swallowing of operative and endoscopic intubation

|                                          | Surgical intubation | Endoscopic intubation |
| ---------------------------------------- | ------------------- | --------------------- |
| Hospital mortality (%)                   | 40                  | 8.6                   |
| Mean hospital stay (days)                | 13.0                | 6.9                   |
| Restoration of normal swallowing (%)     | 15.3                | 33.3                  |

# Laser Therapy

The increasing use of the neodymium-YAG laser has led to its application to the palliation of inoperable obstructive oesophageal tumours (Fleischer 1981). Several reports have alluded to the quality of palliation achieved by this form of therapy (Swain and Bown 1984; Krasner and Beard 1984), although multiple treatments are necessary and there is a risk of perforation. Carter and Smith (1986) compared quality of palliation between 10 patients undergoing laser therapy and 10 undergoing fibreoptic endoscopic intubation, and concluded that the quality of palliation was better with laser therapy. The patients were not randomised and it was acknowledged that several courses of laser therapy were necessary in their patients in whom mean survival was only 6 months.

On the available evidence, it appears that the possibility of superior palliation needs to be weighed against the necessity of patients with a limited life span returning regularly to hospital, and against the capital cost of the equipment. Until the results of randomised prospective controlled trials are known, laser therapy would appear to have most attraction in those patients in whom intubation is not feasible, or has failed due to tumour overgrowth, and in the case of proximally sited tumours, where pharyngeal irritation may preclude patient tolerance of an endoscopic tube (see also Chap. 14).

# Radiotherapy

Palliative radiotherapy may be considered as a relatively non-invasive modality in those patients with squamous lesions which are considered to be locally advanced, or where patients are felt unlikely to withstand major surgery. However, in patients with disseminated metastases or with adenocarcinomas, radiotherapy is of little value. It should be remembered that a course of radiotherapy in frail debilitated patients may be associated with considerable morbidity, and even mortality (Cederquist et al. 1978). Because of the combination of age, general condition and distant metastases, Pearson (1981) found that only half of the patients deemed to have incurable disease were suitable for radiotherapy.

Some have doubted the value of palliative radiotherapy as a concept, as irradiation greater than 5 cm beyond the tumour margin results in an unacceptable reduction of tumour dose, which is likely to be ineffective, and there is little evidence that patients receiving palliative radiotherapy fare better than those receiving no radiation at all (Miller 1962). However, the recent development of intracavitary irradiation (Rowland and Pagliero 1985) may overcome these objections (see Chap. 13).

Palliative radiotherapy may be of more help in the palliation of pain from locally extensive squamous primary tumours or from painful metastases (Werner 1978). However, for the relief of dysphagia it is likely to be ineffective in the majority of patients, resulting in survival for only a few months (Schuchmann et al. 1980), and dilatation or intubation may be a necessary addition to enable nutrition to be maintained (see Chap. 12).

# Chemotherapy

A variety of chemotherapeutic agents have been employed in the management of oesophageal carcinoma, with conflicting, and generally depressing, results of efficacy. The agents principally used include bleomycin (Ravry et al. 1973) and more recently, cisplatinum in combination with bleomycin alone or as a component of regimes including methotrexate, adriamycin, 5-fluorouracil or vincristine (Gisselbrecht et al. 1983; Kelsen 1984). Documented objective response is hard to find, and when it has occurred, this has been of short duration over a few months only. To date, the greatest use of chemotherapeutic agents has been as an adjunct to surgery, either alone or with radiotherapy (Wolfe et al. 1986), but there is little evidence that their efficacy when used in the palliative situation justifies the unpleasant side effects associated with their use.

# Dilatation

Intermittent endoscopic dilatation has been recommended as a palliative procedure for inoperable oesophageal tumours (Graham et al. 1983). As might be expected, recurrent dysphagia usually occurs so rapidly that it has little application beyond that of a temporary measure, or prior to endoscopic intubation.

## Gastrostomy and Oesophagostomy

A feeding gastrostomy and an oesophagostomy to collect saliva used to have a place in the management of inoperable cases with total oesophageal obstruction. However, operative mortality is up to 45%, with no evidence of prolongation of survival (King and Zimmerman 1965). In these circumstances, there is now *no place* for such an unpleasant form of palliation, particularly where more acceptable and less invasive procedures are available which provide better symptomatic relief.

## Conclusions

Until oesophageal carcinoma is detected at an earlier stage in the Western world, palliative procedures will form the mainstay of management in 50%–60% of referred patients. Whilst only 10%–20% of those resected will survive 5 years, resection must be considered to be palliative in the remainder, but it offers better palliation than any other modality, with restoration of reasonable swallowing in over 90% of cases.

Using modern methods of staging, unresectability detected at operation should be a relatively infrequent occurrence, though in these circumstances a palliative bypass procedure or intubation are available alternatives. The former will give better palliation, but with a higher mortality than intubation.

In those patients in whom surgery is considered inappropriate, either by virtue of age, poor general condition or tumour staging, intubation techniques are becoming increasingly used in the United Kingdom, whilst surgical bypass, despite its high mortality, is favoured in the United States and the Far East. Of the intubation techniques available, fibreoptic endoscopic intubation is the least invasive, and associated with the lowest procedure-related mortality and the best palliation. Laser therapy presents a promising alternative to these objectives, and the results of prospective controlled trials are awaited with interest. In the current state of knowledge, there appears little place for palliative radiotherapy or chemotherapy as a sole treatment modality. It is apparent in this distressing disease that our efforts should be directed towards earlier presentation and diagnosis so that the proportion of patients in whom an attempt at curative therapy can be made is increased and our reliance on palliative modalities diminished.

## References

Atkinson M, Ferguson R (1977) Fibreoptic endoscopic palliative intubation of inoperable osophago-
   gastric neoplasms. Br Med J i:266–267
Belsey RHR (1980) Palliative management of esophageal carcinoma. Am J Surg 139:789–794

Belsey R, Hiebert CA (1974) An exclusive right thoracic approach for cancer of the middle third of the esophagus. Ann Thorac Surg 18:1–15

Carter R, Smith J (1986) Oesophageal carcinoma: a comparative study of laser recanalisation versus intubation in the palliation of gastro-oesophageal carcinoma. Laser Med Sci 1:245–252

Cederquist C, Nielsen J, Berthelsen A et al. (1978) Cancer of the oesophagus. II. Theory and outcome. Acta Chir Scand 144:233–240

Celestin LR (1959) Permanent intubation in inoperable cancer of the oesophagus and cardia. A new tube. Ann R Coll Surg Engl 25:165–170

Celestin LR (1978) New techniques of intubation. Proceedings of the world congress of digestive endoscopy p. 97

Diamanetes T, Mannell A (1983) Oesophageal intubation for advanced oesophageal cancer: the Baragwnath experience. Br J Surg 70:555–557

Earlam R (1984) Oesophageal cancer treatment in North-East Thames Region, 1981: medical audit using hospital activity analysis data. Br Med J 288:1892–1894

Earlam R, Cunha-Melo JR (1980) Oesophageal squamous cell carcinoma. I. A critical review of surgery. Br J Surg 67:381–390

Fleischer D (1981) Palliative therapy for esophageal carcinoma by endoscopic Nd-YAG laser. Laser Endosc 2:17–20

Gisselbrecht C, Calvo F, Mignot L (1983) Fluorouracil, adriamycin and cisplatin: combination chemotherapy of advanced esophageal carcinoma. Cancer 52:974–977

Graham DY, Dodds SM, Zubler M (1983) What is the role of prosthesis insertion in esophageal carcinoma? Gastrointest Endosc 29:1–5

Gunnalaugsson GH, Wychulis AR, Rowland C et al. (1970) Analysis of the records of 1657 patients with carcinoma of the esophagus and cardia of the stomach. Surg Gynecol Obstet 130:997–1005

Heimlich HJ, Winfield JN (1955) The use of a gastric tube to replace or bypass the esophagus. Surgery 37:549–559

Johnson CL, Clagett OT (1970) Palliative esophagus gastrostomy for inoperable carcinoma of the esophagogastric junction. J Thorac Cardiovasc Surg 60:269–274

Keeling T, Gillen P, Hennessy TP (1988) Oesophageal resection in the elderly. Ann R Coll Surg Engl 70:34–36

Kelsen D (1984) Chemotherapy of esophageal cancer. Semin Oncol 11:159–168

King TC, Zimmerman JM (1965) Gastrostomies in patients with incurable cancer. Ann Surg 31:251–254

Krasner N, Beard J (1984) Laser irradiation of tumours of the oesophagus and gastric cardia. Br Med J 288–829

Lishman AH, Dellipiani AW, Devlin HB (1980) The insertion of oesophagogastric tubes in malignant oesophageal strictures: endoscopy or surgery? Br J Surg 80:257–259

Miller C (1962) Carcinoma of the thoracic oesophagus and cardia. A review of 405 cases. Br J Surg 49:507–522

Mousseau M, LeForestier J, Barbin J et al. (1956) Place de l'intubation à demeure dans le traitement palliative du cancer de l'oesophage. Arch Mal Appar Digest 45:208–216

Ogilvie AL, Dronfield M, Ferguson R et al. (1980) Outlook with conservative treatment of peptic oesophageal stricture. Gut 21:23–25

Ong GB, Lam KH, Wong J et al. (1978) Factors influencing morbidity and mortality in esophageal carcinoma. J Thorac Cardiovasc Surg 76:745–749

Pearson JG (1981) Radiotherapy for esophageal carcinoma. World J Surg 5:489–493

Postlethwait RW (ed) (1979) Surgery of the esophagus. Appleton-Century-Crofts, New York

Proctor DS (1980) Esophageal intubation for carcinoma of the esophagus. World J Surg 4:451–454

Ravry M, Moertell CG, Schutt AJ et al. (1973) Treatment of advanced squamous cell carcinoma of the gastro-intestinal tract with bleomycin. Cancer Chemother Rep 57:493–496

Rowland CG, Pagliero KM (1985) Intracavitary irradiation in palliation of carcinoma of oesophagus and cardia. Lancet II:981–982

Schuchmann JF, Heydorn WH, Hall RV et al. (1980) Treatment of esophageal carcinoma. A retrospective review. J Thorac Cardiovasc Surg 79:67–71

Skinner DB (1983) En-bloc resection for neoplasms of the esophagus and cardia. J Thorac Cardiovasc Surg 85:59–69

Skinner DB, Little AG, Ferguson MK et al. (1986) Selection of operation for esophageal cancer based on staging. Ann Surg 204:391–401

Swain CP, Bown SG (1984) Laser recanalisation of obstructing foregut cancer. Br J Surg 71:112–115

Watson A (1982) A study of the quality and duration of survival following resection, endoscopic intubation and surgical intubation in oesophageal carcinoma. Br J Surg 69:585–588

Watson A (1984) Therapeutic options and patient selection in the management of oesophageal carcinoma. In: Watson A, Celestin LR (eds) Disorders of the oesophagus. Pitman, London, pp 167–186

Watson A (1985) Palliative intubation in inoperable esophageal neoplasms. Ann Thorac Surg 39:501–502

Watson A (1987) Management of carcinoma of the oesophagus. In: Misiewicz JJ, Pounder RE, Venables CW (eds) Diseases of the gut and pancreas. Blackwell Scientific, Oxford; pp 179–192

Watson A (1988) Pathologic changes affecting survival in esophageal cancer. In: Delarue NC, Eschapasse H (eds) International trends in general thoracic surgery. Saunders, Philadelphia

Werner ID (1978) The palliative management of squamous carcinoma of the intrathoracic and intra-abdominal oesophagus. In: Silber W (ed) Carcinoma of the oesophagus. Balkema, Cape Town, pp 445–448

Wolfe WG, Burton GV, Seigler HF et al. (1986) Early results with combined modality therapy for carcinoma of the esophagus. Ann Surg 205:563–571

Wong J (1981) Management of carcinoma of the oesophagus: art or science? J R Coll Surg Edin 26:138–148

Wong J, Lam KH, Wei W et al. (1981) Results of the Kirschner operation. World J Surg 5:547–552

Wong J (1987) Esophageal resection for cancer: the rationale of current practice. Am J Surg 153:18–24

# Chapter 12

# Radiotherapy and Cytotoxic Therapy

S. J. Arnott

## Historical

Radiotherapy was first used in the treatment of oesophageal cancer soon after the discovery of radium. In a few cases radium was used to give external irradiation gaining temporary relief of symptoms in patients with tumours in the root of the neck. However, it was only when treatment was given using radium inserted into the oesophagus either within a bougie or carried in grooves of a vulcanite tube that cures were obtained (Einhorn 1904; Exner 1904; Guisez 1925; Dufourmental 1930). In the 1930s, techniques were developed to enable radium needles and radium seeds to be implanted directly into oesophageal tumours (Souttar 1934). These techniques were all associated with a number of serious problems and the overall results of treatment were dismal. Perforation of the oesophagus was a major hazard. In addition, the distribution of the sources was often poor, especially when there was significant narrowing of the oesophagus at the upper end of the tumour. This led to inadequate irradiation of some parts of the growth and the delivery of very high doses to others.

The development of radiotherapy equipment capable of producing beams of X- or gamma-rays which would adequately irradiate the oesophagus led to the virtual abandonment of endo-oesophageal treatment although there has been recent renewed interest in its potential (Chap. 13). The radiotherapy apparatus initially available produced only relatively low energy orthovoltage X-rays. However, megavoltage treatments, usually delivered by linear accelerators, are now routinely employed. The beams of X-rays produced by these machines are precise and can be directed to give the maximum dose of irradiation to the tumour-bearing area in the oesophagus whilst at the same time avoiding vital normal structures. The morbidity associated with these treatments is low.

Unfortunately, the considerable technical advances in radiotherapy equipment have not led to significant improvements in the results of treatment and the outlook for most patients with oesophageal cancer remains poor. One of the main reasons for this is that the majority of patients in Western Countries present with advanced tumours and frequently have metastatic disease when the diagnosis is made. This fact naturally influences the results achieved by both surgery and radiotherapy. However, there is probably an additional factor of patient selection which has some bearing on the poor results of radiotherapy. The reasons for choosing surgical or radiotherapeutic management are often unclear. On the whole, patients treated surgically are younger, fitter and have smaller tumours. In spite of this the outcome following surgery can be disastrous especially if an inexperienced surgeon has performed the operation (Matthews et al. 1986). This suggests that selection of treatment should be based on rational parameters in order that patients may receive optimum therapy.

# Radical Radiotherapy

Radiotherapy may be given with curative or palliative intent but the criteria used for the selection of the most appropriate treatment are often unclear. However, there is information now available which can help in formulating these decisions.

When radiotherapy is given with curative intent, doses are employed which are close to the limit that normal tissues can withstand. Only in this way is there a reasonable chance of achieving tumour eradication. However, there is no clear evidence to indicate what is the optimal dose of treatment. The techniques of irradiation must take into account knowledge of the extent of disease together with the known patterns of submucosal and lymphatic spread. As a result an attempt is made to achieve a 5-cm margin both above and below the radiographic limits of the tumour. Laterally, a 2-cm margin beyond the gross definable tumour is included in the treatment field in order to encompass the majority of para-oesophageal nodes. Larger tumours are more likely to have associated wide local infiltration and nodal metastases. However, there is a need to restrict the treatment volume because of the limitations of normal tissue tolerance and the maintenance of dose level. This will mean that the margin around larger tumours is smaller and cure will only be possible for such lesions if they are not widely infiltrating (Pearson 1966). In practice, this dictates that an attempt at cure is only possible if the tumour is of limited extent.

Other factors which must be taken into consideration when planning radical radiotherapy are the age and general condition of the patient, the site of the tumour and its histological grade. Factors which preclude the possibility of radical treatment are the presence of metastases, involvement of the trachea or bronchi, and invasion of adjacent structures such as the thyroid gland and vertebrae.

## Criteria for Radical Radiotherapy

### Age, Sex and General Condition

Age *per se* is not a contraindication to radical radiotherapy as long as the patient is considered fit to undergo high-dose irradiation. In an analysis of 444 patients given radical radiotherapy in Edinburgh, age did not influence the outcome for either male or female patients (Newaishy et al. 1982). On the other hand, survival following surgery is closely determined by age, the operative mortality rising steeply in patients over the age of 70 years. In Western countries oesophageal cancer is mainly a disease of the elderly, the mean age of incidence being 68 years (Waterhouse 1974). Therefore, age is a factor to be considered closely when choosing treatment.

Assessment of the general condition of the patient must take into account medical conditions which are likely to affect the response to irradiation. These include serious cardiopulmonary disease and hypertension.

The sex of the patient has a highly significant effect on the results of radiotherapy. The crude 5-year-survival rates for male patients following radical treatment is approximately 5.7% whereas it is 11.6% for females. The pattern of survival is similar for both males and females during the first two years after irradiation, but thereafter the outlook for females improves and is statistically significantly better at 5 years (Newaishy et al. 1982). Similar survival differences between male and female patients have been described in surgical series but they appear to be less marked (Matthews et al. 1986).

## Tumour Size

The size of the primary tumour is perhaps the most important factor affecting the outcome of treatment. Assessment of the true size of the lesion is difficult in oesophageal cancer although newer techniques of imaging have improved the accuracy of this considerably. The majority of patients referred for radiotherapy have cancers greater than 5 cm in length as determined radiologically. Only about 35% of those given radical treatment will have tumours smaller than 5 cm.

Size would appear to be less influential in determining the outcome of treatment in women than in men. In the Edinburgh series the crude 5-year-survival rate for females with tumours less than 5 cm in length was 12.64% and this fell to 10.95% in those with larger lesions. However, the male survival rate was 11.11% when the tumour was less than 5 cm but only 2.97% if it was larger. There were virtually no long-term survivors, irrespective of the sex of the patient, when the tumour was greater than 8 cm in length (Newaishy et al. 1982).

The importance of tumour size as a predictor of radio-responsiveness has been confirmed by other workers. At the Princess Margaret Hospital in Toronto a 100% tumour response was found in patients with growths less than 5 cm. This fell to 66% for lesions 5–10 cm in size and was only 29% when the tumour was larger than 10 cm (Beatty et al. 1979).

## Tumour Site

Identifying the exact site of origin of an oesophageal cancer is not necessarily straightforward in patients given radiotherapy as often the lesion is too extensive to determine this accurately. The method of classification recommended by the Union Internationale Contre le Cancer (UICC) (1978) takes these difficulties into consideration. When the tumour extends beyond one defined region it is classed as "extensive". Approximately half of all patients receiving radical radiotherapy will have "extensive" cancers. However, it is possible to identify tumours in certain sites which appear to respond better to radiotherapy. Pearson (1977) showed that patients with cancers of the cervical oesophagus and postcricoid region had a much better outlook following radiotherapy than did those with lesions of the intrathoracic oesophagus. This finding was confirmed in a later review from the same centre (Newaishy et al. 1982). The five-year-survival rate for males with cervical oesophageal tumours was 15.38% and for females 20.83%. A report from the University of Florida has described a similar improved response for patients with cervical oesophageal cancer with four out of a total of 16 patients surviving disease-free for more than two years (Mendenhall et al. 1982). A further two patients in this series who died at less than two years were free from any evidence of tumour. Although there have been reports to the contrary, the majority view is that cervical oesophageal tumours do have a better response to radiotherapy (Hancock and Glatstein 1984). The morbidity from irradiating tumours in this site is low.

## Histological Grade

The vast majority of patients referred for radiotherapy will have squamous oesophageal cancers. Most adenocarcinomas arise in the lower third of the oesophagus, many being of gastric origin. Such tumours are much more difficult technically to irradiate and they are more amenable to surgical management.

Over half of the squamous cancers in patients given radiotherapy will be poorly differentiated. However, there is no clear evidence of a relationship between tumour differentiation and outcome of treatment (Andersen et al. 1984).

### Selection of Treatment

A number of factors have been clearly shown to influence the outcome following radiotherapy for squamous oesophageal cancer. Some degree of rational treatment selection is thus possible taking this information into account.

The factors most clearly affecting the outcome following treatment are tumour size and site, and the sex and age of the patient. Many of these are interrelated. For example, men with tumours larger than 5 cm in size do particularly badly following radiotherapy. Perhaps surgery is preferable for these patients. On the other hand, operative mortality rises steeply in patients over 70 years of age. For this age group radiotherapy may be the treatment of choice. Tumours in the cervical oesophagus respond better to radiotherapy and the morbidity of treatment is considerably less than that following surgery. Radiotherapy is probably the preferred treatment for such lesions.

When the extent of radiotherapy is being considered these factors are also important. High-dose treatment should continue to be recommended in female patients whose tumours are no greater than 8 cm in length. This form of radiotherapy can only be justified in men when the lesion is less than 5 cm in length. Patients whose tumours are more advanced are suitable only for palliative measures.

## Treatment Technique and Dose

Many techniques are available for the treatment of oesophageal cancer. To some extent the technique will be determined by the anatomical site of the tumour. Lesions in the cervical oesophagus require a different approach to intrathoracic cancers. No one technique has been shown to be superior. However, all must take into account the need to irradiate the oesophagus uniformly whilst avoiding surrounding vital normal tissues as much as possible. The tolerance doses of the spinal cord and lung are clearly defined but this is not so with the heart (Hancock and Glatstein 1984). Controversy also exists regarding the optimum dose which is necessary in radical radiotherapy. There is general acceptance that the minimum dose that will achieve tumour control in a satisfactory proportion of patients is 5000 cGy. However, doses as high as 7000 cGy have been used (Yang et al. 1983). There is no clear evidence that the higher doses achieve better levels of tumour control. However, in the series reported from Edinburgh 11% of patients received a tumour dose of 5500 cGy compared with the usual dose of 5000 cGy (Newaishy et al. 1982). The five-year survival in females who received this dose was 25% whereas it was only 9.9% in those given 5000 cGy. There was no comparable benefit in male patients. The reasons why patients received the higher dose are not clear and some of the apparent improvement in survival in females may have been due to patient selection. What is of concern is that higher doses may be associated with a greater incidence of complications. In addition high-dose regimens require a longer period of overall treatment time for delivery. In a disease where the one-year-survival rate following radical radiotherapy is only 39%, it is difficult to justify protracted treatment techniques (Arnott 1986).

Tumours arising in the cervical oesophagus or thoracic inlet require special techniques to cope with rapidly changing dimensions of the body at the root of the neck. In addition, the shoulders may have to be avoided in order to achieve homogeneity of dose distribution. The presence of lung will affect attenuation of the beam in the lower part of the treatment field. The most satisfactory techniques employ anterior oblique fields with appropriate use of compensators or wedges (Fig. 12.1) and the use of four-field box treatment plans (Fig. 12.2). These are successful in achieving dose homogeneity in the tumour-bearing area and in avoiding the spinal cord.

Intrathoracic lesions are satisfactorily treated by the use of three-field beam-directed techniques using an anterior and two posterior oblique fields (Fig. 12.3). Other techniques, such as rotational therapy, may also be used but are more complicated and do not achieve a superior dose distribution. Often considerable volumes of lung are traversed by the posterior oblique beams. This can lead to overdosage unless allowance is made for the reduced attenuation of these beams. Compensation must also be made for the changing contour of patients between the upper and lower limits of these fields (Fig. 12.4a,b). CT scanning is of great value in accurately assessing lung volume and permitting the appropriate dose corrections to be made. Modern radiotherapy planning systems are able to incorporate direct transfer of CT images, so improving accuracy.

Although the treatment volumes generally employed encompass the primary tumour and an appropriate surrounding margin, as has already been discussed, more extended techniques have been described (Pierquin et al. 1966; Doggett et

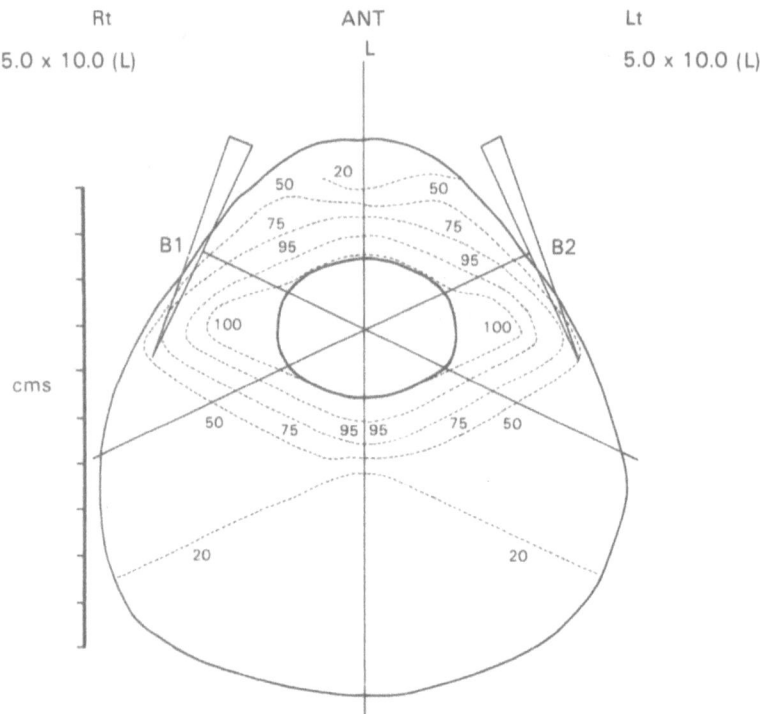

**Fig. 12.1.** Transverse section of upper oesophageal tumour showing distribution of radiation achieved by the use of two anterior oblique fields with wedges.

al. 1970). These have incorporated treatment of the whole mediastinum and even the supraclavicular region and coeliac axis. There is no evidence that these extended irradiation techniques achieve better levels of local tumour control or improved survival. When the supraclavicular region and coeliac axis are irradiated there is considerable associated morbidity affecting principally the heart

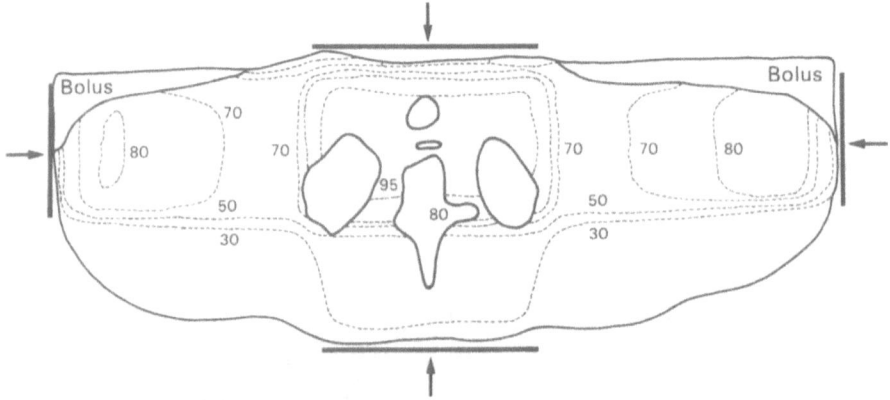

**Fig. 12.2.** Transverse section of upper oesophageal tumour treated by four-field box technique.

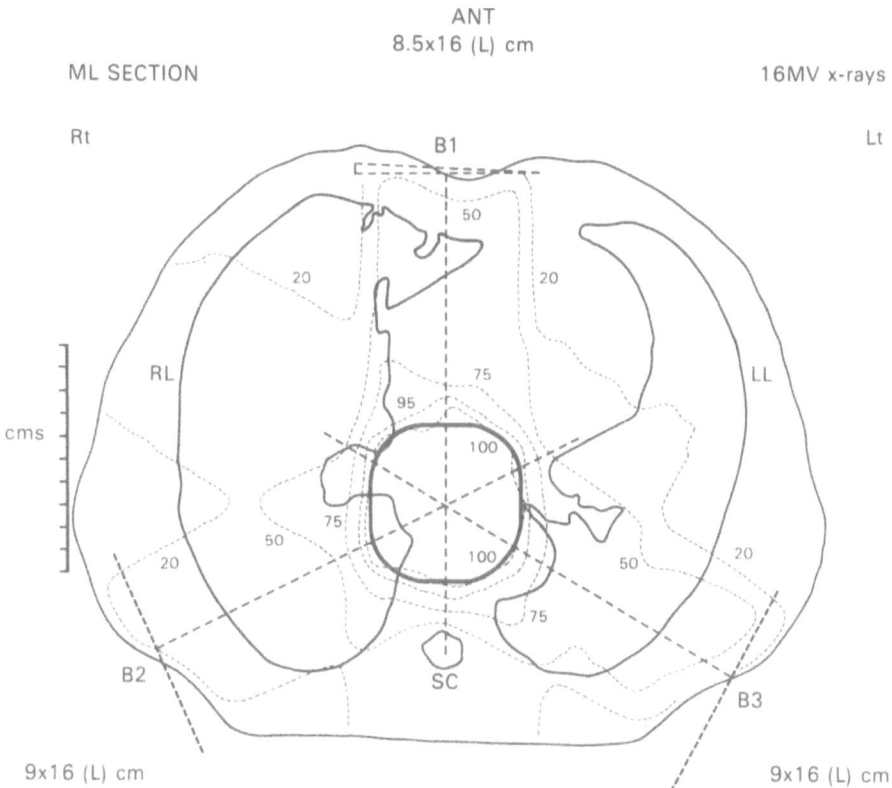

**Fig. 12.3.** Transverse section of midthoracic oesophageal tumour showing distribution of radiation achieved by using three-field technique.

and lungs (Doggett et al. 1970). The study conducted at the Princess Margaret Hospital in Toronto also found that survival was worse in patients treated with extended fields, probably largely due to normal tissue morbidity (Beatty et al. 1979). It is unlikely that extended radiotherapy techniques can offer any benefit over more conventional treatments since they are still loco-regional in extent and will not deal with metastatic disease, which remains the major problem in the management of patients with oesophageal cancer. It has been estimated that, even when the tumour is less than 5 cm in length, 35% of patients will have metastases. When it is greater than 5 cm this proportion rises to 75% (Thompson 1983). Therefore, it would seem most appropriate to recommend the use of limited treatment volumes and doses of 5000–5500 cGy given in 20 daily treatments over a period of four weeks.

## Treatment Morbidity

Serious morbidity following modern radiotherapy treatments is rare and death is exceptional. Erythematous skin reactions are no longer a problem when using

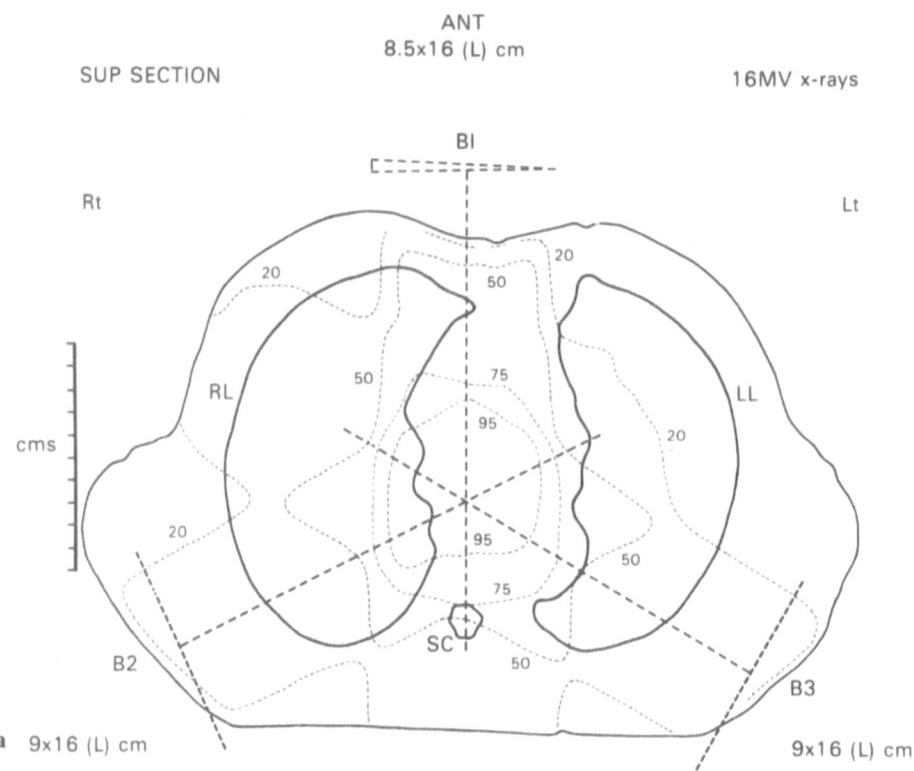

ANT
8.5x16 (L) cm

SUP SECTION                                                                16MV x-rays

**Fig. 12.4a.** Transverse section through superior portion of radiation field showing relatively large volumes of lung included and distribution of radiation achieved.

high energy X-ray apparatus since the dose at the skin is only of the order of 10% of that delivered to the tumour. The most commonly encountered late complication is stricture formation. This is seen in approximately 40% of patients following radical radiotherapy although it is often difficult to distinguish between tumour recurrence and irradiation strictures. Radiation pneumonitis and subsequent fibrosis are seen infrequently after carefully applied treatment. This is a serious complication and requires energetic treatment with steroids and antibiotics. It most usually follows the delivery of high doses of radiotherapy to large volumes of lung as in extended field treatment techniques.

The tolerance limits of the spinal cord are now well known and, as a result, radiation damage to the cord should not occur in properly planned radiotherapy. It has already been indicated that invasion of the trachea or bronchi is a contraindication to radical radiotherapy. However, fistula formation or sometimes massive haemorrhage may occur following treatment, due to shrinkage of tumour that had invaded these organs or adjacent large blood vessels when the true extent of the tumour had not been appreciated prior to therapy. Most commonly, fistulae and haemorrhage are associated with persistent or recurrent tumour.

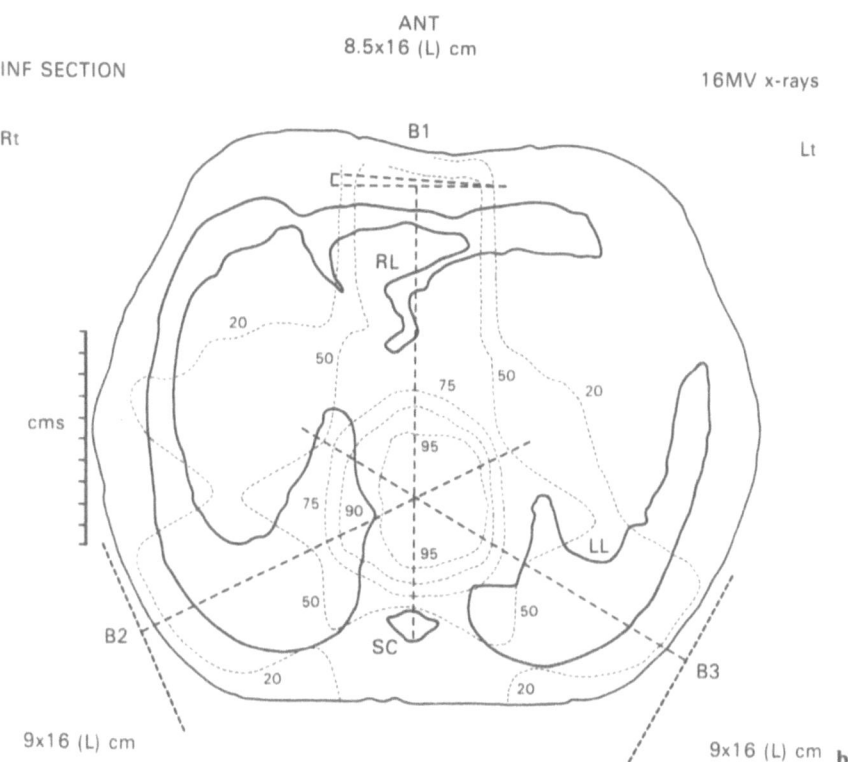

INF SECTION

ANT
8.5x16 (L) cm

16MV x-rays

Rt

B1

Lt

RL

20

50

75

50

20

cms

95

75    90

95

LL

50

50

B2

SC

B3

20

20

9x16 (L) cm

9x16 (L) cm  b

**Fig 12.4** (*continued*) **b.** Transverse section through lower margin of radiation field showing reduced amount of lung present in this situation and slightly different distribution of radiation achieved using similar three-field technique.

## Results of Radiotherapy

Dysphagia will be improved in the majority of patients following radical radiotherapy. The improvement may not be complete and some restriction in dietary practices may be necessary. The development of a stricture must always be considered if dysphagia returns as dilatation is usually of great benefit.

Survival following radiotherapy is poor, the crude 5-year survival being of the order of 9%. This would appear to be similar to that achieved by surgery (Earlam and Cunha-Melo 1980).* To what extent selection bias influences the results of radiotherapy is unclear. However, bearing this in mind, it is important that the selection criteria already described are carefully applied so that high-dose treatment is given only to those who are likely to gain benefit. Patients with very advanced disease whose life expectancy is short and who are unlikely to derive benefit should be treated purely palliatively.

---

*But see p. 16 – Editor.

# Recent Developments in Radiotherapy

Numerous attempts have been made to improve the results of radiotherapy. These have included alteration of treatment fractionation, the use of hypoxic cell sensitisers, fast neutron irradiation and the combination of intracavitary and external beam treatments.

The use of unconventional schedules of X-ray therapy is currently of great interest. Two main possibilities are available. One is to use fewer treatments, with a larger dose per treatment. The other is to employ several small fractions of radiotherapy given each day during courses of treatment. The giving of fewer larger dose treatments has often been a measure of expediency to cope with large patient workloads in overworked departments (Dvivedi and Pradhan 1978). However, there is biological evidence to suggest that large fractions do produce a greater degree of tumour cell kill (Steele and Courtenay 1983). Studies which have examined this form of radiotherapy in oesophageal cancer have largely investigated patients with advanced disease and have found it well tolerated and effective as palliation (Dvivedi and Pradhan 1978). However, there is real concern that this approach may be less effective when used in early tumours and may be associated with a greater incidence of normal tissue complications (Ydrach et al. 1982). The general consensus is that this type of treatment is not suitable for a radical approach but may be of value in palliation.

The application of several fractions of radiotherapy each day attempts to exploit differences in cellular repair mechanisms which are believed to exist between tumour and normal tissues. The hope is that this type of treatment will enhance the difference in response between actively proliferating tumour tissues and the slowly proliferating normal tissues involved in the production of chronic radiation injury (Withers et al. 1982). One disadvantage is that acute normal tissue reactions may be increased since the normal tissues involved in this process are also actively proliferating. This technique has not so far been investigated in oesophageal cancer. However, promising early results have been described when it has been employed in the treatment of patients with head and neck tumours and lung cancer (Saunders and Dische 1987).

The possible advantage in the use of hypoxic cell sensitisers is derived from the theory that all tumours greater than 1 cm in diameter contain a significant proportion of hypoxic cells which may, in part, account for radio-resistance. Research is currently being conducted to investigate drugs which mimic the effect of oxygen in selectively sensitising hypoxic cells. The response of normally oxygenated cells is unaffected (Adams et al. 1976). One of the first of these compounds to be investigated was metronidazole. Subsequently, a number of related compounds have been developed, all with less toxicity and increased sensitising action. The property of these drugs which determines their sensitising effect is their electron affinity. The reason that they are able to sensitise cells in the depth of a tumour is because they are not rapidly metabolised and can therefore diffuse deeply into the tumour. Unfortunately, even the more recent drugs such as misonidazole do have dose-limiting neurotoxicity. A number of newer compounds are now being examined and may offer hope in the future.

The use of hypoxic cell sensitisers has not been extensively investigated in patients with oesophageal cancer. Those reports which have appeared have not demonstrated any significant improvement compared with conventional radio-therapy. A study conducted at the National Cancer Institute in America largely assessed the ability to deliver radiotherapy in conjunction with misonidazole (Schwade et al. 1984). Neurotoxicity was not a problem, nor were the acute radiation reactions produced. However, local tumour control and survival did not appear to be significantly different from that achieved by radiotherapy alone. A study organised in America by the Radiation Therapy Oncology Group (RTOG) found that when large fraction size treatments were combined with misonidazole a very poor result was achieved (Ydrach et al. 1982). The conclusion from this investigation was that the type of radiotherapy and the schedule of misonidazole employed could not be recommended in the treatment of oesophageal cancers. This type of treatment is only likely to influence local control rates and is unlikely to have a significant effect on overall survival. What proportion of treatment failures are solely due to persistent local tumour is not clear. However, it almost certainly is small. Nevertheless, improvements in local tumour control do benefit patients and further investigation of this form of therapy is certainly worthwhile.

The rationale for using fast neutrons rather than conventional X-ray or gamma-ray beams is based on radiobiological studies which have shown that neutron irradiation is more effective, by a factor approaching three, in the destruction of hypoxic tumour cells. Furthermore, the ability of cells to recover from sublethal radiation injury is greatly reduced following neutron therapy. Thus the use of neutrons theoretically should overcome the two main factors believed to be responsible for radio-resistance. Unfortunately, the neutron therapy work which has been carried out has proved disappointing. For example, in the United States an evaluation of 39 patients with inoperable squamous cell cancers organised by the RTOG found that the projected two-year survival was less than 10%, which was worse than would have been expected from conventional radiotherapy. In addition, serious normal tissue morbidity was seen in 50% of the patients. This consisted of severe damage to the oesophagus, lungs and heart. From this and other evidence it seems unlikely that neutron therapy offers any advantage in the treatment of carcinoma of the oesophagus.

An alternative approach to improving local tumour control rates is the combination of intracavitary irradiation and external beam treatments. Renewed interest in intracavitary treatments followed the development of afterloading techniques which virtually abolished the risk of staff radiation exposure (Bottrill et al. 1979). In most instances, the technique has been used for palliation (Rowland and Pagliero 1985). However, the success of this has encouraged its use in earlier cases when combined with external beam radiotherapy. This allows the delivery of a higher local dose of treatment without, at the same time, giving unacceptable doses to surrounding normal tissues. A two-year-survival rate of 37% has been reported from the Princess Margaret Hospital in Toronto using radium and external beam treatment (Rider and Diaz Mendoza 1969). However, there is some evidence that patient selection may have played a part in achieving such good results. A further series of 24 patients were treated in a similar manner at the University of Southern California (George 1980). Patients initially received 4000–5000 cGy of external beam radiotherapy followed by 1500–3000 cGy of intracavitary irradiation. Only two failed to gain significant relief of dysphagia and the survival rate and the quality of life compared favourably with more conventional methods of treatment. Recent reports from Japan have also claimed improved local tumour control in a series of 43 patients given intracavitary and external beam irradiation (Hishikawa et al. 1987). This approach obviously merits further investigation. However, a degree of caution is necessary. Local tissue damage may be increased in inappropriately applied treatments resulting in a higher incidence of ulceration, fistula formation and stricture. It would seem that the tolerance dose of intracavitary irradiation is of the order of 2000 cGy when it is given after external beam treatments of 6000 cGy (Hishikawa et al. 1987).

# Chemotherapy

Chemotherapy has been investigated widely in oesophageal cancer. However, the response to cytotoxic drugs has been poor although in selected patients relief of symptoms may be achieved. There is no evidence that the use of chemotherapy improves survival.

A major problem in oesophageal cancer is the assessment of response of disease. Yet many studies simply describe response rates without indicating whether there has been any symptomatic benefit to the patient or prolongation of life. Frequently results are presented of groups of patients who are non-homogeneous in character and in whom response has been assessed in a variety of ways. A further difficulty lies in the character of the population of patients in whom the disease develops. Many patients with oesophageal cancer are too old or frail to be given cytotoxic chemotherapy.

The most reliable ways in which response of disease may be measured are by CT scanning, barium studies and endoscopy with biopsy. Improvement in dysphagia is unreliable as only a very small reduction in tumour size may be associated with marked improvement in swallowing.

Single agent and combination drug regimens have both been evaluated in patients with oesophageal cancer. Unfortunately, the only conclusion which can be drawn from the studies so far carried out is that a drug capable of producing high response rates is not yet available. Few drugs are able to produce even a 20% response rate. Those that are include cisplatinum, vindesine, mitomycin C and bleomycin. Even with these agents the duration of response is brief, being only of the order of 2–5 months (Kelsen 1984).

Various combinations of drugs have also been evaluated. These have usually incorporated those drugs shown to have the best single agent activity. Most have included cisplatinum. The quoted response rates of these combinations varies widely between 15% and 80% (Kelsen 1984). This is indicative not only of the highly selected nature of the patients investigated but also the way in which response has been measured. The largest series is that from the Memorial Hospital in New York which has evaluated the combination of cisplatinum, vindesine and bleomycin (Kelsen et al. 1983). A total of 68 patients was treated. No complete responses were achieved but partial remissions were seen in 53% of patients. The response rate was better in patients with localised disease. In those with extensive disease, 33% obtained a partial response which lasted for 7 months on average. The toxicity of this regimen was considerable, with 20% of patients experiencing renal dysfunction. Other problems which were encountered were leucopenia and thrombocytopenia (which were dose-limiting toxicities), peripheral neuropathy and pulmonary fibrosis. In some patients this regimen was given in combination with radiotherapy and surgery. Even when this combined approach was used the overall survival was poor.

A number of other cisplatinum-containing combinations have also been evaluated in oesophageal cancer. All are toxic and the mean duration of response is only of the order of 6–8 months. At the present time the chemotherapeutic agents available have only a modest effect on carcinoma of the oesophagus and their associated toxicity is considerable. There can be no justification for the general use of cytotoxic chemotherapy in this disease. Since the overall survival is poor and metastatic disease poses a considerable problem there is a need for continued evaluation of chemotherapy. However, careful assessment is required to ascertain the effect both on the quality of life and also on survival. This should be conducted only in specialised units.

# Combined Modality Treatment

The poor results achieved by radiotherapy, even in patients with disease apparently limited to the oesophagus, have led to the introduction of a number of combined treatment programmes. Most of these have investigated various combinations of surgery and radiotherapy. However, newer regimens have also incorporated chemotherapy in the hope that this might improve local tumour control and also deal with possible micrometastatic disease.

### Preoperative Radiotherapy

The most widely used combined treatment approach has been that of giving radiotherapy prior to planned surgical resection. The rationale for this is that the irradiation might increase the proportion of patients in whom a curative resection might be performed and also reduce local recurrence rates, so improving survival. In addition, radiotherapy might possibly eradicate para-oesophageal disease which would not be amenable to surgical removal. The benefit conferred by proceeding to surgery is that a longer length of oesophagus can be removed than could be effectively treated by radiotherapy alone.

Most studies of preoperative radiotherapy have been non-randomised. In many instances the selection criteria used have not been clearly stated and the patient populations differed widely. In addition, the preoperative radiotherapy schedules employed have varied enormously. As a result, it is difficult to draw any firm conclusions from this work in spite of the fact that large numbers of patients have been treated in this way. In many of the investigations the criteria used to define operability have not been described. Therefore, although radiotherapy may have been given to all the patients in the study, only a varying proportion of patients actually had a resection performed. This is further confirmation of the differences in the populations of patients included in these investigations.

One of the largest studies has been performed in Japan on a total of 346 patients with cervical and thoracic tumours (Akakura et al. 1970). Surgery alone was used to treat 229 patients and 117 were given preoperative radiotherapy. Patients included in the surgery-only arm were treated between 1956 and 1968 and those receiving preoperative radiotherapy between 1963 and 1968.

The radiotherapy doses given were 5000–6000 cGy. Surgery was undertaken after a two-to four-week gap. Only 39.7% of the patients in the surgery-alone group had resectable lesions whereas 82.1% of those given preoperative irradiation had a resection performed. The operative mortality for the two groups of patients was similar at 13.2% in the surgery-only arm and 20.8% in the preoperatively irradiated patients. The five-year-survival rates were 13.6% and 25% respectively. Although this would suggest a great benefit for preoperative radiotherapy, it is impossible to draw any meaningful conclusions from these data. Patients in the two groups were recruited at different periods during which time tremendous developments were taking place in the assessment of patients and in their perioperative care. It is quite likely that the two sets of patients were quite dissimilar in many respects and these differences could entirely account for the results achieved.

The results of most of the preoperative radiotherapy studies do not indicate any benefit even in those patients who completed preoperative radiotherapy and subsequently had a resection performed. For example, in another large study, this time performed in the United States, which included 332 patients, the five-year-survival rate was only 13.9% (Marks et al. 1976). In spite of the fact that all patients received preoperative irradiation to a dose of 4500 cGy, only 30.4% had a resection performed. This indicates that in most instances radiotherapy, even in the doses employed in this study, cannot increase resectability rates.

A few prospectively randomised studies have been reported or have recently been completed. These have investigated differing radiotherapy schedules in patients deemed to have clinically operable oesophageal cancer. One such trial carried out in France evaluated the effect of giving a dose of 4000 cGy in eight to twelve days with operation being carried out within a further eight days of the completion of radiotherapy (Launois et al. 1981). A total of 124 consecutive patients was included in the trial, 57 undergoing immediate operation and 67 receiving preoperative irradiation. Disappointingly, no benefit could be demonstrated in those receiving radiotherapy. The resectability rates were the same as were the operative mortality rates although these were considerable at 23% in both groups. The five-year actuarial survival was 9.5% in irradiated patients and 11.5% in those treated by immediate surgery. These were not significantly different. What is of concern, is that long-term sequelae may yet be encountered in the patients given such a short course of high-dose radiotherapy in spite of the fact that acute morbidity was not increased. This has certainly been the experience in other investigations where high doses of radiotherapy have been employed (Guernsey et al. 1979). The European Organisation for Research on the Treatment of Cancer (EORTC) are currently conducting a trial of preoperative radiotherapy in oesophageal cancer using a lower dose of 3300 cGy given in 12 days. Full results are not yet available from this study, although a preliminary report has not shown any benefit from irradiation (Gignoux et al. 1982). What is particularly disappointing about the studies conducted to date is that there is no evidence that radiotherapy has influenced those factors which affect the outcome following surgery such as the incidence of nodal involvement, the presence of tumour at the resection margins and the ability to perform a curative resection. From this it would seem that preoperative radiotherapy has little to offer in patients with carcinoma of the oesophagus.

## Postoperative Radiotherapy

The value of postoperative radiotherapy is even less clearly defined than preoperative irradiation. A randomised trial of this form of therapy has never been conducted. Most reports have been anecdotal in nature, describing the use of postoperative treatment in small proportions of patients who had undergone resection. One from the Mayo Clinic described the use of postoperative radiotherapy in only 24 patients out of a total of 334 who had had a resection performed (Gunnlaugsson et al. 1970). Attempting to assess any benefit from treatment is therefore impossible. In certain well-defined circumstances post-operative radiotherapy might reduce the incidence of local recurrence and possibly improve survival. These are patients in whom a definitive resection has been performed, who do not have lymph node metastases, and who are found to have tumour at the resection margins (Kasai et al. 1978). When lymphatic spread is present, postoperative treatment is unlikely to be of value.

It is also difficult to imagine that giving radiotherapy to patients who are found to be inoperable will confer any benefit. Such patients have advanced disease which, if found to be beyond the scope of surgical treatment, will certainly not be amenable to radiotherapy. There is thus even less evidence to suggest a benefit from postoperative radiotherapy than preoperative irradiation and its routine use cannot be recommended. Only perhaps in certain selected patients might it be of value.

## Chemotherapy, Radiation and Surgery

Various cytotoxic drugs have been used in combination with radiotherapy in the hope of increasing the efficacy of treatment. There has also been the belief that this approach might help in dealing with micrometastatic disease. This form of therapy has been principally used in patients with disease considered to be unresectable or in those who, on medical grounds, have been considered unsuitable for surgery. The drug which has been most widely used has been bleomycin, largely because it has been shown experimentally to have a radio-sensitising effect. A number of reports have described an even more aggressive approach in patients with operable tumours. In these, chemotherapy has been given as preoperative treatment either alone or in some cases combined with radiotherapy.

Many of the studies have examined only small numbers of patients and have been non-randomised. However, more recently, prospectively randomised trials have been reported. A systematic evaluation of bleomycin, adriamycin or both given together with radiotherapy has been described (Kolaric et al. 1980). Very small groups of patients were evaluated. Although responses appeared better in the chemotherapy and radiotherapy treated patients, the toxicity was consider-able. On the other hand a study carried out by the Eastern Cooperative Oncology Group (ECOG) in the USA failed to demonstrate any benefit in patients treated with a combination of bleomycin and irradiation compared with radiotherapy alone (Earle et al. 1980). Similar findings were reported in a large Scandinavian trial comparing irradiation alone with radiotherapy and bleomycin given either as the sole treatment for inoperable patients or as preoperative therapy in those considered to have operable tumours (Andersen et al. 1984). A total of 259 patients was available for evaluation. The groups were comparable in terms of factors likely to affect prognosis. In the surgically treated patients, the operability rates and the proportion having curative resections were the same whether or not patients had received the preoperative treatment regimens. The postoperative mortality rates were the same at 12%. No significant differences in median survival or two-year-survival rates could be discovered in either operable patients or those allocated to the radiotherapy arms.

The disappointing results obtained using bleomycin together with concern about possible pulmonary complications which might follow its use in patients receiving mediastinal radiotherapy have led to the exploration of alternative drug combinations. These have included 5-fluorouracil (5FU), cisplatinum and mitomycin C. So far, a randomised study of these agents has not been performed. It is therefore difficult to draw firm conclusions from the reported findings although many have claimed that the multimodality approach is superior to the use of radiotherapy alone. One American study retrospectively evaluated three different treatment schedules in 57 patients with oesophageal carcinoma. These were treated with curative intent either by radiotherapy alone, radiotherapy combined with 5FU and cisplatinum or by giving combined 5FU, cisplatinum and radiotherapy as preoperative treatment followed by oesophagectomy (Richmond et al. 1987). The numbers of patients included in each group were obviously small and the treatments were not conducted concurrently. Nevertheless, improved local tumour control and survival were found in those receiving either of the multimodality treatments. This led to the question being raised of whether surgery was really necessary. A similar treatment schedule was described in the treatment of 26 patients at the North Western University in Chicago (Kies et al. 1987). In this study, cisplatinum and 5FU were given for three cycles followed by oesophagectomy or radical radiotherapy or both. Once more the numbers of patients evaluated are very small. Yet a benefit from the use of chemotherapy is claimed. What is worrying about this study is that considerable drug toxicity was encountered. A third technique which has been described is the utilisation of a combined regimen that has produced encouraging results in the treatment of patients with anal cancer. This incorporated the use of 5FU by continuous infusion during the first week of a course of radiotherapy, together with mitomycin C given on day one of the treatment schedule (Keane et al. 1985). In this study too small numbers of patients were examined, the total being only 35. Historical control patients treated by radiotherapy alone were used for comparative purposes. Once more, an advantage to the combined treatment was described.

Major problems which exist in the assessment of these enthusiastic reports are that in each only small numbers of patients have been treated and follow-up has been for a relatively short period of time. In addition, the criteria used to select patients are not defined. The study data are compared with historical controls and it is therefore possible that patients with a better prognosis who were younger and fitter were recruited to these investigations. Advances in staging techniques which have taken place mean that many patients excluded from the recent studies by virtue of having metastatic disease may well be included in the historical control group. A further point is that the more recent treatments incorporate advances in other aspects such as improved radiotherapy equipment and better dose distributions obtained from computer planning systems. The toxicity of these treatment schedules makes it likely that only a limited group of patients is likely to be fit enough to benefit from them. Only by conducting a prospective randomised controlled trial will it be possible to assess whether, in potentially curable patients, the promise of these treatment programmes is confirmed.

## Palliative Treatment

Many patients diagnosed as having oesophageal cancer will be found to have disease so extensive as to be incurable by any of the currently available treatment modalities. What is therefore required in these circumstances is a treatment capable of achieving relief of symptoms as quickly as possible in a high proportion of patients. Unfortunately, no one therapeutic modality satisfies these criteria completely. Therefore, great clinical judgement is necessary in order to choose the most appropriate measures for any individual patient.

Radiotherapy has proved to be extremely effective in alleviating the distressing symptoms of this disease. The principal symptom of dysphagia will be relieved in more than 50% of patients (Boyce 1984). However, radiotherapy is less effective in cases where the dysphagia has been produced by a tumour which is deeply infiltrating. When irradiation is used for palliation a useful dose can only by delivered over a period of one to two weeks and it may take a further two weeks before relief is obtained. Therefore, if the life expectancy of the patient is short, alternative treatments may be preferable. Radiotherapy should only be given to relieve specific symptoms and not used as a "placebo" since there can never be any guarantee of freedom from side-effects. Simple treatment techniques are employed in order to reduce to a minimum the daily treatment times. The overall treatment time should not exceed two weeks so that patients may return to their home environment as quickly as possible.

Radiotherapy may also be of great value in the treatment of metastatic disease. The principal sites of metastases are lymph nodes. Occasionally, a node mass causing specific symptoms or causing the patient concern because of its size and situation may warrant palliative radiotherapy. Blood-borne spread mainly occurs in the later stages to the liver, lungs and adrenals. These metastases are unlikely to be helped by radiotherapy. Infrequently, bone deposits may develop. The pain which they usually cause will generally be helped by a short course of palliative treatment. There is little place for chemotherapy in the palliation of oesophageal cancer largely on account of the poor responses achieved and the toxicity caused by the drugs currently available.

## Conclusions

The outlook for patients with oesophageal cancer is poor and is likely to remain so in the foreseeable future. Unless the disease can be detected at an earlier stage, the therapeutic modalities currently available are unlikely to make a major impact on survival. Whether the newer combined modality treatments will make a modest contribution to improved local tumour control is unknown at present. What is clear is that these aggressive approaches are suitable only for carefully selected patients.

# References

Adams GE, Fowler JF, Dische S, Thomlinson RH (1976) Hypoxic cell sensitisers in radiotherapy. Lancet I:186–188

Akakura I, Nakamura Y, Kakegawa T et al. (1970) Surgery of carcinoma of the esophagus with pre-operative radiation. Chest 57:47–56

Andersen AP, Berdal P, Edsmyr F et al. (1984) Irradiation chemotherapy and surgery in esophageal cancer: a randomised clinical study. Radiother Oncol 2:179–188

Arnott SJ (1986) Oesophageal cancer. In: Fielding JWL, Priestman TJ (eds) Gastrointestinal oncology. Castle House, Tunbridge Wells

Beatty JD, DeBoer G, Rider WD (1979) Carcinoma of the esophagus: pre-treatment assessment, correlation of radiation treatment parameters with survival and identification and management of radiation treatment failure. Cancer 43:2254–2267

Bottrill DO, Plane JH, Newaishy GA (1979) A proposed afterloading technique for irradiation of the oesophagus. Br J Radiol 52:573–574

Boyce WH (1984) Palliation of advanced esophageal cancer. Semin Oncol 11:186–196

Doggett RLS, Guernsey JM, Bagshaw MA (1970) Combined radiation and surgical treatment of carcinoma of the thoracic esophagus. Front Radiat Ther Oncol 5:147–154

Dufourmental L (1930) Le traitement curatif du cancer de l'oesophage. Paris Méd 2:87–89

Dvivedi M, Pradhan DG (1978) Immediate results of weekly fractionation in external radiotherapy. Int J Radiat Oncol Biol Phys 4:573–578

Earlam R, Cunha-Melo JR (1980) Oesophageal squamous cell carcinoma. II. A critical review of radiotherapy. Br J Surg 67:457–461

Earle J, Gelber R, Moertel C (1980) A controlled evaluation of combined radiation and bleomycin therapy for squamous cell carcinoma of the oesophagus. Int J Radiat Oncol Biol Phys 6:821–826

Einhorn M (1904) Observations on radium. Med Rec 66:164

Exner A (1904) Uber die Behandlung von Oesophagus-karzinomen mit Radiumstrahlen. Wien Klin Wochenschr 17:96

George FW (1980) Radiation management in esophageal cancer. Am J Surg 139:795–804

Gignoux M, Buyse M, Segol P, Roussel A, Paillot B, Kunlin A, Duez N (1982) Radiothérapie préoperatoire du cancer de l'oesophage. Résultats préliminaires d'un essai randomisé de l'EORTC. Acta Chir Belge 4:373–379

Guernsey J, Doggett RLS, Mason G et al. (1979) Combined treatment of cancer of the esophagus. Am J Surg 117:157–161

Guisez J (1925) Du cancer de l'oesophage. Bull Otorhinolaryngol (Paris) 23:49–87

Gunnlaugsson GH, Wychulis AR, Roland C et al. (1970) Analysis of the records of 1657 patients with carcinoma of the esophagus and cardia of the stomach. Surg Gynecol Obstet 130:997

Hancock SL, Glatstein E (1984) Radiation therapy of esophageal cancer. Semin Oncol 11:144–158

Hishikawa Y, Kamikonya N, Tanaka S, Miura T (1987) Radiotherapy of oesophageal carcinoma: role of high dose rate intracavitary irradiation. Radiother Oncol 9:13–20

Kasai M, Mori S, Watanabe T (1978) Follow-up results after resection of thoracic esophageal cancer. World J Surg 2:543–551

Keane TJ, Harwood AR, Elhakim T et al. (1985) Radical radiation therapy with 5-fluorouracil infusion and mitomycin C for oesophageal squamous carcinoma. Radiother Oncol 4:205–210

Kelsen D (1984) Chemotherapy of esophageal cancer. Semin Oncol 11:159–168

Kelsen KP, Coonley C, Hilaris B et al. (1983) Cisplatin, vindesine and bleomycin combination chemotherapy of local-regional and advanced esophageal carcinoma. Am J Med 75:639–652

Kies MS, Rosen ST, Tsang T-T et al. (1987) Cisplatin and 5-fluorouracil in the primary management of squamous esophageal cancer. Cancer 60:2156–2160

Kolaric K, Maricic Z, Roth A et al. (1980) Combination of bleomycin and adriamycin with and without radiation in the treatment of inoperable esophageal cancer. Cancer 45:2265–2273

Launois B, Delarue D, Campion JP, Kerbaol M (1981) Preoperative radiotherapy for carcinoma of the esophagus. Surg Gynecol Obstet 153:690–692

Marks RD, Scruggs JH, Wallace KM (1976) Preoperative radiation therapy for carcinoma of the esophagus. Cancer 38:84–89

Matthews HR, Powell DJ, McConkey CC (1986) Effect of surgical experience on the results of resection for oesophageal carcinoma. Br J Surg 73:621–623

Mendenhall WM, Million RR, Bova FJ (1982) Carcinoma of the cervical esophagus treated with radiation therapy using a four-field box technique. Int J Radiat Oncol Biol Phys 8:1435–1439

Newaishy GA, Read GA, Duncan W, Kerr GR (1982) Results of radical radiotherapy of squamous cell carcinoma of the oesophagus. Clin Radiol 33:347–352

Pearson JG (1966) The radiotherapy of carcinoma of the oesophagus and post-cricoid region in South-East Scotland. Clin Radiol 17:242–257

Pearson JG (1977) The present status and future potential of radiotherapy in the management of esophageal cancer. Cancer 39:882–890

Pierquin B, Wambersie A, Tubiana M (1966) Cancer of the thoracic oesophagus: two series of patients treated by 22 MeV betatron. Br J Radiol 39:189–192

Richmond J, Seydel HG, Bag Y et al. (1987) Comparison of three treatment strategies for esophageal cancer within a single institution. Int J Radiat Oncol Biol Phys 13:1617–1620

Rider WD, Diaz Mendoza R (1969) Some opinions on the treatment of cancer of the esophagus. AJR 105:514–517

Rowland CG, Pagliero KM (1985) Intracavitary irradiation in palliation of carcinoma of oesophagus and cardia. Lancet II:981–983

Saunders M, Dische S (1987) Treatment of cancer using multiple fractions per day over a continuous period of 12 days. Br J Radiol 60:607

Schwade JG, Kinsella TJ, Kelly B et al. (1984) Clinical experience with intravenous misonidazole for carcinoma of the esophagus: results in attempting radiosensitisation of each fraction of exposure. Cancer Invest 2:91–95

Souttar HS (1934) Radium and cancer. Heinemann, London, p 296

Steel GG, Courtenay D (1983) The radiobiology of human tumour cells. In: Steel GG, Adams GE, Peckham MJ (eds) The biological basis of radiotherapy. Elsevier, Amsterdam, pp 123–138

Thompson WM (1983) Esophageal cancer. Int J Radiat Oncol Biol Phys 9:1533–1565

Union Internationale Contre le Cancer (1978) TNM classification of malignant tumours, 3rd edn. UICC, Geneva

Waterhouse JAH (1974) Cancer handbook of epidemiology and prognosis. Churchill Livingstone, Edinburgh

Withers HR, Peters LJ, Thames HD et al. (1982) Hyperfractionation. Int J Radiat Oncol Biol Phys 8:1807–1809

Yang ZY, Gu XZ, Zhao S et al. (1983) Long-term survival of radiotherapy for esophageal carcinoma: analysis of 1136 patients surviving for more than five years. Int J Radiat Oncol Biol Phys 9:1769–1773

Ydrach AA, Marcial VA, Parsons J et al. (1982) Misonidazole and unconventional radiation in advanced squamous cell carcinoma of the esophagus: a phase II study of the Radiation Therapy Oncology Group. Int J Radiat Oncol Biol Phys 8:357–359

# Chapter 13

# Brachytherapy (Intracavitary Irradiation)

K. M. Pagliero

Although external beam radiotherapy has a well-established role in the management of oesophageal cancer, its potential to cure is extremely low. A review by Earlam and Cunha-Melo (1980) gives survival rates of 18% at one year, 8% at 2 years and 6% at 5 years. Temporary relief of dysphagia is achieved but local recurrence occurs in 80% of cases and an unpleasant death with aspiration pneumonia results either from malignant obstruction of the oesophagus or from tracheo-oesophageal fistula (Flores et al. 1988).

In an attempt to improve on these poor results, attention has turned to brachytherapy. The concept is not new, for as long ago as 1915 radium bougies were inserted into oesophageal cancer with good effect, but the hazards to the patients and the staff of this uncontrolled radiation caused it to be abandoned (Knox 1915). However, renewed enthusiasm for brachytherapy for carcinoma of the oesophagus (Rowland and Pagliero 1985) has been stimulated lately by the development of "after loading" techniques in the management of carcinoma of the cervix (Fletcher 1971). The discovery of leak-proof radioactive materials such as caesium 137, cobalt 60 or iridium 192 has resulted in safer application. These substances have a higher specific activity than radium and this has cut treatment times dramatically. The use of the after loading method while the patient is in a screened room has eliminated harmful irradiation of the staff.

## Technique

The remote after loading system of Nucletron of Holland has been used. This comprises a 6-channel low dose rate machine that employs 48 pellets of caesium

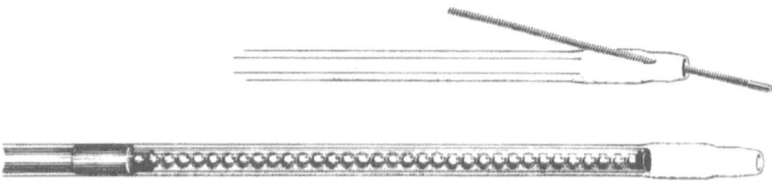

**Fig. 13.1.**   The applicator.

137, each with 40 mCi activity. A pneumatic transfer of these sources down flexible tubing into previously inserted applicators is controlled by computer. The sources are automatically withdrawn into a special safe whenever staff have to enter the treatment room. When treatment is restarted, the computer programs the remaining dose to be administered. The applicator (Fig. 13.1) is of 8-mm external diameter and is introduced under X-ray control over a previously inserted guide wire. The caesium sources are transferred along an insert tube that is locked within the external tube. During the positioning of the applicator an insert containing non-radioactive marker pellets is used so that precise localisation can be visualised on the X-ray screen. During the treatment, the insert tube receives sources to the terminal 12 cm of the applicator. This gives a treatment length of 13 cm so that if it is necessary to irradiate the entire oesophagus this can be achieved with two consecutive applications at the same session. In this series, 2 cm above and below the tumour was treated as well as the tumour itself.

# Insertion

General anaesthesia has usually been used, but the procedure may be done quite satisfactorily under simple sedation and local anaesthesia. The lesion is viewed through the fibreoptic endoscope (Fig. 13.2). It is important to visualise the upper and lower extent of the tumour endoscopically and to demonstrate these two positions on the X-ray screen. Having localised the tumour, a guide wire is passed into the stomach and the endoscope removed. The applicator is then threaded over the guide wire into an appropriate position straddling the tumour (Fig. 13.3). If the whole oesophagus is to be treated in two applications then the lowermost position is treated first before withdrawing the applicator 13 cm to treat the upper half of the oesophagus. Having positioned the applicator, it is

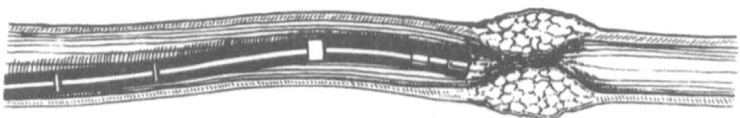

**Fig. 13.2.**   Viewing the lesion endoscopically.

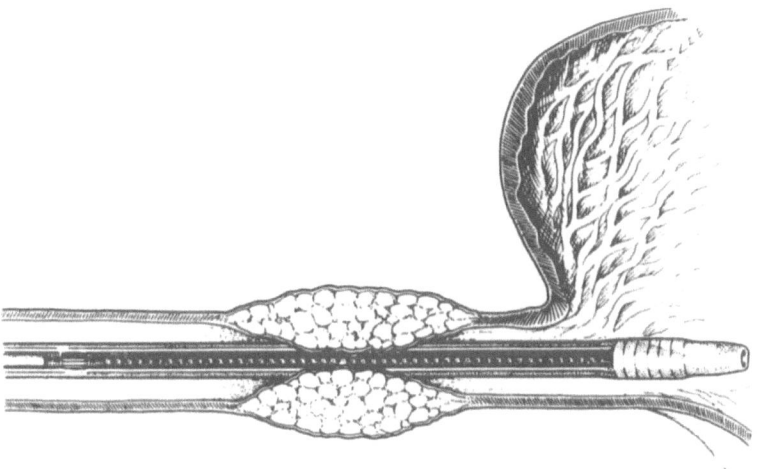

**Fig. 13.3.** Applicator "straddling" the tumour.

easily maintained by fixing it to a simple face-mask which is strapped to the patient's head (Fig. 13.4). The patient is then transferred to the treatment suite without fear of dislocation of the applicator. Once there, the patient can be continuously visualised on closed circuit television (Fig. 13.5). If staff need to enter, the door is wired to the Selectron machine so that as it opens sources are pneumatically withdrawn into the safe. When the time comes to restart treatment, the machinery programs itself with regard to treatment times (Fig. 13.6).

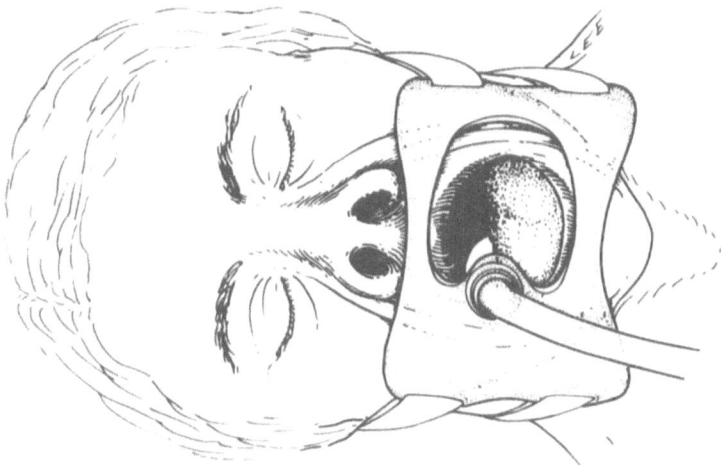

**Fig. 13.4.** Face-mask used to maintain the position of the applicator.

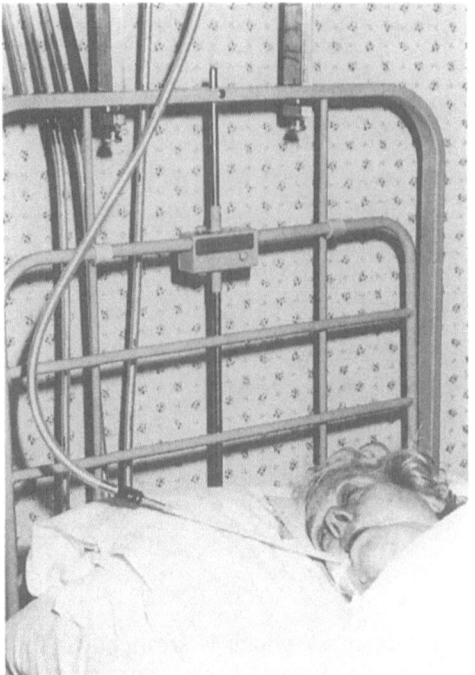

**Fig. 13.5.**   The patient is continuously observed from outside the screened treatment suite.

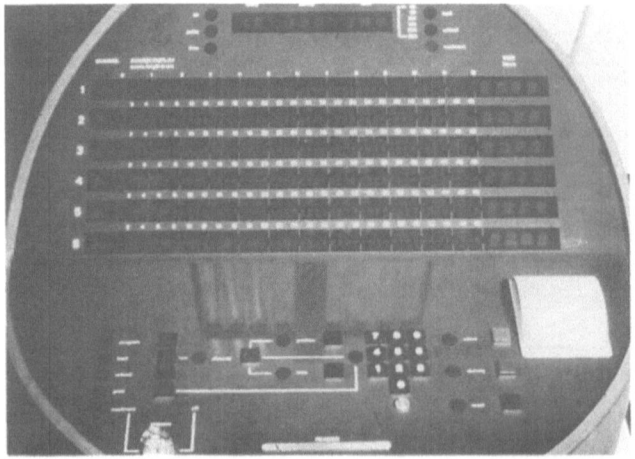

**Fig. 13.6.**   The machine housing the radioactive sources, the machinery to transfer the sources, the "safe" and the computerised controls.

# Dose

In our initial study we chose to use all 48 caesium sources available in a moderately high single dose fraction, to try and gain tumour response with rapid palliation. It was thought that this would be economical both in terms of Health Service resources and also with respect to the use of the limited life expectancy of the patient. A dose of 1500 cGy at 10 mm of central axis was chosen. This was achieved in approximately 1.14 h. The effective treatment volume is thus represented by a cylinder 2 cm in diameter and 13 cm in length. It gives a surface dose of approximately 3500 cGy and beyond 3 cm the dose is subtherapeutic. We were gratified to find that this seemingly large dose obtained a high incidence of therapeutic response with few undesirable tissue side effects and this same dose has been used up to the present time.

# Patient Selection

It is our view that carcinoma of the oesophagus can be cured and therefore all patients who appear to have localised disease and who are considered fit for major surgery are offered resection. However, those that have unresectable disease, who are too old and frail for major operation or who decline surgery are palliated in our unit with brachytherapy as the first option. The only exclusions are patients with tracheobronchial mucosal involvement – one such case developed a fistula following brachytherapy. In addition, some patients present so late and are so debilitated that it is better not to interfere with the inevitable outcome.

# Results

In the first study, 72 patients were treated. The median age was 76 years and the sex distribution was equal. Two-thirds of the patients were considered resectable but not fit for major surgery and one-third were assessed as having unresectable disease. Of the 72 patients, three found they could not complete the treatment, though one withstood it for a sufficient length of time to gain a therapeutic response. Twelve others found the treatment unpleasant, but tolerated it.

The hospital stay was very short, 70% of the patients leaving hospital within 3 days. It is possible to perform this treatment on an outpatient basis, but for social reasons many patients are kept in for 2–3 nights. The hospital stay is considerably shorter than after pulsion or traction intubation. Dysphagia was graded as follows:

0, total dysphagia
1, able to swallow liquids

2, able to swallow puréed mince or soft food
3, eating normally

The effects on dysphagia are illustrated in Fig. 13.7a,b. The majority of patients
responded to treatment. It should be pointed out that the initial benefit is as a

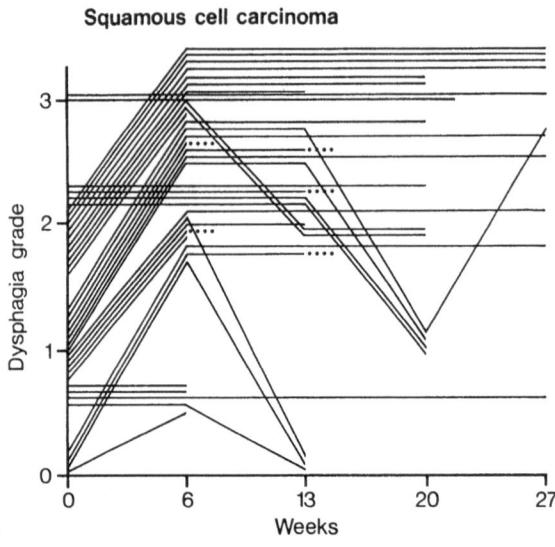

a

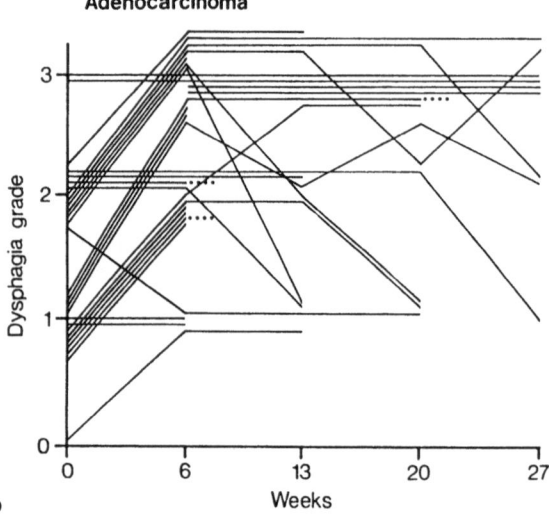

b

**Fig. 13.7a,b.** The effect of brachytherapy on relief of dysphagia in squamous cell carcinoma of the
oesophagus (**a**) and adenocarcinoma of the oesophagus (**b**). 0, total dysphagia; 1, able to swallow
liquids; 2, able to swallow puréed mince or soft food; 3, eating normally. The line for each patient
starts immediately prior to the treatment.

result of the dilatation to enable endoscopic examination of the tumour. Experience with simple bougienage for carcinoma suggests that this benefit is short-lived and that the persistent benefit that is seen in many cases is as a result of brachytherapy.

In those patients who had a recurrence of dysphagia, only one case was noted of benign stricture thought to be the result of irradiation. All the remaining cases developed dysphagia because of recurrence of tumour. When a useful response was achieved for a reasonable length of time before recurrence occurred, brachytherapy was repeated. When there was no initial or subsequent response intubation was carried out and this has been performed in one-fifth of patients. In fitter patients, a good response to brachytherapy has been augmented by the addition of external beam irradiation.

The single most important advantage of brachytherapy has been in patients unable to cooperate with advice about diet. Whereas indwelling tubes are satisfactory in intelligent patients who can understand the principles of management, many less intelligent and debilitated patients do not comply, develop frequent bolus obstruction and often require readmission. No patient developed bolus obstruction after brachytherapy. The response of adenocarcinoma was almost as good as squamous cell carcinoma, an effect which is not usually found after external beam radiotherapy. The side effects were few. Of the 69 patients undergoing full treatment, two suffered sore throats, two developed oesophagitis, five had mild epigastric pain and one had nausea and diarrhoea. One patient was thought to have developed radiation stricture. Finally, one patient who had tracheobronchial involvement developed a fistula following treatment and such a patient would not now be so treated.

There is no doubt that brachytherapy is a kinder treatment than external beam irradiation to these unfortunate patients, both in terms of their well being, the insignificant morbidity of the treatment and the extremely modest demand on their limited time. Not all patients can withstand the rigours of external beam radiation and no patient has been considered too frail for brachytherapy.

A pleasing improvement in survival using brachytherapy rather than intubation has been noted. The 40% six-month and 5% one-month survival in this series has been improved upon by Flores et al. (1988) who, by adding 4000 cGy in 15 treatments in 3 weeks of external beam irradiation, have achieved a 67% six-month and a 25% one-year survival. The addition of external irradiation will provide a better dose in depth to the most peripheral better-oxygenated parts of the tumour and is clearly a logical addition. Unfortunately, not all patients are fit enough to withstand this extra treatment.

There is no doubt that the advent of brachytherapy has made a significant impact on the palliation of carcinoma of the oesophagus. There is much to learn in terms of permutations of the radiation doses. Furthermore, a more effective response may be anticipated with the use of sensitising chemotherapeutic agents such as 5-fluorouracil (Byfield et al. 1980), methotrexate (Roussel 1977), bleomycin (Kolarick et al. 1976) or adriamycin (Kolarick et al. 1977). In addition, work is being performed on the combination of brachytherapy with hyperthermia which is reported to cause "tumour stabilisation" (Storm et al. 1987).

There is no doubt that brachytherapy is kind treatment to these unfortunate patients and is to be highly recommended as the first line of palliative treatment for carcinoma of the oesophagus. There is no mortality, a trivial incidence of side effects, a quick return home, a symptomatic benefit in terms of dysphagia and little of the patient's remaining time is spent in hospital, either as an outpatient or an inpatient.

In those patients where there is little response or the tumour recurs, brachytherapy does not preclude any of the other forms of palliation available.

# References

Byfield JE, Barone RM, Mendelsohn J et al. (1980) Infusional 5-flourouracil and x-ray therapy for non-resectable esophageal cancer. Cancer 45:703–708

Earlam R, Cunha-Melo JR (1980) Oesophageal squamous cell carcinoma. II. A critical review of radiotherapy. Br J Surg 67:457–461

Fletcher G (1971) Cancer of the uterine cervix. Janeway lecture, 1970. Am J Roentgenol Rad Ther Nucl Med 111:225–242

Flores AD, Stoller JL et al. (1988) Combined primary treatment of cancer of the esophagus and cardia by intracavitary and external irradiation. In: International trends in general thoracic surgery, vol 4. CV Mosby Co, St Louis, pp 368–377

Knox R (1915) Radiography, X-ray therapeutics and radium therapy. A and C Black, London, pp 374–375

Kolarick M, Maricic Z, Dujmoric I et al. (1976) Therapy of advanced oesophageal cancer with bleomycin, irradiation and in combination. Tumori 62:255–262

Kolarick M, Maricic Z, Roth A et al. (1977) Adriamycin alone and in combination with radiotherapy in the treatment of inoperable oesophageal cancer. Tumori 63:485–491

Roussel A (1977) Treatment of nonoperable cancer of the oesophagus. Digestion 16:271

Rowland CG, Pagliero KM (1985) Intracavitary irradiation in palliation of cancer of the oesophagus and cardia. Lancet II:981–983

Storm FK, Scanlon FF, Baker HW et al. (1977) Tumour stabilisation after hyperthermia. An important criterion of response to thermal therapy. J Surg Oncol 34:143–149

*Chapter 14*

# Laser Therapy

K. Matthewson

## Background

A review of the literature on the surgical treatment of oesophageal cancer in
83 783 patients found that 58% were explored, 39% were resected, 26% survived
to leave hospital, but only 4% survived for 5 years (Earlam and Cuhna-Melo
1980a).* With such a low expectation of a surgical cure the main aim of treatment
is often palliation. Good palliation will give maximum relief from symptoms
whilst inflicting the minimum of morbidity and mortality, and for oesophageal
cancer this will involve restoration of swallowing to as near normal as possible,
with as little time spent in hospital as possible. Each form of palliation has its
merits and also its disadvantages. Surgery probably produces the best palliation,
but with the cost of considerable morbidity and mortality (Watson 1982).
Radiotherapy can be effective but there is a prolonged morbidity and the
amelioration of dysphagia can be slow (Earlam and Cuhna-Melo 1980b).
Bougienage may need to be frequently repeated (Tytgat and den Hartog Jager
1983) and endoscopic insertion of an endoprosthesis produces a questionable
degree of palliation and is not universally applicable (Lux et al. 1986).

Endoscopic laser therapy was first used on humans in West Germany in 1975
for the treatment of bleeding peptic ulcers (Kiefhaber et al. 1977) but it
subsequently became apparent that it could be used to destroy endoscopically
accessible upper and lower gastrointestinal tumours. Many authors have now
reported that endoscopic laser treatment can re-establish luminal patency in

---

*But see p. 16 – Editor.

oesophageal cancer patients and reasonable consensus is developing on the type of patient who can be treated with benefit. The technique has been principally used as a palliative therapy.

# Lasers

The first laser was constructed by T. Maiman in the Howard Hughes Research Laboratories in 1960 (Maiman 1960). It was built from polished ruby and emitted powerful pulses of red light. The word "laser" is an acronym for "light amplification by the stimulated emission of radiation". The light produced by this process of "stimulated emission" has a number of properties which make it a useful therapeutic tool. The two most important are monochromaticity and collimation. Monochromaticity implies that the light consists of a single wavelength which depends upon the nature of the substance in which the laser light is generated. Different wavelengths of light can cause different effects in living tissue and an appropriate wavelength must be chosen for a particular task. Collimation implies that the beam of light is not divergent or convergent but retains its cross-sectional profile over large distances. The beam is pencil-thin and the laser light power per unit cross-sectional area can be enormous. This property of collimation allows the light to be passed through a lens and focused onto the end of a thin, flexible, optical fibre which transmits the light along its length by multiple internal reflections, and from which it emerges in a divergent cone. Such optical fibres can readily be passed along the biopsy channel of standard fibreoptic endoscopes and they represent a highly convenient means of delivering energy into endoscopically accessible living tissue.

# Interaction between Laser Light and Living Tissue

Several important changes occur in living tissue as it is rapidly heated: coagulation occurs in the region of 60°C depending upon the length of exposure to that temperature and involves conformational changes to structural proteins with thermal contraction and the development of oedema; at 100°C tissue water boils and evaporates; and between 250°C and 400°C tissue becomes carbonised and vaporised. Most medical lasers can produce all these effects if the power density of the laser light incident on the tissue is sufficient. However, the depth to which these effects can be produced depends upon the wavelength of light being used. If laser light is directed at the stomach wall with just sufficient power to cause vaporisation of the superficial layer of cells there will be histological damage apparent below this. With carbon dioxide laser light (wavelength 10 600 nm, far infrared) the depth of this damage is about 0.1 mm, whereas with argon ion laser light (wavelengths 488 and 510 nm, visible blue-green) it is about 1 mm and with neodymium yttrium aluminium garnet (Nd YAG) laser light (wavelength 1064 nm, near infrared) it is of the order of 5 mm (Bown 1983). There is theoretically a greater risk of perforation with the Nd YAG laser than the argon ion laser because of its deeper penetration but this disadvantage is more than outweighed by its ability to coagulate deeper vessels, so minimising any risk of bleeding as tumour tissue is destroyed. Endoscopic laser treatment of oesophageal cancer is currently almost exclusively performed using the Nd YAG laser.

# Indications and Aims

The principal indication is symptomatic, inoperable oesophageal cancer. Patients are usually incurable either because of metastatic disease or local invasion, they may have other major pathology which precludes surgery, or they may have had a local recurrence following attempted curative surgery. Dysphagia will have been caused by intraluminal tumour bulk; it is not possible with the current state of the art to treat dysphagia caused by extrinsic compression (Bown et al. 1987). It is not essential to be able to pass a guide wire through the lesion and it is possible to treat tumours at any level within the oesophagus, although high cervical lesions may be technically difficult. Some authors consider bleeding from an inoperable cancer to be a further indication (Mathus-Vliegen and Tytgat 1986). The basic aim of laser therapy is to destroy intra-oesophageal tumour bulk, thereby relieving dysphagia, improving nutrition and restoring the quality of life.

# Equipment

The equipment (Fig. 14.1) required for endoscopic laser therapy includes the Nd YAG laser itself with a suitably prepared fibre delivery system. This usually consists of a central optical fibre 400 or 600 μm in diameter which is enclosed in a Teflon cannula approximately 2.5 mm in diameter. There is a metal tip glued close to the tip of the fibre which holds it and the cannula together, preventing them from moving relative to one another. The surrounding cannula protects the fibre and allows coaxial carbon dioxide to be passed along the fibre delivery system. This is usually in the form of a slow background flow which blows debris from the tip of the fibre to keep it clean, and a more rapid flow when the footswitch is partially depressed. This serves to cool the tip of the fibre during therapy and also blows away debris and smoke to keep the treatment field clearly visible.

Also required is a standard forward viewing fibreoptic endoscope with a biopsy channel diameter of at least 2.8 mm. Preferably this should have a suitable filter fitted to the eyepiece to prevent laser light reflected from the mucosa passing back up the endoscope and causing an eye injury. If no protective filter is fitted, then the operator and anyone viewing via a side arm must wear protective goggles during treatment. It is also convenient to have a nasogastric tube connected to an underwater seal drain available. The nasogastric tube can be fed down the

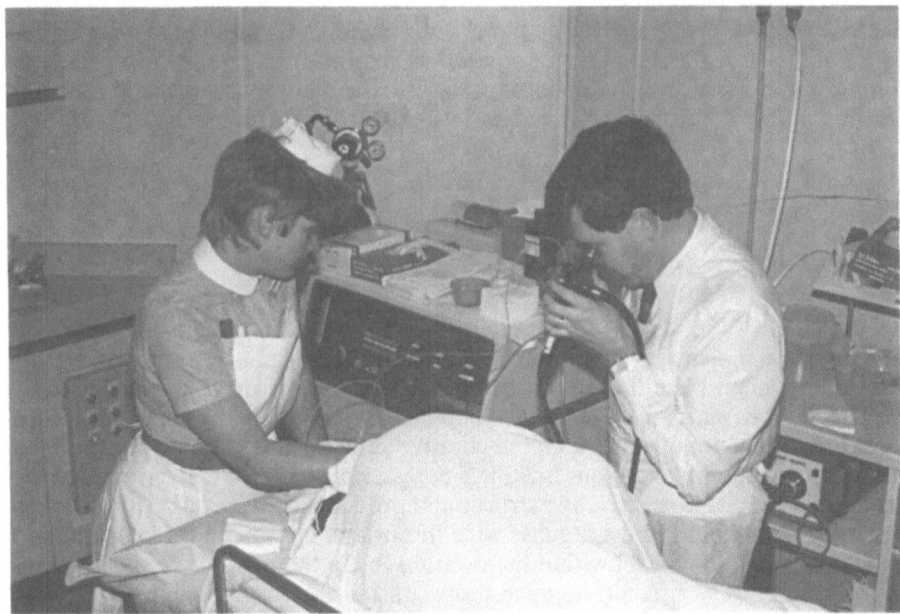

**Fig. 14.1.** Laser photocoagulation in progress. The laser is a Fibreglass 100 (Pilkington Medical Systems) in the centre of the figure and the laser fibre is the fine catheter passing through the biopsy channel of the endoscope. No protective goggles need be worn if there is a safety filter fitted into the endoscope. The patient has been sedated but not anaesthetised.

oesophagus alongside the endoscope and acts as an exhaust for the coaxial carbon dioxide and the smoke which is produced.

## Endoscopic Technique

Prior to the endoscopy the laser is calibrated to give about 70 watts at the distal end of the fibre with an exposure duration of 1 s. The patient is sedated with intravenous diazepam emulsion and pethidine, although some patients remain comfortable without pethidine. Standard oesophagoscopy is performed and the laser fibre can be advanced through the biopsy channel until it appears in the endoscopic field of view. The fibre tip is generally held about 1 cm above the tumour for treatment as greater separation may result in little tissue effect and too small a separation risks the fibre touching the tumour during exposure. This frequently results in the fibre tip "burning out" and it will then need to be reprepared.

The aim is to vaporise tumour which is protruding into the oesophageal lumen. Vaporisation is immediately recognised by black discoloration of tissue with the production of smoke and this is accompanied by a layer of coagulation beneath. Different tumours respond differently to the same quantity of laser light because

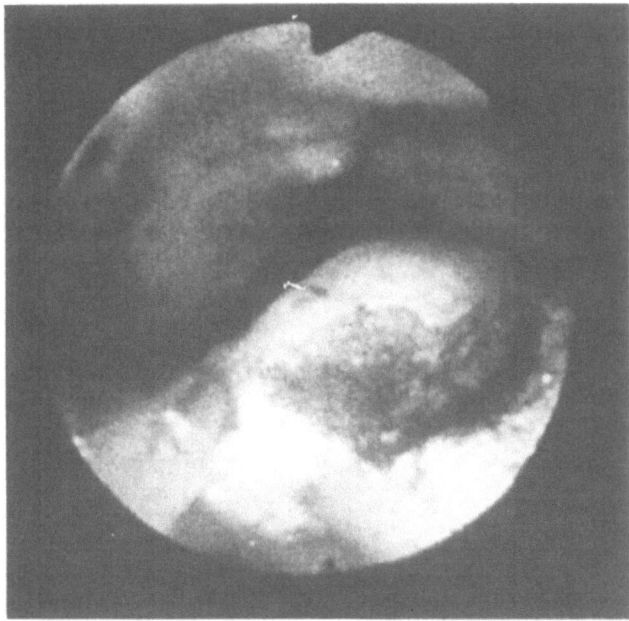

**Fig. 14.2.** Partially
lasered nodule of
oesophageal cancer.

of their different optical properties. It may take only a small quantity of light to
vaporise a soft red tumour which absorbs the light strongly, whilst a white fibrous
tumour which scatters the light but absorbs poorly may require much more. If
there is no tissue effect or only a small white patch of coagulation then the fibre
can be advanced closer to increase the power density on the tissue or the laser
power or exposure duration may be increased. If the laser effect is too fierce then
the power setting may be decreased. Repeated pulses of laser light on tumour
protruding into the lumen are then used to progressively "shave" the tumour
back (Fig. 14.2).

  If it is possible, it is preferable to begin treating the tumour at its distal margin
and work proximally. This is because the oesophageal lumen is then clearly
defined and the therapy can proceed much more rapidly (Fig. 14.3a). If the
endoscope cannot be passed directly through the tumour, but a guide wire can, it
is better to dilate and then pass the endoscope through to begin distally. If even a
guide wire cannot be passed then treatment should begin at the proximal end and
proceed distally, but taking great care not to create false passageways which could
lead to a perforation (Fig. 14.3b). Slough and carbonised necrotic tumour can be
brushed away periodically using an endoscopic brush to keep the treatment field
clear. Coagulated tumour continues to slough off over a period of a few days
following the endoscopy, and if necessary further treatment may be given at 3- to
4-day intervals. Some patients may require 3 or 4 treatment sessions to get an
optimal response, particularly if treatment has to begin at the proximal margin.
The end point of therapy is when all tumour protruding into the lumen has been
destroyed (Fig. 14.4a,b).

  As an adjuvant to "conventional" non-contact laser therapy, an alternative
technique has been described. This involves the use of artificial probes, usually
sapphire, attached to the distal end of the laser fibre. They can withstand

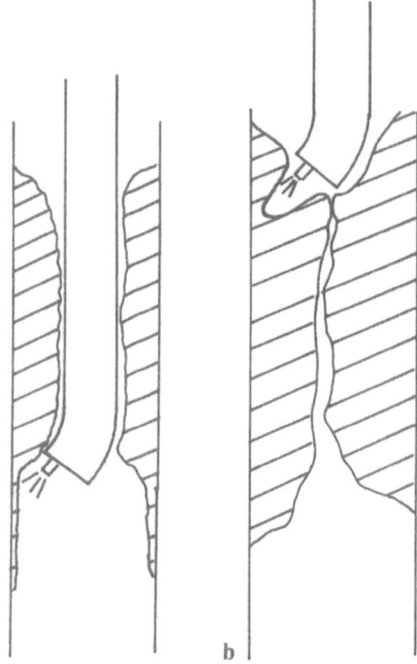

**Fig. 14.3a.** Line drawing illustrating easier laser treatment of oesophageal cancer when the distal margin is accessible and, **b**, greater risk of perforation when treating from proximal margin.

temperatures of up to 2000°C, are available in a variety of shapes (hemispherical, wedge-shaped, chisel-shaped) and are used in direct contact with the tissue being treated (Steger and Hira 1987). Such probes are generally used with a lower power setting of the order of 15 W with exposure durations of up to 5 s. The probe can be pressed against the tumour surface and held in position during exposure or

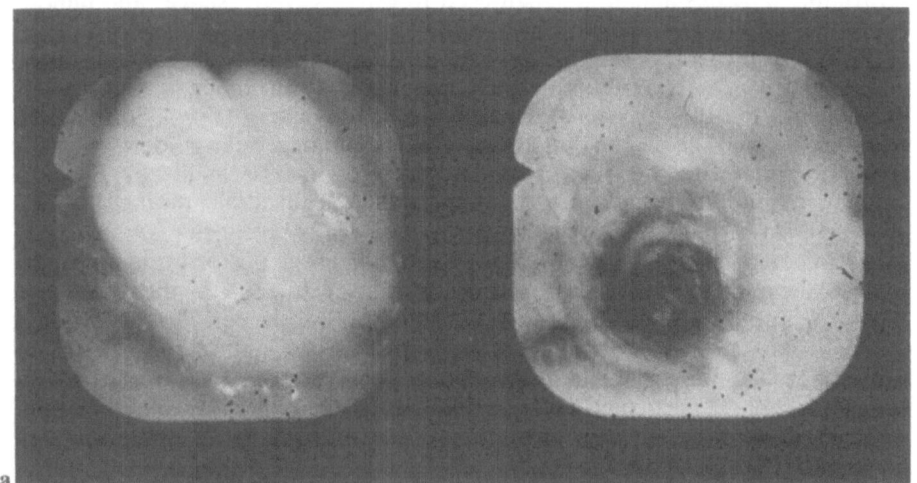

**Fig. 14.4a,b.** Oesophageal cancer before laser therapy (**a**) and following a course of laser therapy (**b**). Courtesy of Dr SG Bown and Mr H Barr.

can be moved over its surface with to and fro movements. The contact probe may prove useful when trying to define an indistinct oesophageal lumen. Coaxial carbon dioxide gas or water can be used to cool the probe which does require removal from time to time to remove adherent debris. The total energy used during a single treatment session using a contact probe (approximately 500–2000 J) is usually less than with the non-contact technique (approximately 2000–10 000 J). Advantages of the contact technique include the lack of uncomfortable gaseous intestinal distension which may accompany the non-contact technique, the lack of laser induced oedema and the greatly reduced risk of heat damage to the fibre tip (Ell et al. 1986a). Disadvantages include adherence of the sapphire to tissue during exposure and the difficulty in keeping the probe in contact with the tumour when the angle of approach is acute and there is a large respiratory excursion. Advantages of the non-contact technique are that the treatment field is always in view allowing the amount of vaporisation occurring to be continually reassessed, and it is possible to treat large tumours rapidly with a "paint brush" type movement of the laser beam over the tumour rather producing a single punctate lesion and then having to resite the probe.

# Results

There are now many reports of series of patients with inoperable oesophageal cancer who have been treated using endoscopic laser therapy and all claim that some such patients benefit from this treatment. These reports describe the treatment of these patients in an open, non-randomised, uncontrolled fashion. Claims of success for therapy are based on comparisons of individuals before and after therapy has been given. It is clearly important under these circumstances to predefine and quantify the variables which will be compared with their pretreatment levels. The variables which have been used include oesophageal patency assessed endoscopically, luminal diameter assessed by barium meal (Fig. 14.5a,b), degree of dysphagia, severity of pain and quality of life or functional assessments. All these are difficult to quantify accurately.

Fleischer and Kessler (1983), in one of the earlier reports, described the treatment of 14 patients with inoperable squamous cell cancer of the oesophagus. Tumours ranged from 5 to 11 cm in length and in 11 patients "luminal" occlusion was stated to be >90%, although how this was measured was not described. The mean number of treatment sessions required to alleviate symptoms was 5.3, although this would now be considered to be excessive. The average energy used per treatment session was 4615 J and the mean total energy per patient was 24 394 J. Destruction of a major part of intraluminal tumour was achieved in all patients. Oesophageal dilatation was undertaken at the conclusion of therapy in half of the patients. Arbitrary scoring systems for dysphagia, odynophagia and spontaneous chest pain were used to compare symptoms before and after treatment. All patients who had any of these particular symptoms had improved by completion of therapy and all could eat solid food. Eleven of the 14 patients left hospital and their mean survival was 14 weeks.

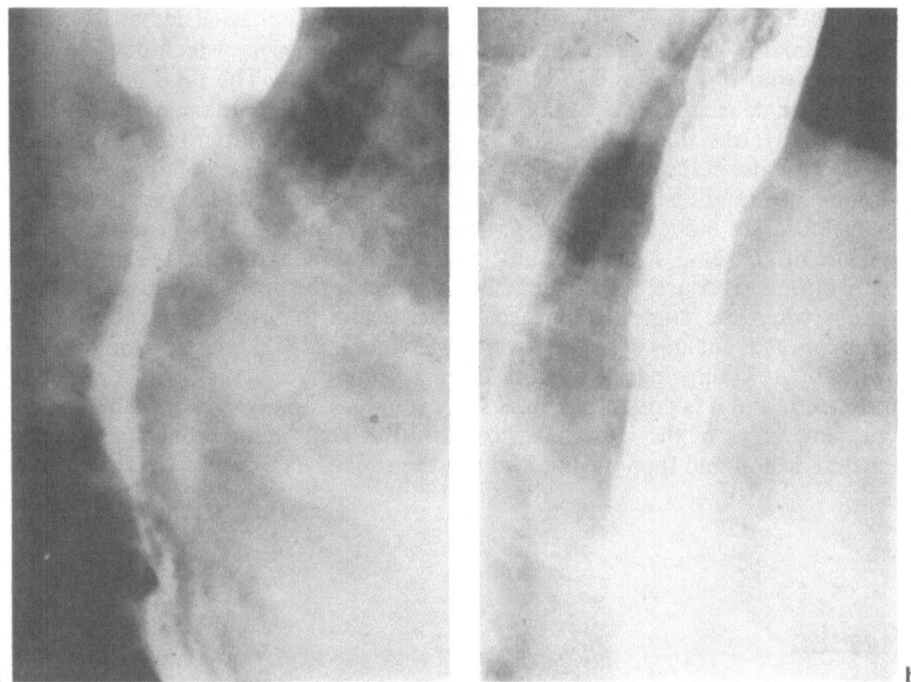

a                                                                                              b

**Fig. 14.5a,b.**    Barium swallow showing oesophageal cancer (**a**) and after completion of laser therapy (**b**). Courtesy of Dr SG Bown.

Another early series (Swain et al. 1984) reported the treatment of 6 patients with obstructing foregut cancer with either the argon ion or Nd YAG laser. The tumours were occluding up to 90% of the lumen and were between 7 and 13 cm in length. Two to six sessions of 2000–10 000 J were required to relieve dysphagia. Quantitative barium studies showed a significant improvement in minimum luminal diameter and all patients could eat solids at completion of therapy. No attempt was made to quantify dysphagia.

Fleischer and Sivak (1984) specifically studied the treatment of 15 patients with advanced adenocarcinoma of the gastric cardia. Four of these were patients who developed a recurrence following surgery and 7 had been found to be inoperable at laparotomy. All but 3 had had at least one form of palliative therapy before laser therapy was attempted. Tumour length ranged from 3 to 10 cm. Patients were treated with a mean of 2.8 treatment sessions. Minimum luminal diameter improved from a mean of 3.3 mm before therapy to 12.1 mm afterwards and all patients had an improvement in their dysphagia and could take at least some solids afterwards.

A consecutive series of 30 patients with inoperable cancer of the oesophagus and gastro-oesophageal junction were treated by Mellow and Pinkas (1985). Although "luminal patency" was achieved in 97%, dysphagia improved in only 83% and the disparity was attributed to pharyngeal dysphagia, possibly as a consequence of previous radiotherapy. Of these patients 70% were able, following the treatment, to eat all foods and were able to go home (functional success). The best predictor of such functional success was the patient's pretreatment performance status as assessed by their mobility and activity. Neither age, histological type, tumour length, extent of occlusion, weight loss or degree of dysphagia were predictive of functional success or failure, although lesions in the very proximal oesophagus appeared to fare worse than more distal lesions. Fleischer and Sivak (1985) also studied parameters affecting the initial outcome in a retrospective series of 60 patients. The best response occurred for tumours in a straight segment of mid or distal oesophagus, particularly if they were <5 cm in length. Results were least good and the technical difficulties greatest for tumours of the cervical oesophagus. It was technically easier to treat mucosal rather than submucosal tumours and the outcome was better for mucosal tumours. The tumour histology had no bearing on the outcome. Table 14.1 summarises data from a number of reported studies. It does not include all published studies, and, where authors have published multiple series, only the largest one containing the necessary data was used unless it is clear that the series were clearly separate.

**Table 14.1.** Data on treatment parameters, success rates and complication rates for some published trials

| | No. of patients | Initial success | No. of sessions | Energy per session (J) | Energy per course (J) | No. of perforations | No. of fistulae | No. of bleeds | No. of deaths |
|---|---|---|---|---|---|---|---|---|---|
| Bown et al. (1967) | 34 | 29 | 2.7 | 4 400 | 12 000 | 2 | 0 | 0 | 1 |
| Buset et al. (1983) | 10 | 10 | 2.6 | 10 112 | 26 121 | 0 | 0 | 1 | 0 |
| Carter and Smith (1986) | 10 | 8 | 3.6 | 3 212 | 11 564 | 0 | 0 | 0 | 0 |
| Fleischer and Kessler (1983) | 14 | 14 | 5.3 | 4 615 | 24 394 | 1 | 1 | 0 | 0 |
| Fleischer and Sivak (1984) | 15 | 15 | 2.8 | 6 129 | 17 570 | 0 | 0 | 0 | 0 |
| Krasner et al. (1987) | 76 | 71 | 4.0 | 3 586 | 13 941 | 3 | 1 | 0 | 3 |
| Mathus-Vliegen and Tytgat (1986) | 9 | 7 | 2.4 | 2 842 | 7 105 | 0 | 0 | 0 | 0 |
| Mellow and Pinkas (1985) | 30 | 23 | 3.3 | 5 455 | 18 000 | 0 | 2 | 1 | 1 |
| Rieman et al. (1985) | 18 | 14 | 3.5 | 3 362 | 8 673 | 1 | 0 | 0 | 1 |
| Total | 216 | 191 (88%) | 3.5 | 4 329 | 15 152 | 7 (3.2%) | 4 (1.9%) | 2 (1%) | 6 (2.7%) |

A major problem with the above studies is that they all considered the response to therapy shortly after it had been completed, a time when the beneficial effects of therapy were likely to be maximal. Even simple oesophageal dilatation can produce a good, albeit temporary alleviation of dysphagia and many of the patients in the foregoing studies had oesophageal dilatation in addition to laser therapy. The duration of symptomatic relief, the need for further therapy and the late outcome are clearly important in the assessment of any technique for palliation of oesophageal cancer but few studies have looked at these in detail. Of the 34 patients treated by Bown et al. (1987), significant initial improvement was achieved in 29 following a mean of 2.7 treatment sessions. Of these, 18 required further intervention because of recurrent dysphagia after a mean of 6 weeks (range 2–15), 10 of whom were successfully managed by a repeat course of laser therapy alone. Repeat courses of laser therapy were well tolerated, often as an outpatient, were easier to perform than the initial course and required a mean of 1.6 sessions. Insertion of an endoprosthesis was necessary in 8 patients who had recurrent dysphagia due to extrinsic tumour. The mean survival in this group of patients was 19 weeks.

# Complications

The most important potential complications of laser therapy are perforation, tracheo-oesophageal fistula formation and bleeding. These are relatively infrequent and the relative risk can only be gauged from large numbers of patients. The frequency of these complications in 216 patients from a number of published series is shown in Table 14.1. No life-threatening bleeding occurred as a result of therapy and when any bleeding did occur during therapy it could almost always be controlled by further pulses of photocoagulation. Minor post-treatment bleeding was observed in only 2 patients. Perforation occurred in 5 (3.4%) and tracheo-oesophageal fistulae in 3 (2.0%) giving an occurrence of major complications in 5.4% of patients treated. There were 4 deaths thought to have been related to laser therapy (2.7%). Ell et al. (1986b) conducted a survey of 20 centres which had each treated more than 15 patients, giving information on a total of 1184. The overall complication rate was 4.1%, of which 2.1% were perforations, 0.8% were fistulae, 0.7% had haemorrhage and 0.6% developed some form of sepsis. The overall mortality rate was 1%.

Other less important side effects and complications have also been noted such as pain during therapy, mild fever and leucocytosis.

# Comparisons with Other Techniques

The technique most directly comparable with laser recanalisation is the endo-scopic insertion of an endoprosthesis. Neither technique is applicable to all cases of inoperable oesophageal cancer. Laser therapy cannot be used in patients with extrinsic tumour compression whereas endoprostheses can. Endoprostheses cannot be used in very high tumours or in those through which a guide wire cannot be passed whereas lasers can. Many tumours may be treated by either technique, but few studies have addressed the question of which technique provides superior palliation. Carter and Smith (1986), in a non-randomised study, compared 10 patients treated by intubation with 10 patients treated by laser. All subjects were considered inoperable. Of the intubation patients, 6 had a

Celestin tube inserted by the traction method at laparotomy, 3 had Nottingham tubes inserted by the pulsion method and 1 died soon after an attempted unsuccessful Nottingham tube insertion. Of the intubation patients, 8 returned to a soft diet, although 5 deteriorated, 3 because of tumour overgrowth and 2 because of tube dislodgement. Of the patients treated by laser, 8 returned to a solid diet and improvement was apparent in 8 only 12 h after the initial treatment session. Repeated laser sessions were required to maintain the benefit. Mean survival in laser patients was 6.1 months compared with 3.9 months in intubation patients. Complications were more frequent in the intubation group: 1 patient died shortly after an unsuccessful attempt to insert a Nottingham tube; in 2 patients the tube became displaced; 6 had troublesome acid regurgitation; and terminal tube obstruction occurred in 3. One patient died within a week of successful laser therapy and 1 developed a tracheo-oesophageal fistula which was thought to be due to radiotherapy rather than laser therapy as it occurred below the treated area.

An examination of the literature on endoprostheses for gastrointestinal malignancies suggests that the complication rate is rather higher than for laser therapy. Combining the results of 2 surveys on endoprosthesis insertion (Tytgat 1980; Bennett 1981) to give information on about 2667 procedures suggests a perforation rate of 9%, and a tube migration rate of 10%. In the Tytgat study, tube obstruction occurred in 5% and procedure-related deaths occurred in 4.5%.

# Combination Therapy

The different techniques for palliation of oesophageal cancer are not necessarily mutually exclusive (Fig. 14.6). Oesophageal dilatation, as described previously,

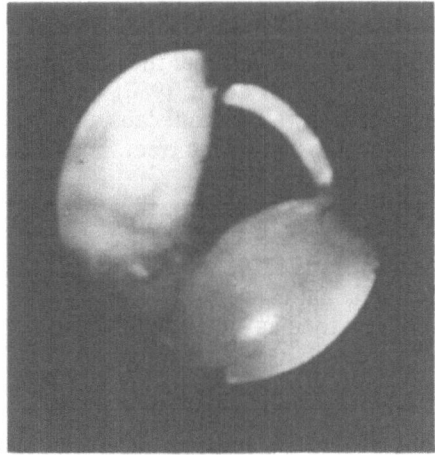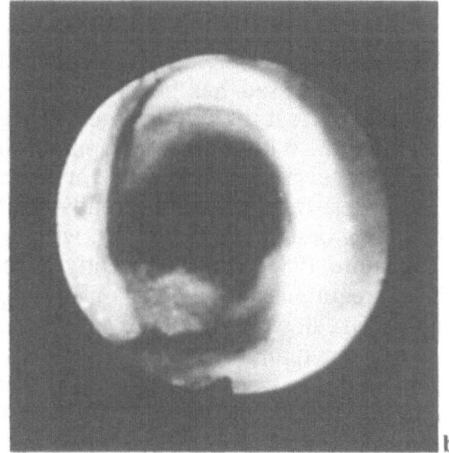

**Fig. 14.6a,b.** Oesophageal cancer overgrowing an endoprosthesis (a) and following laser therapy (b). Courtesy of Mr H Barr.

often facilitates laser treatment of oesophageal cancer. Laser therapy may make the insertion of an endoprosthesis possible where otherwise it would not have been, although a study by Barr et al. (1987) suggests that this may increase the complication rate and offer a poorer quality of palliation. A combination more likely to improve the outlook is that of laser therapy and radiotherapy. Radiotherapy may slow the regrowth of tumour into a recanalised oesophagus and may destroy extrinsic tumour. Bader et al. (1986) reported 48 patients treated by laser and then by after loading therapy. After laser recanalisation an afterloading tube was inserted via the nose and positioned close to the tumour. The tube was then connected to the radiation source which in this case was [192]iridium, and which was then passed down the tube to irradiate the tumour. The high activity of the iridium meant that it needed to be applied for about 10 min only, and this was used for adenocarcinomas as well as squamous carcinomas. Complete relief from dysphagia was obtained in 37 (77%) of the patients, with only 11 of these developing recurrent dysphagia. This represents a considerably smaller restenosis rate than with laser therapy alone. Complications occurring in the after loaded patients included 2 tracheo-oesophageal fistulae, 2 and 5 months after therapy, a cervical fistula after endoscopic bougienage in preparation for boost radiotherapy, and two endoscopy-related deaths. Mean survival time was 5.9 months.

# Early Oesophageal Cancer

Most oesophageal cancers are at a fairly advanced stage at the time of diagnosis and curative therapy is not possible. For those which are detected early a cure may be possible, particularly if there is no lymphatic spread. Currently, the best prospect of a cure is by surgical resection, but endoscopic laser techniques are improving and it is becoming increasingly possible to gauge accurately the depth of invasion of the tumour, particularly by endoscopic ultrasound (Tio et al. 1986). The relationship between the depth of laser-induced damage and the amount of laser energy used has been carefully quantified (Bown et al. 1980) and it is possible to treat the full thickness of the oesophageal wall without causing a free perforation. With these developments it may become justified to treat those who are poor surgical risks because of concomitant disease.

Japanese workers have already treated early upper gastrointestinal cancers, including oesophageal growths, with the Nd YAG laser (Maryuama et al. 1984; Takemoto 1986) with apparently encouraging results. Takemoto reported the laser treatment of 962 cases of upper gastrointestinal cancer, of which 49 were oesophageal, with the aim of a cure. All were regarded as inoperable because of severe concomitant disease. In the 427 who were followed up for a year, 347 appeared free from recurrence. Further work with more prolonged follow-up is required to establish whether the cure rates by laser therapy in such patients are sufficiently high to be able to provide a viable alternative to surgery, which may result in a higher cure rate at the cost of greater perioperative morbidity and mortality.

# Laser Hyperthermia

The Nd YAG laser may be used, with power settings far smaller than those previously described, to induce tissue necrosis. Narrow-gauge optical fibres (without the protective Teflon sheath) may actually be inserted into the tissue to be treated. Power settings of 1–2 W can then be used for very long exposure durations of the order of 500 to 1000 s, and in rat liver produce well-defined and reproducible necrotic zones of up to 16 mm in diameter (Matthewson et al. 1987). Necrosis is caused by occlusion of small and large blood vessels within the treated area and healing is by granulation and fibrosis. Temperature changes in the treated area are consistent with damage by a purely thermal means. The technique has also been evaluated in normal and neoplastic colon in rats (Matthewson et al. 1988). Full thickness thermal damage can be induced in the normal colonic wall without perforation and treated tumours necrose and slough off over a few days leaving an ulcer which rapidly heals (Fig. 14.7). Although not yet used in man, the technique could easily be applied to oesophageal cancers. Large tumours might be precisely treated by multiple insertions of the laser fibre with multiple prolonged exposures. It might even become possible to insert the fibre through the oesophageal wall to treat extrinsic tumour demonstrated by endoscopic ultrasound.

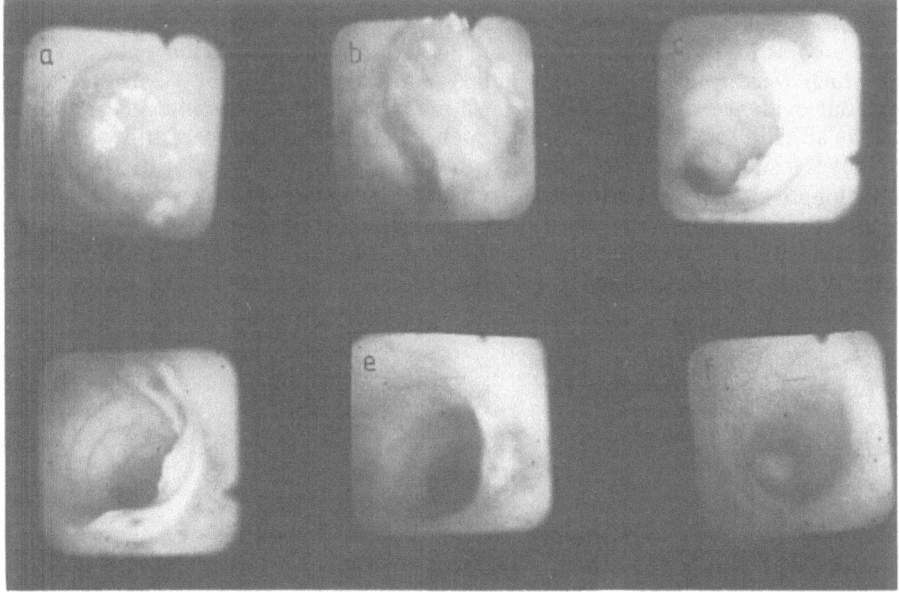

**Fig. 14.7a,b,c,d,e,f.** Colonoscopic photographs of colonic cancer in a rat. **a**, Before therapy, **b**, immediately after low power interstitial Nd YAG laser photocoagulation, **c**, 4 days post-therapy, **d**, 7 days post-therapy, **e**, 14 days post-therapy and **f**, 28 days post-therapy.

# Photodynamic Therapy (PDT)

PDT is a technique which has been the subject of considerable investigation in recent years. It is based on the parenteral administration of sensitising drugs which are selectively retained by cancerous tissue. The most extensively studied drugs are haematoporphyrin derivatives and the phthallocyanines. These have important properties, including fluorescence under ultraviolet light, and activation by light at a wavelength corresponding to one of their absorption peaks, producing cytotoxic substances such as singlet oxygen. Dye lasers are available which can be tuned to precisely the wavelength required to activate the sensitising drug. Usually visible red light is required, which can be delivered to the tumour via an optical fibre in much the same way as Nd YAG laser light. Illumination of the tumour being treated is at a very low power (<1 W) for prolonged periods of time (>600 s) and may be performed with the laser fibre tip held above the tumour, or inserted interstitially. The mechanism of PDT tumour necrosis is probably through tumour vasculature shutdown, although laser hyperthermia probably also contributes.

There are a number of theoretical risks which may accompany PDT. Firstly, the technique causes extensive necrosis of tumours without residual fibrosis and if tumour has replaced the full thickness of the oesophageal wall, the necrotic process may simply result in a large perforation. It may, therefore, only be suitable for attempted curative surgery of superficial tumours but not for advanced tumours. Secondly, whereas the Nd YAG laser technique coagulates large vessels as it destroys tumour, PDT does not and there may, therefore, be problems with bleeding.

Endoscopic PDT was used to treat 19 cases of early upper gastrointestinal cancer by Tajiri et al. (1987). They included 6 superficial oesophageal cancers, 3 of which were followed up by regular endoscopic biopsy for 1.3 to 3.9 years without evidence of recurrence. The other 3 underwent oesophagectomy 6–12 weeks after PDT. One had three independent superficial cancers and was found to have residual islands of cancer, one had been irradiated with the wrong wavelength and no PDT effect occurred, and no cancerous tissue was found in the resected oesophagus of the third. It is this author's opinion that such work should proceed with extreme caution, and that good surgical candidates should not be deprived of their best chance of a cure, which in the present state of the art is undoubtedly surgery.

# Summary

Many cases of oesophageal cancer are inoperable at the time of diagnosis and a number of techniques are available for palliation. In patients whose gullet is obstructed by intraluminal tumour, endoscopic Nd YAG laser therapy, after 2 or 3 treatment sessions, can restore normal or near normal swallowing in 70% to 80%. The technique can be used in tumours not treatable by intubation, such as high cervical lesions, and those through which a guide wire cannot be passed, and the quality of palliation is probably superior. The technique requires a degree of expertise and in experienced hands major complications will occur in 5% of cases or fewer. About 50% of patients will develop recurrent dysphagia and require further intervention, either further laser therapy or an endoprosthesis. Laser therapy should be regarded as complementary to other palliative techniques, and its use can be combined with bougienage, intubation and radiotherapy.

In the future, with improved assessment of local invasion and spread of tumours, it may become possible to cure some early oesophageal cancers either with the Nd YAG laser or by photodynamic therapy. This will require much careful study with cautious assessment before it can become a demonstrable reality.

# References

Bader M, Dittler HJ, Ultsch B, Ries G, Siewert JR (1986) Palliative treatment of malignant stenoses of the upper gastrointestinal tract using a combination of laser and afterloading therapy. Endoscopy 18 (suppl 1):27–31

Barr H, Krasner N, Raouf A, Walker RJ (1988) Laser therapy or intubation for palliation of malignant dysphagia. Gut 29:740 (abstract)

Bennett JR (1981) Intubation of oesophageal malignancies: a survey of current practice in Britain, 1980. Gut 22:336–338

Bown SG (1983) Phototherapy of tumours. World J Surg 7:700–709

Bown SG, Salmon PR, Storey DW et al. (1980) Nd YAG laser photocoagulation in the dog stomach. Gut 21:818–825

Bown SG, Hawes R, Matthewson K et al. (1987) Endoscopic laser palliation for advanced malignant dysphagia. Gut 28:799–807

Buset M, Dunham F, Baize M, de Toeuf J, Cremer M (1983) Nd YAG laser, a new palliative alternative in the management of oesophageal cancer. Endoscopy 15:353–356

Carter R, Smith J (1986) Oesophageal carcinoma: a comparative study of laser recanalization versus intubation in the palliation of gastro-oesophageal carcinoma. Lasers Med Sci 1:245–251

Earlam R, Cunha-Melo JR (1980a) Oesophageal squamous cell carcinoma. I. A critical review of surgery. Br J Surg 67:381–390

Earlam R, Cunha-Melo JR (1980b) Oesophageal squamous cell carcinoma. II. A critical review of radiotherapy. Br J Surg 67:457–461

Ell C, Hochberger J, Lux G (1986a) Clinical experience of non-contact and contact Nd-YAG laser therapy for inoperable malignant stenoses of the oesophagus and stomach. Lasers Med Sci 1:143–146

Ell C, Rieman JF, Lux G, Demling L (1986b) Palliative laser treatment of malignant stenoses in the upper gastrointestinal tract. Endoscopy 18 (Suppl 1):21–26

Fleischer D, Kessler F (1983) Endoscopic Nd YAG laser therapy for carcinoma of the esophagus: a new form of palliative treatment. Gastroenterology 85:600–606

Fleischer D, Sivak MV (1984) Endoscopic Nd:YAG laser therapy as palliative treatment for advanced adenocarcinoma of the gastric cardia. Gastroenterology 87:815–820

Fleischer D, Sivak MV (1985) Endoscopic Nd:YAG laser therapy as palliation for esophago-gastric cancer. Parameters affecting initial outcome. Gastroenterology 89:827–831

Kiefhaber P, Nath G, Moritz K (1977) Endoskopische blutstillung gastrointestinaler blutungen mit einem leistungsstarken Neodym-Yag laser. (Endoscopic haemostasis of gastrointestinal haemorrhages using high power neodymium Yag laser.) Chirurgie 48:198–203

Krasner N, Barr H, Skidmore C, Morris AI (1987) Palliative laser therapy for malignant dysphagia. Gut 28:792–798

Lux G, Groitl H, Ell C (1986) Tumour stenoses of the upper gastrointestinal tract – therapeutic alternatives to laser therapy. Endoscopy 18 (Suppl 1):37–43

Maiman T (1960) Stimulated optical radiation in ruby. Nature 187:493–494

Maryuama Y, Sasako M, Takami M, Iwasaki M, Hashimoto D (1984) Nd YAG laser endoscopy for early gastric cancer. Lasers Surg Med 3:341

Mathus-Vliegen EMH, Tytgat GN (1986) Laser photocoagulation in the palliative treatment of upper digestive tumors. Cancer 57:396–399

Matthewson K, Coleridge-Smith P, O'Sullivan J, Northfield TC, Bown SG (1987) Biological effects of intra-hepatic Nd YAG laser photocoagulation in rats. Gastroenterology 93:550–557

Matthewson K, Barton T, Lewin M, O'Sullivan J, Northfield TC, Bown SG (1988) Low power interstitial Nd YAG laser photocoagulation in normal and neoplastic rat colon. Gut 29:27–34

Mellow MH, Pinkas H (1985) Endoscopic laser therapy for malignancies affecting the esophagus and gastro-oesophageal junction. Analysis of technical and functional efficacy. Arch Int Med 145:1443–1446

Rieman JF, Ell C, Lux G, Demling L (1985) Combined therapy of malignant stenoses of the upper gastrointestinal tract by means of laser beam and bougienage. Endoscopy 17:43–48

Steger AC and Hira N (1987) The palliative endoscopic treatment of inoperable oesophago-gastric and rectal cancer: a low power direct contact laser technique. Ann R Coll Surg Engl 69:166–168

Swain CP, Bown SG, Edwards DAW, Kirkham JS, Salmon PR, Clark CG (1984) Laser recanalization of obstructing foregut cancer. Br J Surg 71:112–115

Tajiri H, Daikuzono N, Joffe SN, Oguro Y (1987) Photoradiation therapy in early gastrointestinal cancer. Gastrointest Endosc 33:88–90

Takemoto T (1986) Laser therapy of early gastric cancer. Endoscopy 18 (Suppl 1):32–36

Tio TL, den Hartog Jager FCA, Tytgat GNJ (1986) The role of endoscopic ultrasound in assessing local resectability of oesophagogastric malignancies. Accuracy, pitfalls and predictability. Scand J Gastroenterol 21 (Suppl 123):78–86

Tytgat GN (1980) Endoscopic methods of treatment of gastrointestinal and biliary stenosis. Endoscopy supplement, review of the European congress of gastro-intestinal endoscopy, pp 57–68

Tytgat GN, den Hartog Jager FCA (1983) To dilate or intubate. Gastrointest Endosc 29:58

Watson A (1982) A study of the quality and duration of survival following resection, endoscopic intubation and surgical intubation in oesophageal cancer. Br J Surg 69:585–588

# Chapter 15

# Management of Complications of Intrathoracic Resection

R. S. Bonser and P. Goldstraw

## Introduction

Considerable morbidity and not infrequent mortality attends the surgical treatment of oesophageal carcinoma. Clinical impression would suggest that patients
either have a relatively trouble-free postoperative recovery or a prolonged and
morbid postsurgical course. Two major factors in postresection morbidity –
pulmonary complications and anastomotic leakage – will be reviewed in some
detail in this chapter, and other complications will be mentioned briefly. Specific
complications relating to individual types of oesophagectomy technique, e.g.,
stricture formation, have been dealt with in previous chapters and will not be
discussed here.

Both major causes of morbidity are associated with infection and thus it is
pertinent to discuss the microbiology of the normal and obstructed oesophagus.

## The Influence of Bacterial Flora on Postoperative Morbidity

Although at birth the intestinal tract is sterile, colonisation by aerobic and
anaerobic organisms soon occurs and the adult microbial flora of the gullet is

dependent on the organisms contained in swallowed saliva and food (Jawetz et al. 1972). The bactericidal acid pH of the stomach and the periodic nature of oesophageal transit keep the number of micro-organisms to a minimum. In the presence of gastro-oesophageal obstruction these checks on bacterial prolife-ration are lost and the obstructed conduit acts as a reservoir of potentially pathogenic bacteria, thus increasing the dangerous consequences of periopera-tive aspiration pneumonia, wound contamination and postoperative anastomotic leakage. The spectrum of organisms found in the obstructed oesophagus is similar to that of the mouth and includes alpha- and non-haemolytic *Streptococci*, coliforms including *Pseudomonas* and *Bacteroides fragilis*, *Melaninogenicus* and other species (Finlay et al. 1982; Gatehouse et al. 1978) (Table 15.1). Although the pathogenicity of individual organisms of this oral-type flora may be low, mixed inoculation may be more than additive in its pathogenic potential. Resections for gastro-oesophageal carcinoma are more commonly associated with sepsis than are operations for non-obstructive gastric lesions, and the wound infection rate is related to the organism count within the viscus at operation (Gatehouse et al. 1978; Keighley and Burdon 1979).

**Table 15.1.** Microbial flora in carcinoma of the oesophagus (adapted from Finlay et al. 1982)

*Aerobes*
   Alpha-haemolytic streptococci
   Non-haemolytic streptococci
   Coagulase-negative staphylococci
   *Lactobacilli* spp.
   *Corynebacterium* spp.
   *Branhamella catarrhalis*
   *Escherichia coli*
   *Proteus mirabilis*

*Anaerobes*
   *Bacteroides melaninogenicus*
   *Bacteroides fragilis*
   Other bacteroides spp.
   Anaerobic cocci
   *Clostridium* spp.

In the light of this bacteriological information and the data on wound infection rates, it is appropriate to consider antibiotic prophylaxis against wound infection for patients undergoing oesophageal resection. Antibiotics effective against anaerobes, coliforms and gram-positive cocci could be expected to reduce endogenous infection rates. Appropriate prophylaxis should, therefore, include metronidazole in combination with gentamicin or a broad spectrum cephalos-porin (Little et al. 1981). *Staphylococcus aureus*, despite its paucity in the oesophageal flora, is present in approximately a quarter of positive wound infection isolates (Gatehouse et al. 1978). Contamination by this organism may be either exogenous or from the patient's own nose or skin. The frequent appearance of *Staphylococcus aureus* in wound isolates would indicate the inclusion of gentamicin in the prophylaxis regimen or the addition of a penicillinase-resistant penicillin.

# Pulmonary Complications

Postoperative pulmonary complications remain a cause of significant morbidity and mortality after major surgery and particularly after intrathoracic resection for oesophageal carcinoma (Eikhoff 1980; Postlethwait 1983). Reviews estimate an incidence of up to 27% (Jackson et al. 1979; Ong et al. 1978). The mortality of such postoperative pulmonary complications varies between 20% and 68% (Postlethwait 1983; Jackson et al. 1979; Ong et al. 1978). The incidence of pulmonary complications may be lower if oesophagectomy is performed without thoracotomy (Orringer 1984).

In obstructive oesophageal carcinoma, postoperative pulmonary problems may arise due to aspiration pneumonitis occurring pre-, peri- or postoperatively or may be due to pulmonary infection. Overspill of oesophageal contents into the lungs leads to a mechanical and chemical pneumonitis. The colonisation of oesophageal contents by large numbers of potentially pathogenic organisms would appear to increase the incidence and seriousness of an infective pneumonitis including anaerobic pulmonary infection (Editorial, 1976). These dual pathologies may occur alone or interact with one another to contribute to postoperative pulmonary complications. In addition, advancing age, smoking, preoperative chronic respiratory disease, and long operation times are all risk factors for postoperative pulmonary morbidity (Garibaldi et al. 1981; Wightman 1968). During anaesthesia and surgery, care should be taken during intubation, extubation and recovery to prevent silent spill of oesophageal contents into the airways, especially during surgical manipulation. In the postoperative period this potential for spill is increased by gastric atony, gastric distension and abdominal distension due to paralytic ileus or pneumoperitoneum. This may be aggravated if the patient is sedated by analgesia. Atelectasis and loss of surfactant occurs during anaesthesia due to the use of low tidal volumes and elective single lung ventilation (Vickers 1982). Further pulmonary injury may occur with surgical manipulation and retraction. Inadequate expansion of the lower lung zones will be exacerbated by diaphragmatic paralysis due to surgical division and reconstruction. Atelectasis leads to intrapulmonary shunting with impairment of gas exchange, and profound degrees of arterial hypoxaemia have been demonstrated after thoraco-abdominal oesophageal procedures (Kasai et al. 1971; Bainbridge and Matthews 1980). The upper abdominal and thoracic incisions of oesophageal surgery greatly increase the risks of postoperative pulmonary complications (Garibaldi et al. 1981). It appears that separate abdominal and thoracic incisions affect postoperative pulmonary function less than a single thoraco-abdominal incision, possibly because of the absence of diaphragmatic and costal arch disruption (Craig 1981). Reduced diaphragmatic activity after surgery, possibly by reflex neural inhibition, may be seen without disruption, and appears independent of the site of incision (Ford and Guenter 1984). Such reflex inhibition largely disappears within 24–48 hours of surgery, supporting the practice of elective positive pressure ventilation postoperatively in selected patients (Editorial 1984).

Postoperatively the inability of a patient to cough and clear his own tracheo-bronchial secretions is increased by poor preoperative nutritional state, inhibition of cough by postoperative pain, and diaphragmatic palsy. The cough reflex is suppressed by opiate administration. Dry gas anaesthesia and the use of atropine increase the viscosity of secretions, and endotracheal and endobronchial tubes may disturb normal bronchial ciliary function (Vickers 1982). There is a reduction in the ability to produce adequate cough pressures following thoracotomy and this is greater after oesophagectomy than after pulmonary resection (Byrd and Burns 1975; Sugimachi et al. 1982). All these factors may lead to the creation of a vicious cycle of respiratory failure, and careful monitoring and early intervention are required.

## Management

Management of these difficult problems should begin before surgery. Complete dysphagia must be treated expeditiously because of the potential risk of aspiration pneumonitis. It is well recognised that breathing exercises and postural drainage reduce exacerbations of chest infections in chronic pulmonary sepsis, and exercises have also been shown to be helpful in reducing postoperative pulmonary complications after major chest surgery in patients over 60 years of age, who have been heavy smokers and have reduced performance on preoperative lung function tests (Palmer and Sellick 1953; Vriu and Vriu 1977). Physiotherapy, both pre- and postoperatively, is beneficial to patients with chronic bronchitis but not to those with normal lung function (Laszlo et al. 1973). Patients may derive some benefit from the use of incentive spirometry which is both free of complications and inexpensive (Celli et al. 1984).

The role of prophylactic antibiotics in preventing postoperative pulmonary sepsis remains unclear. The results of the majority of clinical trials have shown no benefit, but some reports have shown a reduction in the frequency of postoperative chest infections (Palmer and Sellick 1952; Thulborne and Young 1962; Collins et al. 1968; Morran et al. 1978). As antibiotic prophylaxis is desirable in oesophageal resection for other reasons, it is appropriate that the antimicrobial agents chosen should adequately cover likely respiratory pathogens. The usual organisms incriminated in exacerbations of chronic lung disease are *Streptococcus pneumoniae* and *Haemophilus* species. Although gram-negative organisms such as *Klebsiella* and *Pseudomonas* are commonly seen in postoperative sputum cultures, their appearance may be related to the use of broad-spectrum antibiotics and need not necessarily indicate the need for further, wider antibiotic therapy (Collins et al. 1968). The guidelines of antibiotic prophylaxis proposed in the earlier section should adequately cover *Haemophilus* and *Streptococci*, although resistant strains are becoming more common. Expert microbiological advice should be obtained in the management of clinically apparent postoperative infections.

Bacterial filtration of anaesthetic equipment does not reduce postoperative pulmonary infection (Collins et al. 1968; Editorial 1977; Feeley et al. 1981). However, the anaesthetist has a major role in preventing perioperative aspiration, and intubation must be performed with the risks of aspiration in mind. Anaesthetic induction should be performed with an elevated head position and with suction facilities immediately at hand. Extubation should only take place when the patient is awake and erect. Postoperatively, patients should be nursed with the head and shoulders elevated at all times, and physiotherapists should be warned of the risks of postural changes. Routine use of bronchodilator therapy is unhelpful (Collins et al. 1968).

Adequate pain relief is essential following thoracic operations as it may lead to more effective clearing of sputum even without restoring lung mechanics to preoperative values. Cryoanalgesia of two or three intercostal nerves above and below the thoracotomy space, to include drain insertion sites, has been found useful in the management of post-thoracotomy pain in this unit and others (Maiwand and Makey 1981). Each intercostal nerve is exposed close to the intercostal foramen, proximal to the collateral branch, and freezing undertaken for 30 seconds. During defrosting the nerve will remain adherent to the probe until thawing is complete, and premature tugging on the probe may lead to nerve damage. A single 30 s freeze period produces analgesia for about a month and numbness should clear within six weeks (Maiwand et al. 1986). This is in contrast to the three-month period of post-cryoanalgesia numbness following longer freezing or multiple freeze/thaw cycles (Maiwand and Makey 1981; Maiwand et al. 1986). Intercostal nerve blocks using local anaesthetic agents have been shown to improve post-thoracotomy respiratory function (Toledo-Pereyra and De Meester 1979; Faust and Nauss 1976). This advantage is also seen with cryoanalgesia, vital capacity returning to an average of 65% of preoperative values within 48 hours (Maiwand et al. 1986). Alone, cryoanalgesia may not confer optimal analgesia and additional analgesia is usually necessary (Orr et al. 1981; Roxburgh et al. 1987). The authors' practice involves the use of cryoanalgesia and postoperative opiate analgesia administered as a continuous infusion of pethidine. Our practice is to administer pethidine in a dose (mg) equivalent to bodyweight × 2 (kg) added to 100 ml of 5% dextrose in water infused intravenously at a rate of 0–20 ml/hour, thus giving a maximum dose of pethidine of 10 mg/kg/24 hours. This infusion is adjusted by nursing staff and physiotherapists according to analgesic requirement. The regimen is flexible and safe and does not cause respiratory depression.

We are convinced that physiotherapy and incentive spirometry are also important in the postoperative period although their benefits remain unproven (Celli et al. 1984; Van de Water et al. 1971). The prevention of fluid overload is also essential, especially in patients with pre-existing cardiac disease, since contused lungs are particularly susceptible to pulmonary oedema.

The inability to evacuate tracheobronchial secretions effectively must be recognised early and appropriate measures undertaken. If this is not adequately dealt with by physiotherapy and optimum analgesia, a minitracheostomy inserted through the cricothyroid membrane may prevent deterioration into respiratory failure and the consequent need for artificial ventilation (Matthews and Hopkinson 1984). The minitracheostomy should always be supplemented by physiotherapy and is less effective in dealing with accumulated secretions in the left bronchial tree. The preoperative insertion of a minitracheostomy tube may be helpful in certain patients in dealing with the consequences of aspiration. Caution must be used during insertion of this device if a cervical anastomosis has been constructed.

# Anastomotic Leakage

The development of anastomotic leakage can be a catastrophic complication of oesophageal resection. Its development will be discussed in terms of anatomical considerations, nutritional status and anastomotic technique.

## Anatomical Considerations

The oesophagus does not possess a serosal coat and has a segmental blood supply (Swigart et al. 1950). The cervical oesophageal blood supply is derived from the inferior thyroid artery. The thoracic portion is supplied by branches of intercostal, tracheal and bronchial arteries and the oesophageal branches of the descending aorta (Swigart et al. 1950; Shapiro and Robillard 1950). The intra-abdominal oesophagus receives its blood supply from branches of the left gastric and inferior phrenic arteries. This segmental arterial arrangement allows the technique of blind dissection of the oesophagus without thoracotomy with minimal blood loss (Orringer and Sloan 1978). Venous drainage is similarly segmental with drainage into the inferior thyroid vein from the cervical oesophagus, the azygos and hemiazygos veins in the chest and into the left gastric vein in the abdomen. In addition venae comitantes of the vagi enable a venous connection along the adventitia to be developed. Both arterial and venous systems are connected to abundant submucosal vascular channels (Potter and Holyoke 1950; Butler 1951) fed by larger trunks penetrating the muscle layers at intervals of about 2 cm. There is an extensive intramural arterial and venous collateral circulation. Despite this, during surgical mobilisation of the oesophagus it is widely held that the portion of the oesophagus not to be resected should be left undisturbed as much as possible to minimise ischaemia and venous obstruction, and the length of proximal oesophagus to be mobilised for the anastomosis should be kept as short as practicable. Clearly, if the oesophageal blood supply is marginal, perioperative manipulation, hypoxia and hypotension may lead to impairment of anastomotic healing. However, this intramural anastomotic network does allow procedures requiring extensive mobilisation to be performed. Methods of management of oesophageal varices have been developed in which large lengths of oesophagus are devascularised, divided and subsequently re-anastomosed (Sugiura and Futagawa 1977). Other workers have been able to mobilise the whole length of oesophagus on its pharyngeal vascular connections in order to perform anterior chest wall oesophagostomy without ischaemic problems (Williams and Payne 1982). The oesophagus, therefore, although having a segmental blood supply, may not be the organ incriminated if ischaemia results in anastomotic problems, and anastomotic leakage is more likely to be the result of impaired blood supply of the viscus used as an oesophageal substitute (Payne and Ellis 1975; Le Roux and Knothe 1962).

The use of the stomach as an oesophageal substitute takes advantage of its rich arterial supply, with many anastomotic and collateral networks within the gastric wall. It has been established both by clinical practice and anatomical demonstration that the gastric fundus can remain viable when supplied by the right gastric and right gastro-epiploic arteries even when the extra-gastric portion of the left gastric artery or its branches have been divided (El-Eishi et al. 1973; Thomas et al. 1979). If the right gastric supply is compromised, ischaemia of the medial edge of the gastric fundus may occur (D'Abreu 1963). Gastric mucosal cellular metabolism can tolerate a 60% reduction in total gastric blood flow and can thus withstand surgical mobilisation well (Bowen et al. 1977). Even this margin of safety does not allow inattention to intraoperative haemodynamic changes and circulating blood volume. Blood viscosity in the perioperative period may also be important (Tagart 1981) and increased viscosity may impair blood flow through the microcirculation. In colonic surgery higher haemoglobin levels are associated with a higher incidence of anastomotic leakage (Tagart 1981). Similarly, preoperative irradiation may impair the microcirculation. Preservation of venous drainage is also important. The right gastro-epiploic vein is at risk during mobilisation and must be protected during surgery. The potential problems of jejunal or colonic reconstruction will not be discussed in detail. However, both these substitutes carry the risk of postoperative infarction if blood supply is compromised (Postlethwait 1983). The colon may have a dubious vascular arcade in some patients, and may be an unsuitable choice of conduit in the elderly. The arterial supply of the colon has a variable marginal system at the splenic flexure and the venous drainage of the right colon may not have adequate marginal continuity (Nicks 1967).

## Nutritional Status

There is little doubt that poor preoperative nutritional status must affect the postoperative morbidity of patients undergoing oesophageal resection (Editorial 1979). This is not only in terms of healing potential but also in terms of physical strength needed to co-operate with postoperative physiotherapy. In a study of 48 patients with oesophageal carcinoma, Conti et al. (1977) demonstrated that a preoperative weight loss greater than 15% of premorbid bodyweight led to a substantially higher morbidity and mortality rate. The majority of deaths and complications in these patients were sepsis-related. Malnutrition in oesophageal cancer patients has been associated with a depression of cellular immunity (Haffejee and Angorn 1979). In biological terms, nutritional support of such patients can suppress gluconeogenesis, decrease nitrogen excretion, decrease skeletal muscle proteolysis and increase protein synthesis (Burt and Brennan 1984). If these biochemical improvements were reflected in reduced postoperative complications, preoperative nutritional support would be mandatory. However, whether nutritional support affects clinical outcome is questionable. Retrospective clinical studies have suggested clinical benefit (Daly et al. 1982; Piccone et al. 1979), but randomised clinical controlled trials have not shown any advantage to adjuvant parenteral nutrition. Muller et al. (1982), in a study of patients with gastrointestinal carcinoma divided into groups having a ten-day preoperative nutritional support and no support, found improved results in terms of mortality and major morbidity in the treated group. However, this study included many patients with carcinomas other than oesophageal and there was a high mortality in the control group. The benefits of preoperative nutrition in oesophageal cancer patients cannot be ascertained with certainty. In another randomised prospective study of patients awaiting surgery for gastro-oesophageal cancer (Heatley et al. 1979), one group received additional nutrition with 2800 kcal and a moderate nitrogen load for 7–10 days prior to surgery whilst another group received no additional nutritional support. Both the mortality and morbidity were reduced in the treated group but this reached statistical significance only in terms of wound sepsis. The collected data of several studies are shown in Table 15.2. Except for the two studies mentioned above, parenteral nutrition prior to surgery has not been shown to influence mortality or major morbidity rates. There does appear to be a trend towards decreased mortality in the treated groups and further larger studies are required to define the role of preoperative adjuvant nutrition. At present, the evidence for clinical benefit is lacking and it is doubtful if surgery should be delayed by a possibly futile attempt to improve nutritional status.

**Table 15.2.**  Results of randomised trials of adjuvant preoperative total parenteral nutrition (TPN) in patients with oesophageal carcinoma (adapted from Burt and Brennan 1984)

| | No. patients Control TPN | Duration TPN (days) | Wound infection (%) Control TPN | Major comp. (%) Control TPN | Mortality (%) Control TPN |
|---|---|---|---|---|---|
| Heatley et al. (1979) | 36  38 | 7–10 | 31  8[a] | NA[b]  NA | 22  16 |
| Moghissi et al. (1977) | 5  10 | 13–14 | 20  0 | NA  NA | NA  NA |
| Muller et al.[c] (1982) | 59  66 | 10 | NA  NA | 17  32 | 19  4.5 |
| Simms et al. (1980) | 10  10 | 7–10 | NA  NA | NA  NA | 10  0 |
| Lim et al. (1981) | 10  10 | 28 | 50  30 | 40  10 | 20  0 |
| | | | 33  10 | | 20  6.5 |

[a]p 0.05
[b]NA – data unavailable
[c]includes other gastrointestinal carcinomata

## Anastomotic Technique

Apart from impaired blood supply of oesophagus or oesophageal substitute, technical errors in construction of the anastomosis are important. Poor apposition of mucosa to mucosa, the absence of a serosal coat, the poor suture holding of the muscular layers and anastomotic tension may all contribute to anastomotic failure (D'Abreu 1963; Yun-K'an et al. 1964, 1965; Huang 1963; Collis 1952; Katz et al. 1981). The choice of suture technique and material will depend upon individual preference and the training of the surgeon. Braided sutures have superior handling qualities compared to monofilament materials but tend to be more irritant, may saw or tear through tissues and may potentiate local infection by bacterial adherence (Katz et al. 1981). Absorbable sutures such as catgut and polyglycolic acid may lose strength within a few days of surgery and thus may not be ideal when such a deterioration in suture strength may occur at a time when anastomotic strength is several days short of its maximum (Fontaine and Dudley 1978; Postlethwait et al. 1952). Orringer et al. (1977) compared the use of polypropylene, silk and wire in a series of single layer anastomoses in animal experiments. Polypropylene was superior because of its handling characteristics and minimal tissue reaction. Subsequent single layer anastomoses in 71 patients resulted in 7 anastomotic leaks. Other workers have found single layer wire preferable to polypropylene in animal experiments (Senyk and Rank 1978). Concern exists that a continuous suture technique may lead to stricture formation. In a report of a variety of suture techniques and materials in animal experiments Postlethwait et al. (1950) found an inner mucosal layer of interrupted runs of continuous chromic catgut and an outer layer of interrupted silk to be the most satisfactory. A single layer of interrupted sutures has been found satisfactory by other workers (Orringer et al. 1977), whilst an everting anastomotic technique seems unsatisfactory (Wesselhoeft et al. 1968). If a double layer of sutures is used, care must be taken to include submucosal tissue in the mucosal layer (Akiyama et al. 1978). Our preference is for a single continuous suture of polypropylene through all layers of the viscera to be anastomosed.

Whatever suture materials or techniques are used it is probable that meticulous conduit preparation, mucosal apposition and prevention of tension are the most important factors. Certainly excellent clinical results can be obtained with sutured anastomoses (Akiyama et al. 1978) and the question as to whether mechanical stapling devices will reduce anastomotic failure remains unanswered. Although some workers feel that the incidence of leak is reduced if mechanical stapling is performed, stricture rates are increased and the best results of sutured anastomoses are comparable (Pearlstein et al. 1978; Wilson et al. 1982; Chassin 1978; Akiyama et al. 1978).

Tension can be reduced by careful mobilisation of an adequate length of oesophageal substitute and by fixing this to the mediastinum or chest wall following completion of the anastomosis. An adequate gastric drainage procedure (e.g., pyloromyotomy) may reduce tension further by preventing gastric distension after vagotomy (Yun-K'an et al. 1965), but if the pylorus is normal and the vagotomised stomach is transposed high into the chest or neck, gastric drainage has been shown to be unnecessary (Goldstraw and Bach 1981). But if the pylorus is scarred by previous coincident ulceration, formal pyloric drainage is mandatory.

It is not known if sepsis adjacent to a disrupted suture line is the cause or effect of leakage. In colonic surgery adequate mechanical preparation of bowel is thought to reduce the incidence of anastomotic dehiscence. Oesophageal mechanical preparation is not feasible in obstructive lesions and should be unnecessary in non-obstructive lesions. Attempted sterilisation of the oesophagus with antibiotics may, however, be helpful. In animal experiments, systemic administration of antibiotics has been found to decrease anastomotic leak rates (Hopkins et al. 1984).

Cervical anastomoses are probably more likely to leak than intrathoracic anastomoses because of the additional conduit mobilisation, possible resultant ischaemia, and additional factors such as intermittent tension during neck extension and swallowing. Fixation of the anastomosis to the cervical tissues may reduce tension and reduce the incidence of leak (Sugimachi et al. 1983). These factors are offset by the less devastating consequences of a leak occurring in the neck.

An increased incidence of anastomotic dehiscence has been reported to occur in patients undergoing oesophagectomy in whom adequate proximal resection has not been performed (Keighley et al. 1981). Whilst the authors therefore recommend intraoperative frozen section analysis, the influence of this factor on the frequency of anastomotic leak has been contested (Papachristou and Fortner 1979; Hermreck and Crawford 1976). Palliative procedures, where extra-

**Table 15.3.** Influence of conduit on anastomotic leak rates for intrathoracic anastomoses

| | Oesophagojejunostomy | | | Oesophagogastrostomy | | | Oesophagoduodenostomy | | |
|---|---|---|---|---|---|---|---|---|---|
| | Number | Leaks | % | Number | Leaks | % | Number | Leaks | % |
| Inberg et al. (1971) | 74 | 3 | 4 | 65[a] | 8 | 12 | 8 | 3 | 38 |
| Papachristou et al. (1979) | 254 | 30 | 11.8 | 91 | 8 | 8.7 | 4 | 1 | 25 |
| Hermreck et al. (1976) | 20 | 2 | 10 | 28 | 5 | 18 | 3 | 1 | 33 |
| Wilson et al. (1982) | 9 | 2 | 22 | 153 | 13 | 8.5 | 0 | 0 | 0 |
| | 357 | 37 | 10.4 | 337 | 34 | 10.1 | 15 | 5 | 33 |

[a]represents oesophagogastrostomy following proximal gastrectomy

oesophageal disease cannot be totally extirpated, have been found to have higher failure rates than potentially curative resection in some series but not in others (Wilson et al. 1982; Papachristou and Fortner 1979; Hermreck and Crawford 1976).

Hypoxia and hypotension in the perioperative period may compromise intrathoracic oesophagogastric anastomoses if the blood supply is marginal. In a series of 5 patients developing shock or hypovolaemia in the first 48 hours following surgery (with no evidence of anastomotic failure at this time) no fewer than 4 (80%) developed anastomotic dehiscence a mean of 4 days later (Hermreck and Crawford 1976). This was in comparison with an overall incidence of anastomotic leak of 11% in this series.

The choice of oesophageal substitute may have some role in the development of anastomotic leakage. Table 15.3 represents the cumulative results of four studies and demonstrates that although oesophagogastric and oesophagojejunal anastomoses have been found satisfactory in many patients, oesophagoduodenal anastomoses have an unacceptably high failure rate, probably because of the unavoidable tension created with such a reconstruction (Wilson et al. 1982; Papachristou and Fortner 1979; Hermreck and Crawford 1976; Inberg et al. 1971). End-to-side oesophagogastric anastomoses are preferable to an end-to-end technique (Papachristou and Fortner 1979). Results following oesophago-colonic anastomoses are mixed. Postlethwait (1983), using the right colon as the oesophageal substitute in a series of 34 colonic interpositions, described 7 anastomotic leaks resulting in 4 deaths with 5 cases of colonic infarction.

The following factors are important in the prevention of anastomotic leak.

Minimal mobilisation of proximal oesophagus

Maintenance of vascular supply of oesophageal substitute

Avoidance of tension on anastomosis

Mucosal apposition and avoidance of eversion

Prevention of perioperative hypoxia and hypotension

Antibiotic prophylaxis

Avoidance of incomplete resection

Gastric drainage, e.g. pyloromyotomy when necessary

Fixation of conduit to adjacent tissues

# Clinical Presentation and Management of Anastomotic Leakage

## Incidence

The incidence of anastomotic leak in several studies has been reviewed by Chassin (1978) and estimated as between 0% and 41%. In a review of 1232 postoperative deaths following resection for oesophageal carcinoma (Postlethwait 1986), anastomotic dehiscence was identified as the cause of 300 cases, approximately one quarter of all deaths. In a further review (Wilson et al. 1982) with an overall mortality of 12.6%, three quarters of all deaths could be attributed to anastomotic leak. The incidence of anastomotic leak was 34.1%, 7.6%, and 3.7% in one series (Postlethwait 1983) following palliative bypass, palliative resection and curative resection respectively. Anastomotic leak would appear to increase in frequency with advancing age. In one series (Inberg et al. 1971), the leak occurred two and a half times more frequently in patients over 70 years old than in those aged 60–69 years, and was twice as likely to be fatal in the older group. The risk of death from anastomotic leak is substantial and does not seem to decrease with increasing experience with the complication (Le Roux and Knothe 1962; Papachristou and Fortner 1979). The incidence of anastomotic leak does not seem to be influenced by the seniority of the surgeon performing resection unless longer operation times are involved (Keighley et al. 1981; Papachristou and Fortner 1979). Table 15.4 identifies the incidence of leak and mortality in a number of studies and demonstrates the grave prognostic significance of this complication.

**Table 15.4.** Anastomotic failure rates and mortality from oesophagogastrectomy with intrathoracic anastomoses

| | No. of patients | Leakage | | Mortality from leak | |
|---|---|---|---|---|---|
| | | No. | % | No. | % |
| Le Roux et al. (1961) | 408 | 41 | 10 | 38 | 93 |
| Inberg et al. (1971) | 207 | 19 | 9 | 10 | 53 |
| Hermreck et al. (1976) | 63 | 13 | 21 | 7 | 54 |
| Ong et al. (1978) | 92 | 21 | 23 | 9 | 43 |
| Papachristou et al. (1979) | 91 | 8 | 9 | 7 | 87 |
| Wilson et al. (1982) | 167 | 19 | 11 | 4 | 21 |
| Postlethwait (1983) | 164 | 6 | 3.6 | 3 | 50 |
| | 1408 | 135 | 9.6 | 84 | 62 |

## Presentation

Anastomotic leak may be appreciated within the first few days after surgery when it is associated with either technical error in anastomotic construction or avascular necrosis of the viscus used as the oesophageal substitute. The oesophagus itself is rarely the viscus incriminated (Payne and Ellis 1975; Le Roux and Knothe 1962). More commonly the leak occurs after the first week (Le Roux and Knothe 1962). Intrathoracic leaks are often heralded by the persistence of a low grade fever, leucocytosis and the onset of atrial fibrillation. Some patients will have sudden development of chest or abdominal pain occurring during the first exposure of parietal pleura or peritoneum to alimentary content. Pain may also occur on swallowing. In some patients the leak is only diagnosed at post mortem. Some patients may be relatively asymptomatic apart from the development of a pleural effusion which is subsequently found to contain oesophageal flora. Although relatively well at this stage of presentation, rapid deterioration is likely without intervention. In patients with cervical anastomoses, the leak presents as a pyrexial illness with the development of a fluctuant abscess, surgical emphysema or spontaneous discharge from the neck incision.

Early detection of anastomotic leak is essential if morbidity and mortality are to be minimised. Meticulous attention to clinical examination in the postoperative period with regular chest X-rays to detect the development of pleural effusion or hydropneumothorax is important, coupled with a high index of suspicion if the surgeon is less than totally satisfied with the anastomosis. Early contrast radiology of the oesophagus following surgery has been recommended in order to detect subclinical leaks (Desbleds et al. 1975). Contrast swallows should be performed 4–7 days after surgery prior to the institution of oral diet or earlier if leak is suspected. This will define the degree of anastomotic dehiscence and the extent of mediastinal, pleural or peritoneal contamination.

## Management

Once diagnosed, attention should be paid to the following factors: nutrition; antibiotics; drainage of infected space; reoperation; dilatation.

### Nutrition

All studies of anastomotic leak have highlighted the importance of adequate nutrition. If the leak is small, especially if the anastomosis is cervical, oral feeding need not be discontinued as long as distal obstruction is not present and the patient remains well and non-toxic (Orringer and Lemner 1986). For larger leaks, nutrition must be maintained by other means. Positive nitrogen balance can be achieved with long-term total parenteral nutrition (TPN) (Dudrick et al. 1968), and successful management of gastrointestinal fistulae has been achieved with TPN (Miller and Taylor 1975; Jorgensen et al. 1979). This is facilitated by a hospital nutrition team consisting of pharmacist, dietitian and clinicians. Jorgensen (1979) used a nutritional regimen of TPN in the management of anastomotic dehiscence following oesophago-gastrostomy. Total parenteral nutrition was continued for 10–62 days (mean 33.6 days) and during this period patients were able to maintain their weight. Other workers have recommended jejunostomy feeding and advocate the routine insertion of a small-bore jejunostomy feeding tube during all oesophageal resection procedures (Orringer and Lemner 1986). The use of the gastrointestinal tract via nasogastric, nasoduodenal or jejunostomy tube for enteral nutrition is preferable in terms of ease, cost and complications (Hatfield 1982; Anon 1986). The insertion of a fine-bore tube, tunnelled through the muscle layers of the jejunum, adds little time to the operative procedure and can be used in the early postoperative period as soon as ileus has settled. Patency and accurate positioning should be confirmed 48–72 hours postoperatively by a contrast tube-jejunogram, prior to the institution of feeding. Alternatively, tube-jejunostomy can be performed as part of a salvage procedure should anastomotic dehiscence occur. In many units, early reintroduction of oral feeding following cervical anastomoses obviates the need for additional nutritional measures in uncomplicated patients.

## Antibiotics

Systemic antibiotics should be commenced as soon as the diagnosis is confirmed. Agents will be selected on the basis of the likely organisms present in the oesophagus (p. 268) and the results of culture and sensitivities of the intrathoracic collection of fluid. Antibiotics cannot be a substitute for effective surgical drainage but may reduce the patient's toxicity and control bacteraemia.

## Drainage of infected space

As most intrathoracic leaks become evident after the initial postoperative intercostal drains have been removed, further drainage procedures will be required. Even if the original drains remain in situ they may not provide adequate drainage of the mediastinal or pleural fluid. The practice of leaving drains in place until contrast swallow has been performed or oral feeding recommenced is not recommended, both for this reason and because of the immobilisation that prolonged drainage entails. Some leaks, including the majority of those associated with cervical anastomoses, are small and localised and have the appearance of a diverticulum at the anastomosis on contrast radiology. In such cases, no drainage will be required as long as the patient remains well and non-toxic and contrast radiology does not demonstrate any distal obstruction (Desbleds et al. 1975; Orringer and Lemner 1986). If these requirements are met, such leaks will heal spontaneously with conservative treatment. The radiological appearances should demonstrate the potential for the juxta-anastomotic collection to drain into the anastomotic lumen. Oral feeding can be reintroduced at an early stage and Orringer (1986) recommends that swallowing should be instituted with the patient sitting upright, positioned to hold the site of the leak uppermost. Oral diet need not be restricted to fluids only, as in the absence of distal obstruction, solid or semisolid food will be less likely to leak through a small area of dehiscence (Orringer and Lemner 1986). Hermreck and Crawford (1976) described five cases of leak in eleven cervical anastomoses. These were successfully managed by local drainage and irrigation with anastomotic revision in certain cases. No leaks were fatal and all eventually healed. In another series (Chassin 1978), four patients with minor intrathoracic leaks presented as small sinus tracks or pockets on contrast radiology. These patients were asymptomatic and were managed by nasogastric suction or a nil-by-mouth regimen. Serial contrast swallows revealed satisfactory healing without further intervention. In other cases there will be pleural and mediastinal collections of contaminated fluid with hydropneumo-thorax and the appearance of mediastinal fluid levels on lateral chest films. Drainage may be provided initially by the insertion of large (32–36 French gauge) intercostal catheters under local anaesthesia. Correct drain positioning is critical and must be carefully monitored by daily chest X-ray examinations. The presence of persistent fluid levels indicates inadequate drainage and, if the situation cannot be improved by closed drain insertion, thoracotomy will be necessary. Signs of continuing sepsis almost certainly indicate the presence of unidentified loculae of infection and require urgent re-operation. The possibility of a coexistent subphrenic collection should be considered in patients whose fever does not respond to closed drainage (Chassin 1978). In some instances of chronic leak, posterior rib resection at the most dependent part of the pleural cavity may be required (Orringer and Lemner 1986). This is in order to form an efficiently draining oesophago-cutaneous fistula and to prevent systemic sepsis. Whilst it is attractive to avoid re-operation, this rarely proves feasible and most patients fall into one or more of the categories mentioned below.

## Re-operation

Urgent re-thoracotomy should be undertaken in the following circumstances:

1. Complete anastomotic dehiscence, as shown by contrast radiology, with uncontrolled contamination of the pleural space by saliva and gastric contents
2. Suspicion of conduit infarction
3. Failure to drain intrathoracic fluid collections adequately
4. Persistence of signs of sepsis.

   Inberg et al. (1971) described their experience in 19 patients with anastomotic failure. Diagnosis was confirmed by water-soluble contrast radiology routinely performed one week postoperatively and led to immediate re-exploration to close or cover the site of the leak, to insert a feeding jejunostomy and to provide adequate drainage. Multiple intercostal drains were also inserted adjacent to the site and anastomotic decompression was achieved by the retrograde passage of a catheter with multiple side holes through the jejunum, proximal to the feeding jejunostomy site. With this aggressive approach 9 of the 19 patients survived. In another series (Keighley et al. 1981) the catastrophic consequences of intra-peritoneal contamination were demonstrated and 11 of 13 patients died despite aggressive management. In the same report intrathoracic leak was managed by re-operation and attempted repair of the anastomosis. Direct suture line repair was performed in 3 patients, of whom 2 survived. If direct repair was judged not feasible, multiple drains were inserted around the anastomosis. Of 9 patients in whom drainage alone was performed, only 2 survived. Late anastomotic-cutaneous fistulae occurring more than one month postoperatively were seen in 2 patients, both of whom survived with conservative management. Hermreck and Crawford (1976) reported their experience of the management of 8 cases of intrathoracic or intra-abdominal leakage. In these patients re-exploration for drainage was performed, along with cervical oesophagostomy for salivary diversion and central venous cannulation or enteral access procedures for nutrition. Seven of the 8 patients died. Based on these discouraging results Hermreck and Crawford altered the management protocols and reported 2 further cases. At re-operation the distal oesophagus was disconnected from the anastomosis and closed using a double layer of mechanically applied staples. Cervical oesophagostomy was not performed. Saliva was removed from the blind-ending oesophageal stump by a sump nasogastric tube with continuous suction applied. The distal limb of the anastomosis was exteriorised as a mucus fistula used for subsequent enteral feeding. Until this was established, TPN was continued. The contaminated pleural space was thoroughly debrided, lavaged and drained. If peritoneal contamination was present, sump and Penrose drainage of the left hypochondrium was performed. The patients were main-tained on positive pressure ventilation for three days following re-operation. Late reconstruction was subsequently performed. This approach resulted in the survival of both patients. Wilson et al. (1982) recommended the routine use of water-soluble contrast radiology 5–7 days after surgery with a nasogastric tube still *in situ*. Small intrathoracic leaks were managed successfully conservatively. Twelve patients suffered severe intrathoracic leak. If the anastomosis did not appear to be severely disrupted, patients were managed by nasogastric suction with intercostal drains carefully positioned either percutaneously or at re-operation, and by parenteral feeding. Major anastomotic disruption was managed by proximal oesophageal closure by the use of a stapling device with continuous nasogastric aspiration of saliva. The gastric remnant was closed and decompressed by a tube gastrostomy. Feeding tube-jejunostomy was performed for nutrition. Late Roux-en-Y jejunal reconstruction was performed once all signs of sepsis had abated and nutritional status had improved. This aggressive approach led to the survival of 15 out of 19 patients. Of the four deaths that occurred, all were attributable to persistent mediastinal or intrapleural sepsis.

The data from the above series and others allow a plan of management to be formulated for these difficult problems. Patients with severe mediastinal, pleural or peritoneal contamination due to a major leak are critically ill and demand intensive monitoring of respiratory and haemodynamic parameters. Early ope-ration allows establishment of properly placed intrapleural drains, complete debridement of infected material within the mediastinum, and an assessment of the state of the oesophagogastric anastomosis. Sump drainage of any associated intrabdominal fluid collections is necessary (Wilson et al. 1982). At thoracotomy, the lung is carefully retracted and cleared of fibrinous peel. Minor leaks can be sutured and covered by omentum or a vascular pedicle of diaphragm, but as indicated previously they will probably heal with conservative drainage pro-cedures alone. Complete dehiscence will not heal and the surgical procedure in such cases will depend on the condition of the patient, the anticipated long-term prognosis (palliative or curative initial procedure) and the availability of alternative viscus as an oesophageal substitute. Re-resection and the perfor-mance of a cervical reconstruction with the conduit positioned away from the area of maximal contamination may salvage the situation. This approach would seem reasonable in patients who have undergone palliative resection and are unlikely to benefit from defunctioning and later reconstruction. In cases of conduit infarction adequate resection and defunctioning is necessary. In most cases of major dehiscence following oesophagogastrectomy the appropriate course of action will combine trimming of the proximal oesophagus and closure, coupled with either defunctioning cervical oesophagostomy or chronic oesophageal intubation with a nasogastric tube applied to continuous low pressure suction to clear accumulations of saliva and prevent aspiration (Wilson et al. 1982). The gastric remnant should be trimmed back to healthy tissue, and closed and defunctioning tube gastrostomy performed (Urschel et al. 1974). A tube jejunostomy can be utilised for feeding once ileus resolves and in the interim parenteral nutrition is commenced. This avoids the problem of using the gastrostomy for feeding purposes in its atonic, vagotomised state. Complete clearance of all infected material, alimentary diversion and the establishment of adequate enteral feeding access is likely to give the best results in anastomotic leak. These measures have been demonstrated to improve prognosis in spontaneous oesophageal perforation (Triggiani and Belsey 1977; Abbot et al. 1970). In cases where defunctioning has been performed with loss of oesophago-intestinal continuity, late reconstruction can be more safely performed when sepsis is controlled and nutritional status is adequate.

## *Dilatation*

In patients with less severe leak in whom adequate drainage of the pleural cavity is achieved, a chronic oesophagopleurocutaneous fistula may develop. Fistula healing may be delayed by the presence of distal anastomotic obstruction due to anastomotic stricture, inflammatory oedema or spasm. In such cases bougienage may be performed safely using large bore Maloney dilators, as the mediastinal inflammatory reaction supports the anastomosis (Orringer and Lemner 1986). In addition to these measures, other workers have recommended local endoscopic treatment of the disrupted area with 20% caustic sodium hydroxide in order to promote a hyperplastic inflammatory fibrotic reaction to aid closure of the leak, although this remains unproven (Gunning and Kingsnorth 1979).

## Conclusion

Anastomotic leak remains a major cause of death following oesophageal resection for carcinoma. Whether the incidence of leak can be reduced by the use of mechanical stapling devices or pedicled omental wraps remains unknown (Dudrick et al. 1968). Although a good prognosis can be anticipated with cervical anastomotic failure or small intrathoracic leaks, major intrathoracic or intraperitoneal contamination carries an extremely high mortality. Early diagnosis is essential. Once the diagnosis is confirmed, intensive management is indicated with accurate and complete drainage of the contaminated cavities, maintenance of nutrition, assessment of the degree of dehiscence, selective use of re-operation for oesophageal closure, decompression of the oesophageal substitute and direct placement of drainage and feeding catheters. With this aggressive approach patient salvage may be possible.

    The management of this difficult problem and the multiple factors affecting the choice of treatment are shown in Fig. 15.1.

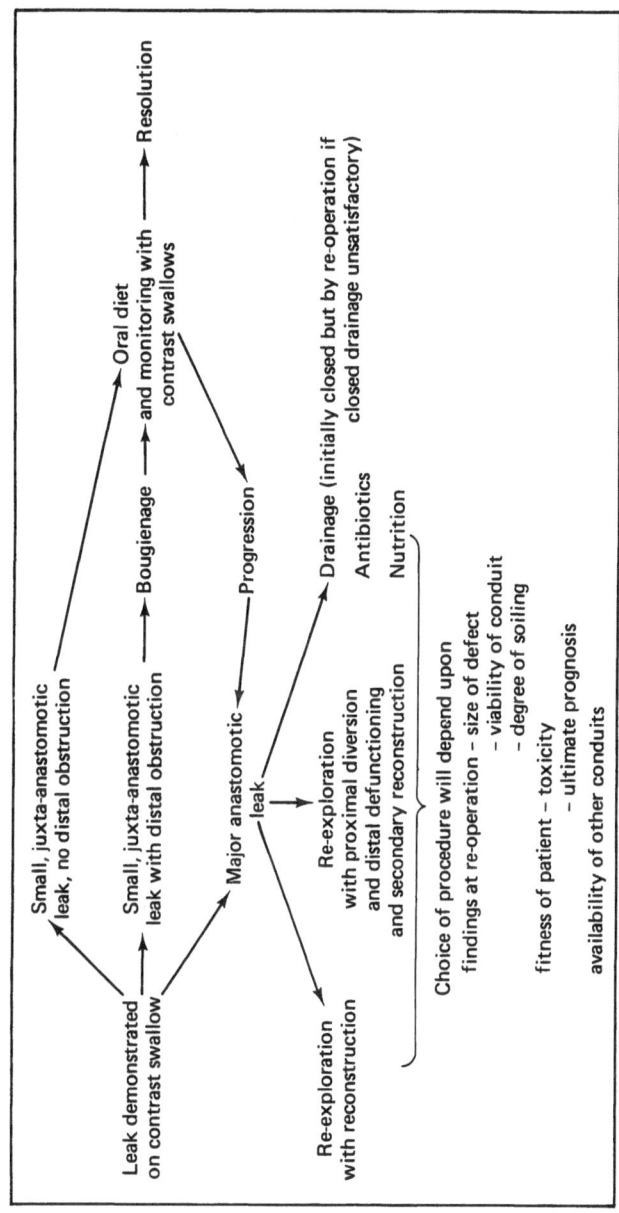

**Fig. 15.1.** Flow chart for management of intrathoracic anastomotic failure.

# Other Complications Related to Infection

Although anastomotic dehiscence is commonly associated with mediastinitis and empyema, both these complications can occur without demonstrable anastomotic failure. However, occult leak is probably the aetiology in the majority of cases. Contrast radiology is essential to confirm the integrity of the anastomosis although false negative results occasionally occur. Diagnosis of empyema will be made by the aspiration and drainage of infected pleural fluid. Although empyema drainage should not require continued antibiotic therapy, culture of the infected material will be helpful should systemic signs of sepsis develop.

Wound infection occurs more commonly in operations on the upper gastro-intestinal tract when obstruction is present (Gatehouse et al. 1978) and occasionally may manifest as an aggressive and extending anaerobic gangrenous infection. In such an event antibiotic therapy is mandatory and wound debridement will be necessary. The incidence of wound infection is reduced by antibiotic prophylaxis (Little et al. 1981).

Fatal erosion of the aorta or heart has been reported as a consequence of intrathoracic resection (Ong et al. 1978; Le Roux and Knothe 1962). In one series, aortic erosion following anastomotic dehiscence accounted for 8% of all deaths associated with resection. The presentation of such a complication is rapidly fatal and unlikely to be retrievable. Although such a complication may be related to the inadvertent misplacement of a suture, it is thought most commonly to be the result of infection or acid erosion of the aortic wall at the site of an occult leak.

# Chylothorax Following Oesophagectomy

The close and variable anatomical relationship of the thoracic duct to the oesophagus makes it vulnerable to intraoperative injury. The duct after draining the cysterna chyli passes between the crura of the diaphragm to the right of the aorta. It passes cranially, coming to lie on the right side of the oesophagus, medial to the azygos vein before crossing from right to left, behind the oesophagus at the level of the 5th or 6th thoracic vertebra just inferior to the tracheal bifurcation. The duct then ascends in the superior mediastinum into the neck where it passes behind the carotid sheath, eventually draining into the union of the left internal jugular and subclavian veins. These anatomical paths are variable and the duct may be multiple (Van Perris 1949; Kausel et al. 1957). Injury to the duct in the lower chest would thus usually present as a right chylothorax and injury to the duct above the level of the carina would result in a left chylothorax (Ross 1961). However, this rule of thumb is unreliable and any previous operation will allow efflux of chyle to the same side.

The consequences of chylothorax are threefold: pulmonary; nutritional; immunological.

## Pulmonary Consequences

The development of a postoperative pleural effusion of any size will compress underlying lung tissue, predisposing to pulmonary infection. If large, effusions may cause mediastinal shift leading to respiratory failure even in the most robust patient. In frail patients with limited respiratory reserve, small effusions may have a disproportionate effect on the adequacy of ventilation and the ability to cough.

## Nutritional Consequences

A chyle leak has severe nutritional consequences. The thoracic duct returns to the vascular system a variable amount of protein and more than half of the ingested fats, in the form of chylomicrons (Ross 1961; Roy et al. 1967). In addition to the severe loss of fluid (up to 2.5 l/day) chyle leak, therefore, results in loss of protein, fats and fat-soluble vitamins with documented decreases in body weight, total serum protein and serum albumin levels (Ross 1961; McIrvine and Mannick 1983).

## Immunological Consequences

The loss of lymphocytes (over 1 million/day), results in immunological deficiency which, compounded by poor nutritional status, may cause death due to infective complications (Ross 1961; Ferguson et al. 1985). In postsurgical patients, lymphocyte counts fall within 24 hours of operation and recover within the first 5 days (McIrvine and Mannick 1983). In patients with chylothorax, total lymphocyte counts remain at a low level as long as the leak persists. Significant immunodeficiency from this occurs within two weeks, the minimum period that elective thoracic duct drainage leads to satisfactory immunosuppression when used to reduce graft rejection in transplantation (Niblack and Richie 1983).

The incidence of thoracic duct injury has been estimated at 0.5% after oesophageal resection (Lam et al. 1979). The diagnosis, easy in theory, is often delayed in practice. The development of a large milky pleural effusion is usual, but clearer effusions may occur in the fasting patient. There may be a latent period following duct injury. The relatively intact mediastinal pleura may be sealed by adhesions over the pleural breach, leading to either delayed rupture into the pleural cavity or progressive mediastinal enlargement (Ross 1961; Bressler et al. 1953). Elevated triglyceride levels and stainable fat may be found in the effusion, but are not necessarily specific for chylothorax. Fat-laden discharge may issue from a chest drain following a fatty meal as a consequence of direct anastomotic leak rather than from thoracic duct injury (Roy et al. 1967; Lam et al. 1979). Lymphangiography has been used by several workers to confirm the presence of chylothorax and allow assessment of the site and degree of extravasation, thus aiding management decisions (Ferguson et al. 1985; Lam et al. 1979).

The management of chylothorax following oesophagectomy is a subject of considerable controversy. That significant nutritional and immunological deficiencies occur after about two weeks following thoracic duct drainage is suggested by elective drainage procedures for transplantation immunosuppression (Lam et al. 1979). It would, therefore, seem inadvisable to persist with conservative management beyond this period. In addition, spontaneous resolution of chylous leak following resection for malignancy is unlikely in view of the extensive disruption of minor lymphatic channels during surgical dissection and possible pre-existing lymphatic obstruction due to malignancy.

The earliest report of chylothorax complicating oesophageal resection was by Bressler et al. (1953). The patient was successfully managed by closed chest drainage until spontaneous resolution occurred. Brewer et al. (1955) employed anastomosis of the thoracic duct to the hemiazygos vein in a case of post-oesophagectomy chylothorax. Subsequent authors, however, have employed simple tube thoracostomy (Ferguson et al. 1985; Lam et al. 1979; Rubin et al. 1977), pleurodesis (Wu et al. 1955; Gingell 1965) or re-operation with duct ligation (Ferguson et al. 1985; Lam et al. 1979). None of these methods has been uniformly successful and the mortality of the complication approaches 50%. Undoubtedly this reflects the high potential for infective complications in immunosuppressed and nutritionally depleted patients. Duct ligation alone may not be successful because persistent distal lymphatic obstruction allows continued leakage of lymph generated within the thorax (McIrvine and Mannick 1983).

Although, on theoretical grounds, it would seem appropriate to commence patients with chylothorax on low fat diets with medium chain triglycerides which are absorbed into the bloodstream directly (Lichter et al. 1968; Hashim et al. 1964), this may not result in satisfactory control of chyle production and loss, and total parenteral nutrition is preferable.

Once the diagnosis of postoperative chylothorax is confirmed, management will include tube thoracostomy to monitor nutritional losses and to help prevent secondary pulmonary complications. Ideally, the site of leakage should be investigated by lymphangiography. With pleural drainage established it would seem reasonable to undertake a short trial of conservative management with parenteral nutritional support for 3–4 days. If, during this time, there is no appreciable decrease in drainage then re-operation is necessary. At thoracotomy the site of leak can often be identified if careful inspection is made along the expected course of the thoracic duct. Techniques used to highlight the leak, such as the oral administration of cream stained with a lipophilic dye, are of little value. If attempts to identify or control the leak locally prove unsuccesful then mass ligation of the duct above the diaphragm can be performed via a lateral thoracotomy from either side. Multiple suture ligation of the tissue between the oesophagus, aorta and azygos vein is undertaken immediately above the hiatus.

# Cardiological Complications

Approximately 10% of deaths following oesophageal resection are related to cardiac problems (Postlethwait 1986). Patients undergoing oesophageal resection are commonly of an age when coexistent coronary artery disease is present. Perioperative myocardial infarction may occur and expert anaesthetic management is essential in the elderly patient. All patients should have central venous and arterial access to monitor their haemodynamic status and gas exchange. Intraoperative hypotension and hypertension should be avoided, and blood loss replaced with colloid or whole blood, depending on preoperative haematocrit. In the postoperative period careful regard to fluid status is essential to avoid volume and sodium overload. Supraventricular arrhythmias, predominantly atrial fibrillation, are common after thoracotomy, and the incidence increases with age and extent of surgery. Arrhythmias are particularly common if pericardial resection has been performed or if postoperative pulmonary complications develop. Prophylactic administration of digoxin is used by the authors in these circumstances. Digoxin 0.5 mg is administered slowly intravenously during anaesthesia and serum potassium levels checked regularly. Subsequently, a maintenance dose of digoxin is prescribed throughout the early postoperative period. Although digoxin may not prevent the development of atrial fibrillation, prophylactic administration allows a controlled ventricular response should fibrillation supervene. The digoxin may be discontinued after a month to six weeks if the patient maintains sinus rhythm. If atrial fibrillation is unresponsive to digoxin, or if other supraventricular dysrhythmias occur, the choice of treatment will depend on the patient's condition and the haemodynamic consequences of the dysrhythymia. In some cases cardioversion may be necessary or other anti-arrhythmic agents may be tried. Cardiological advice should be taken for complicated arrhythmias.

# Other Complications

As in any major operation, morbidity and mortality will occasionally result from other complications such as pulmonary embolism or renal failure. Pulmonary embolism alone accounts for 9% of reported mortality following oesophageal resection (Postlethwait 1986). The efficacy of specific prophylaxis against pulmonary embolism is not substantiated in such patients and their use cannot be recommended. These complications are not individual to oesophageal resection and their management will follow standard principles.

# Summary

The overall mortality of resection for carcinoma of the oesophagus varies considerably. A range of 0.8–37.5% has been recorded in a survey of recent reports (Postlethwait 1983). The latter figure is unacceptably high, especially as cure rates are low (Earlam and Cunha-Melo 1980).* Every endeavour should be made to reduce mortality to a figure below 10%. This chapter has highlighted some of the more common complications of oesophageal resection and discussed ways in which they may be prevented and treated. A patient undergoing

---

*But see p. 16 – Editor

oesophageal resection requires diligent and skilful management at all stages of his care. Careful evaluation and selection, and optimum preparation are necessary prior to surgery. At the time of operation both the surgeon and anaesthetist have important roles to play in the prevention of aspiration and other pulmonary complications and in the construction of a well-vascularised anastomosis, meticulously performed in a haemodynamically stable, well-oxygenated patient. After operation a high level of care is required by nurses, physiotherapists and surgeons. Diligent and frequent monitoring of the patient's clinical condition, haematological and biochemical parameters and chest X-ray film appearances will allow early detection of potential problems. Once detected, complications should be treated early and aggressively. An attempt has been made in this chapter to make recommendations that will help to minimise morbidity and mortality for this major surgical procedure.

# References

Abbott OA, Mansour KA, Logan WA, Hatcher CR, Symbas PN (1970) Atraumatic, so-called 'spontaneous' rupture of the oesophagus. J Thorac Cardiovasc Surg 59:67

Akiyama H, Miyazono H, Tsurumaru L, Hashimoto C, Kawanura T (1978) Use of the stomach as an esophageal substitute. Ann Surg 188:606

Anon (1986) Enteral feeds for adults: an update. Drug Ther Bull 24:61

Bainbridge ET, Matthews HR (1980) Hypoxaemia after left thoracotomy for benign oesophageal disease. Thorax 35:264

Bowen JC, Dinesh K, Garg BS (1977) Effect of graded mechanical ischaemia on oxygen tension and electrical potential in the canine gastric mucosa. Gastroenterology 73:84

Bressler S, Wiener D, Thomson SA (1953) Traumatic chylothorax following oesophageal resection. J Thorac Surg 26:321

Brewer LA (1955) Surgical management of lesions of the thoracic duct. The technique and indications for retroperitoneal anastomosis of the thoracic duct to the hemiazygos vein. Am J Surg 90:210

Burt ME, Brennan MF (1984) Nutritional support of the patient with esophageal cancer. Semin Oncol 11:127

Butler H (1951) The veins of the oesophagus. Thorax 6:276

Byrd RB, Burns JR (1975) Cough dynamics in the post-thoracotomy state. Chest 67:654

Celli BR, Rodriguez KS, Snider GL (1984) A controlled trial of intermittent positive pressure breathing, incentive spirometry and deep breathing exercises in preventing pulmonary complications after abdominal surgery. Am Rev Respir Dis 130:12

Chassin JL (1978) Stapling technique after esophagogastric resection. Am J Surg 136:399

Collins CD, Darke CS, Knowelden J (1968) Chest complications after upper abdominal surgery: their anticipation and prevention. Br Med J ii:462

Collis JL (1952) Carcinoma of the oesophagus. Lancet II:613

Conti S, West JP, Fitzpatrick HF (1977) Mortality and morbidity after esophagogastrectomy for cancer of the esophagus. Am Surg 43:92

Craig DB (1981) Postoperative recovery of pulmonary function. Anesth Analg 60:46

D'Abreu AL (1963) Some reflections on surgery of the oesophagus. Ann Surg 158:747

Daly JM, Massai E, Giacco G et al. (1982) Parenteral nutrition in esophageal cancer patients. Ann Surg 196:203

Desbleds MT, Desbleds M, Assailly M (1975) Roentgenologic examination seven days after oesophageal anastomosis. Ann Chir 29:841

Dudrick SJ, Wilmore DW, Vars HM, Rhoads JE (1968) Longterm total parenteral nutrition with growth development and positive nitrogen balance. Surgery 64:134

Earlam R, Cunha-Melo JR (1980) Oesophageal squamous cell carcinoma. I. A critical review of surgery. Br J Surg 67:381

Editorial (1976) Anaerobes in pleuropulmonary infection. Lancet I:289

Editorial (1977) Postoperative chest infections. Br Med J ii:1500

Editorial (1979) Parenteral nutrition before surgery. Br Med J ii:1529

Editorial (1984) Are postoperative pulmonary complications preventable? Lancet II:1079

Eikhoof TC (1980) Pulmonary infection in surgical patients. Surg Clin North Am 60:175

El-Eishi HI, Ayoub SF, Abd-El-Khalek M (1973) The arterial supply of the human stomach. Acta Anat 86:565

Faust RJ, Nauss LA (1976) Post-thoracotomy intercostal block. Comparison of its effects on pulmonary function with those of intramuscular meperidine. Anesth Analg 55:542

Feeley TW, Hamilton WK, Xavier B, Moyers J, Eger EI (1981) Sterile anaesthetic breathing circuits do not prevent postoperative pulmonary infection. Anaesthesiology 54:369

Ferguson MK, Little AG, Skinner CB (1985) Current concepts in the management of postoperative chylothorax. Ann Thorac Surg 40:542

Finlay IG, Wright PA, Menzies T, McArdle CS (1982) Microbial flora in carcinoma of oesophagus. Thorax 37:181

Fontaine CJ, Dudley HAF (1978) Assessment of suture materials for intestinal use by an extramucosal implant technique and quantitative histological evaluation. Br J Surg 65:288

Ford GT, Guenter CA (1984) Towards prevention of postoperative pulmonary complications. Am Rev Respir Dis 130:4

Garibaldi RA, Britt MR, Coleman ML, Reading JC, Pace NL (1981) Risk factors for postoperative pneumonia. Am J Med 70:677

Gatehouse D, Dimock F, Furdon DW (1978) Prediction of wound sepsis following gastric operations. Br J Surg 65:551

Gingell JC (1965) Treatment of chylothorax by producing pleurodesis using iodised talc. Thorax 20:261

Goldstraw P, Bach P (1981) Gastric emptying after oesophagectomy as assessed by plasma paracetamol concentrations. Thorax 36:493

Gunning AJ, Kingsnorth A (1979) Treatment of chronic oesophageal perforation with special reference to an endoscopic method. Br J Surg 66:226

Haffejee AA, Angorn IB (1979) Nutritional status and the non-specific cellular and humoral response in esophageal carcinoma. Ann Surg 189:475

Hashim SA, Roholt HB, Babayan VK et al. (1964) Treatment of chyluria and chylothorax with medium chain triglyceride. N Engl J Med 270:756

Hatfield ARW (1982) Hyperalimentation. Br J Hosp Med 220

Heatley RV, Williams RHP, Lewis MH (1979) Preoperative intravenous feeding – a controlled trial. Postgrad Med J 55:541

Hermreck AS, Crawfod DG (1976) The esophageal anastomic leak. Am J Surg 132:794

Hopkins RA, Alexander JC, Postlethwait RW (1984) Stapled esophagogastric anastomoses. Am J Surg 147:283

Huang KC (1963) Analysis of anastomotic leakage following esophageal resection with esophago-gastrostomy for cancer. Zhong-Waike Z 11:859

Inberg MV, Linna MI, Sheinin TM, Vanttinen E (1971) Anastomotic leakage after excision of esophageal and high gastric carcinoma. Am J Surg 122:540

Jackson JW, Cooper DKC, Guvendik L, Reece-Smith H (1979) The surgical management of malignant tumours of the oesophagus: a review of the results of 292 patients treated over a 15-year period (1961–1975). Br J Surg 66:98

Jawetz E, Melnick JC, Adelberg EA (1972) Review of medical microbiology (10th edn). Lange, Los Altos, California

Jorgensen ST, Pederson H, Larsen V (1979) Conservative treatment with total parenteral nutrition in patients with gastro-oesophageal anastomotic leaks. Acta Chir Scand 145:173

Kai Z, Yihua Y (1987) Use of the pedicled omentum in oesophagogastric anastomosis: analysis of 100 cases. Ann R Coll Surg Engl 69:209

Kasai M, Abo S, Watanabe T (1971) Studies on the reduction of operative mortality after radical operations for carcinoma of the thoracic esophagus. Jap J Surg 1:1

Katz S, Izhar M, Mirelman D (1981) Bacterial adherence to surgical sutures: a possible factor in suture induced infection. Ann Surg 194:35

Kausel HW, Reeve TS, Stein AA, Alley RD, Stranahan A (1957) Anatomic and pathological studies of the thoracic duct. J Thorac Surg 34:631

Keighley MRB, Burdon DW (1979) Antibiotic prophylaxis in surgery. Pitman, London

Keighley MRB, Moore J, Lee JR, Mallins D, Thomson H (1981) Preoperative frozen section and cytology to assess proximal invasion in gastro-oesophageal carcinoma. Br J Surg 68:73

Lam KH, Lim STK, Wong J, Ong GB (1979) Chylothorax following resection of the oesophagus. Br J Surg 66:105

Laszlo G, Archer GG, Darrell JH, Dawson JM, Fletcher CM (1973) The diagnosis and prophylaxis of pulmonary complications after surgical operations. Br J Surg 60:129

Le Roux BT, Knothe W (1962) Complications of oesophagogastrectomy for carcinoma. J R Coll Surg Edin 7:132

Lichter I, Hill GL, Nye ER (1968) The use of medium chain triglycerides in the treatment of chylothorax in a child. Ann Thorac Surg 5:352

Lim STK, Choa G, Lam KH et al. (1981) Total parenteral nutrition versus gastrostomy in the preoperative preparation of patients with carcinoma of the oesophagus. Br J Surg 68:69

Little G, Alvin E, Matthews HR (1981) Prophylactic antibiotics in oesophageal resection. Thorax 36:73

Maiwand O, Makey AR (1981) Cryoanalgesia for relief of pain after thoracotomy. Br Med J 282:1749

Maiwand O, Makey AR, Rees A (1986) Cryoanalgesia after thoracotomy: improvement of technique and review of 600 cases. J Thorac Cardiovasc Surg 92:291

Matthews HR, Hopkinson RB (1984) Treatment of sputum retention by minitracheostomy. Br J Surg 71:147

McIrvine AJ, Mannick JA (1983) Lymphocyte function in the critically ill surgical patient. Surg Clin North Am 63:245

Miller HAB, Taylor GA (1975) Management of late cases of oesophageal disruption with intravenous hyperalimentation. Can J Surg 18:41

Moghissi K, Hornshaw J, Teasdale PR et al. (1977) Parenteral nutrition in carcinoma of the oesophagus treated by surgery. Nitrogen balance and clinical studies. Br J Surg 64:125

Morran C, McNaught W, McArdle CS (1978) Prophylactic cotrimoxazole in biliary surgery. Br Med J ii:462

Muller JM, Brenner V, Diesnt C et al. (1982) Preoperative clinical feeding in patients with gastrointestinal carcinoma. Lancet I:68

Nakayama K, Kakaegawa T (1981) Latest management of pulmonary complications following esophageal cancer surgery in Japan. Int Adv Surg Oncol 4:111

Niblack GD, Richie E (1983) Thoracic duct drainage: an overview. Heart Transplant 2:197

Nicks R (1967) Colonic replacement of the oesophagus: some observations on infarction and wound leakage. Br J Surg 54:124

Ong GB, Lam KH, Wong J, Lim TK (1978) Factors influencing morbidity and mortality in esophageal carcinoma. J Thorac Cardiovasc Surg 76:745

Orr IA, Keenan DJM, Dundee JW (1981) Improved pain relief after thoracotomy: use of cryoprobe and morphine infusion. Br Med J 283:945

Orringer MB (1984) Transhiatal esophagectomy without thoracotomy for carcinoma of the thoracic oesophagus. Ann Surg 200:282

Orringer MB, Lemner JH (1986) Early dilation in the treatment of oesophageal disruption. Ann Thorac Surg 42:536

Orringer MB, Sloan H (1978) Esophagectomy without thoracotomy. J Thorac Cardiovasc Surg 76:643

Orringer MB, Appeleman HD, Argenta L et al. (1977) Polypropylene suture in esophageal and gastrointestinal operations. Surg Gynecol Obstet 144:67

Palmer KNV, Sellick BA (1953) The prevention of postoperative pulmonary atelectasis. Lancet I:164

Palmer KNV, Sellick BA (1952) Effect of procaine penicillin and breathing exercises on postoperative pulmonary complications. Lancet I:345

Papachristou DN, Fortner JG (1979) Anastomotic failure complicating total gastrectomy and esophagogastrectomy for cancer of the stomach. Am J Surg 138:399

Payne WS, Ellis FH (1975) Complications of esophageal and diaphragmatic surgery. In: Arte CS, Hardy JP (eds) Management of surgical complications, 3rd edn. Saunders, Philadelphia

Pearlstein L, Azneer IB, Polk HC (1978) An experimental assessment of esophageal anastomotic integrity. Surg Gynecol Obstet 146:53

Piccone VA, Ahmed N, Grosberg S et al. (1979) Esophagogastrectomy for carcinoma of the middle third of the esophagus. Ann Thorac Surg 28:369

Postlethwait RW (1983) Complications and deaths after operations for oesophageal carcinoma. J Thorac Cardiovasc Surg 85:827

Postlethwait RW (1986) Surgery of the oesophagus. Appleton-Century-Crofts, Connecticut, p 408

Postlethwait RW, Deaton WR, Bradshaw HH, Williams RW (1950) Esophageal anastomosis: types and methods of suture. Surgery 28:537

Postlethwait RW, Weinberg M, Jenkins LB, Brockington WS (1952) Mechanical strength of esophageal anastomoses. Ann Surg 133:472

Potter SE, Holyoke EA (1950) Observations on the intrinsic blood supply of the oesophagus. Arch Surg 61:944

Ross JK (1961) A review of the surgery of the thoracic duct. Thorax 16:12

Roxburgh JC, Markland CG, Ross BA, Kerr WF (1987) Role of cryoanalgesia in the control of pain after thoracotomy. Thorax 42:292

Roy PH, Can DT, Payne WS (1967) The problem of chylothorax. Mayo Clin Proc 55:457

Rubin JW, Moore JV, Ellison RG (1977) Chylothorax: therapeutic alternatives. Ann Surg 43:292

Senyk J, Rank F (1978) Oesophageal tissue reaction to different suture materials. Scand J Thorac Cardiovasc Surg 12:263

Shapiro AL, Robillard GL (1950) The esophageal arteries: their configurational anatomy and variations in relation to surgery. Ann Surg 131:171

Simms JM, Oliver G, Smith JAR (1980) A study of total parenteral nutrition in major gastric and oesophageal resection for neoplasia. J Parenter Nutr 4:422

Sugimachi K, Ueo H, Natsuda Y, Kai H, Inokuchi K, Zaitsu A (1982) Cough dynamics in oesophageal cancer: prevention of postoperative pulmonary complications. Br J Surg 69:734

Sugimachi K, Inokuchi K, Natsude Y et al. (1983) Delayed anastomosis of the cervical portion of the oesophagus in bypass operations for unresectable carcinoma of the esophagus. Surg Gynecol Obstet 157:233

Sugiura M, Futagawa S (1977) Further evaluation of the Sugiura procedure in the treatment of oesophageal varices. Arch Surg 112:1317

Swigart LL, Siekert RG, Hambley WC, Anson BJ (1950) The esophageal arteries: an anatomic study of 150 specimens. Surg Gynecol Obstet 90:234

Tagart REB (1981) Colorectal anastomosis: factors influencing success. J R Soc Med 74:111

Thomas DM, Langford RM, Russell RCG, Le Quesne LP (1979) The anatomical basis of gastric mobilisation in total oesophagectomy. Br J Surg 66:230

Thulborne T, Young MH (1962) Prophylactic penicillin and postoperative chest infection. Lancet II:907

Toledo-Pereyra LH, De Meester TR (1979) Prospective randomised evaluation of intrathoracic intercostal nerve block with bupivacaine on postoperative ventilatory function. Ann Thorac Surg 27:203

Triggiani E, Belsey R (1977) Oesophageal trauma: incidence, diagnosis and management. Thorax 32:241

Urschel HC, Razeuk MA, Wood RE et al. (1924) Improved management of esophageal perforation: exclusion and diversion in continuity. Ann Surg 179:587

Van de Water JM, Watring WG, Linton LA, Murphy M, Byron RL (1971) Prevention of postoperative pulmonary complications. Surg Gynecol Obstet 135:229

Van Pernis PA (1949) Variations of the thoracic duct. Surgery 26:806

Vickers MD (1982) Postoperative pneumonias. Br Med J 284:292

Vriu JK, Vriu RA (1977) Effectiveness of breathing exercises in preventing pulmonary complications following open heart surgery. Phys Ther 57:1367

Wesselhoeft CW, Glew DH, Randolph JG, Blades B (1968) Experimental and clinical evaluation of an everting oesophageal anastomosis in the growing subject. J Thorac Cardiovasc Surg 56:658

Wightman JAK (1968) A prospective survey of the incidence of postoperative pulmonary complications. Br J Surg 55:85

Williams DB, Payne WS (1982) Observations on esophageal blood supply. Mayo Clin Proc 57:448–453

Wilson SE, Stone R, Scully M, Ozeran L, Benfield JR (1982) Modern management of oesophageal leak after oesphago-gastrectomy. Am J Surg 144:95

Wu YK, Howe YL, Huong KC et al. (1955) Surgical treatment of carcinoma of the oesophagus and cardia of the stomach. Chin Med J 73:181

Yun-K'an L, Yueh-Min L, Tao-Ming C, Chih-Chiang K (1964) An analysis of mortality and postoperative complications of oesophageal resection for cancer. Chin Med J 83:39

Yun-k'an L, Tzu-Huang T, Yu-Chic K, Yueh-Min L, Tao-Ming C (1965) Surgical considerations in anastomotic leakage following esophageal resection for cancer. Chin Med J 84:612

# Subject Index